369 0246398

Access Professor Wormald's videos for *Endoscopic Sinus Surgery, Third Edition,* online at MediaCenter.thieme.com!

Simply visit MediaCenter.thieme.com **and, when prompted during the registration process, enter the scratch-off code below to get started today.**

X5BG-D5Y4-HC26-N3V9

This book cannot be returned once this panel has been scratched off.

With detailed instruction and careful attention to the relevant anatomy via a generous number of CT scan images, the third edition's 56 videos (see the Video Contents on pages ix-x for a complete listing) demonstrate the endoscopic surgical techniques described in this book. Let Peter-John Wormald's narration guide you to an improved understanding of, and skill in, basic and advanced Paranasal Sinus Surgery, Skull Base Surgery, and Transnasal Intracranial Surgery.

System requirements:

	WINDOWS	MAC	TABLET
Recommended Browser(s)**	Microsoft Internet Explorer 8.0 or later, Firefox 3.x	Firefox 3.x, Safari 4.x	HTML5 mobile browser. iPad — Safari. Opera Mobile — Tablet PCs preferred.
	** all browsers should have JavaScript enabled		
Flash Player Plug-in	Flash Player 9 or Higher* ** Mac users: ATI Rage 128 GPU does not support full-screen mode with hardware scaling*		Tablet PCs with Android OS support Flash 10.1
Minimum Hardware Configurations	Intel® Pentium® II 450 MHz, AMD Athlon™ 600 MHz or faster processor (or equivalent) 512 MB of RAM	PowerPC® G3 500 MHz or faster processor Intel Core™ Duo 1.33 GHz or faster processor 512MB of RAM	Minimum CPU powered at 800MHz 256MB DDR2 of RAM
Recommended for optimal usage experience	Monitor resolutions: • Normal (4:3) 1024×768 or Higher • Widescreen (16:9) 1280×720 or Higher • Widescreen (16:10) 1440×900 or Higher DSL/Cable internet connection at a minimum speed of 384.0 Kbps or faster WiFi 802.11 b/g preferred.		7-inch and 10-inch tablets on maximum resolution. WiFi connection is required.

Endoscopic Sinus Surgery

Anatomy, Three-Dimensional Reconstruction, and Surgical Technique

Third Edition

Endoscopic Sinus Surgery

Anatomy, Three-Dimensional Reconstruction, and Surgical Technique

Third Edition

Peter-John Wormald, MD, FRACS, FCS (SA), FRCS (Ed), MB ChB
Professor and Chairman
Department of Otolaryngology
University of Adelaide
Adelaide, South Australia, Australia

Thieme
New York · Stuttgart

Dedicated with love to Fiona, my wife, without whom this
book would not have been possible, and to Nicholas and Sarah,
my children, who provide my inspiration.

Thieme Medical Publishers, Inc.
333 Seventh Ave.
New York, NY 10001

Executive Editor: Timothy Y. Hiscock
Managing Editor: J. Owen Zurhellen IV
Editorial Assistant: Elizabeth Berg
Editorial Director: Michael Wachinger
Production Editor: Heidi Grauel, Maryland Composition
International Production Director: Andreas Schabert
Senior Vice President, International Marketing and Sales: Cornelia Schulze
Vice President, Finance and Accounts: Sarah Vanderbilt
President: Brian D. Scanlan
Compositor: Maryland Composition
Printer: Everbest Printing Co.
Front Cover Illustration: Hugh Thomas

Library of Congress Cataloging-in-Publication Data

Endoscopic sinus surgery : anatomy, three-dimensional reconstruction, and surgical technique / edited by
Peter-John Wormald. — 3rd ed.
      p. ; cm.
   Includes bibliographical references and index.
   ISBN 978-1-60406-687-6
   I. Wormald, P. J.
   [DNLM: 1. Paranasal Sinuses—surgery. 2. Natural Orifice Endoscopic Surgery—methods. 3. Paranasal Sinus Diseases—surgery.
   4. Paranasal Sinuses—anatomy & histology. 5. Video-Assisted Surgery. WV 340]
   617.5'23—dc23

                                                                                             2012021281

Important note: Medical knowledge is ever-changing. As new research and clinical experience broaden our knowledge, changes in treatment and drug therapy may be required. The authors and editors of the material herein have consulted sources believed to be reliable in their efforts to provide information that is complete and in accord with the standards accepted at the time of publication. However, in view of the possibility of human error by the authors, editors, or publisher of the work herein or changes in medical knowledge, neither the authors, editors, nor publisher, nor any other party who has been involved in the preparation of this work, warrants that the information contained herein is in every respect accurate or complete, and they are not responsible for any errors or omissions or for the results obtained from use of such information. Readers are encouraged to confirm the information contained herein with other sources. For example, readers are advised to check the product information sheet included in the package of each drug they plan to administer to be certain that the information contained in this publication is accurate and that changes have not been made in the recommended dose or in the contraindications for administration. This recommendation is of particular importance in connection with new or infrequently used drugs.

Some of the product names, patents, and registered designs referred to in this book are in fact registered trademarks or proprietary names even though specific reference to this fact is not always made in the text. Therefore, the appearance of a name without designation as proprietary is not to be construed as a representation by the publisher that it is in the public domain.

Printed in China

ISBN 978-1-60406-687-6
eISBN 978-1-60406-688-3

Contents

Video Contents

Foreword

The fact that Peter-John Wormald's book on endoscopic sinus surgery is now entering its third edition speaks volumes about the popularity of his work. Professor Wormald has an exceptional reputation worldwide as a teacher of endoscopic sinus surgery, and his experience is evident throughout this book and the accompanying videos. The first edition had been named "Best Book of 2005" by the British Medical Association amongst other honors, and the second edition was similarly well received. This third edition has been further updated and expanded, with three new chapters (on the anatomy of the sphenoid, surgery of the craniocervical junction, and management of major blood vessel injury) and with many superb anatomic dissection photographs taken by Professor Wormald's resident Rowan Valentine at Albert L. Rhoton, Jr.'s Skull Base Laboratory at the University of Florida.

The hallmarks of Professor Wormald's book are the step-by-step, easy-to-read descriptions of the surgical procedures, and the wealth of illustrations accompanying the text. This aids in understanding the detailed anatomy and the surgical procedures, especially for surgeons with limited experience in this field. The fact that this is a single-authored book by an experienced educational leader results in a pleasing consistency in content and style across all chapters. For this edition, there are more videos of the anatomy and procedures, providing an excellent adjunct to the text.

Endoscopic Sinus Surgery: Anatomy, Three-Dimensional Reconstruction, and Surgical Technique, Third Edition will be of particular value to residents and practicing otolaryngologists who wish to advance their knowledge within the field of endoscopic sinus surgery, improve their surgical techniques, and further their knowledge of the relevant surgical anatomy. As a result, the residents and otolaryngologists who read this book will be grateful to Professor Wormald for helping them to finesse their surgical technique and expand their surgical repertoire into expanded endoscopic techniques.

David W. Kennedy, MD, FACS, FRCSI
Rhinology Professor, Department of
Otorhinolaryngology–Head and Neck Surgery
Perelman School of Medicine
University of Pennsylvania
Philadelphia, Pennsylvania

Preface

This third edition of *Endoscopic Sinus Surgery* continues to refine and improve the concepts and illustrations of the second edition. With time, surgical techniques are refined and adjusted and these have been added to this edition. Each chapter has been thoroughly revised and, while some have required minimal changes, others have undergone extensive revision and adjustment. New chapters on the anatomy, craniocervical junction, and the management of major vascular hemorrhage have been added. Probably the biggest single change in this edition has been the addition of cadaver dissection images done by Rowan Valentine under the guidance of Albert L. Rhoton, Jr. in the latter's laboratory in Gainesville, Florida. Both Rowan and I are immensely grateful to Professor Rhoton for his guidance and mentorship; we hope that the images in this book reflect the high standard of excellence associated with work emanating from his laboratory. In addition, there have been a number of major advances, especially in the realm of endoscopic skull base surgery, that have necessitated updating of the second edition. Closure of large skull base defects has progressed, with pedicled vascularized flaps now the norm, with resultant significant improvement in postoperative cerebrospinal fluid leak closure rates. We have developed a whole new set of skills and expertise in the endoscopic management of major vascular hemorrhage with the development of an animal model the realistically mimics the clinical scenario. This has allowed us to develop specific instructions on how to manage this catastrophe, hopefully with better patient outcomes. These techniques are now detailed in this edition. The addition of the chapter on endoscopic surgery in the craniocervical junction area is also important, as a significant number of clival tumors will invade this area and need to be surgically dealt with, and there are a number of important primary diseases involving this region that can be dealt with endoscopically.

This book differs from many others on anatomy and surgical techniques in that its scope is purely anatomical and operative. No attempt is made to cover the pathology or medical treatment of any the conditions discussed: such information can be found in several excellent texts currently available. Many of the operative techniques presented in this book are novel, but the results achieved with them have been carefully audited and published in peer-reviewed journals and therefore they are presented here. It is hoped that the description of the relevant anatomy and surgical techniques in this text are sufficiently clear that the reader will be able to apply them in his/her everyday practice. The concepts are presented with extensive use of illustrations, CT and MRI scans, and intraoperative and postoperative photographs. In addition, the accompanying videos have exercises which allow the reader to perform three-dimensional reconstruction of the anatomy and subsequently develop a surgical plan. Each of these is followed by an edited video clip of the surgery where the reader can confirm that the reconstructions he or she created reflect the anatomy seen during surgery. This combination of text and videos should reinforce understanding of sinus anatomy and give the surgeon confidence to tackle the many anatomical variations and technical challenges that may occur during endoscopic sinus and skull base surgery.

Acknowledgments

A book of this nature is an accumulation of all knowledge gleaned from many teachers over a number of years. However, I would like to single out the late Mike McDonogh as the teacher who had the greatest influence on my career as a rhinologist. Mike was an exceptional person who was highly innovative and his humor, wit, and intelligence will be greatly missed. His ideas led to the development of the "swing-door" uncinectomy and the "bath-plug" closure of cerebrospinal leaks. I will remain forever indebted to him for his teaching, mentoring, and friendship.

I would also like to acknowledge Rowan Valentine, who is an ENT surgeon with a very bright future. Rowan undertook a nine-month fellowship with Professor Albert L. Rhoton, Jr., during which time he has produced a magnificent set of anatomical dissections on cadavers. The addition of these images to this book has immeasurably enhanced the book and the understanding of the anatomy and, consequently, the surgical techniques described.

Andrew van Hasselt deserves a special mention for his support over many years. In addition, I would like to thank the Australian Society for Otolaryngology Head and Neck Surgery members for making me welcome in Australia and for their ongoing support of the development of academic ENT.

1 Setup and Ergonomics of Endoscopic Sinus Surgery

There has been a significant shift from external and headlight sinus surgery to endoscopic sinus surgery (ESS) in the past quarter-century. This dramatic change was initiated by the pioneering studies of Messerklinger in which he demonstrated that each sinus has a predetermined mucociliary clearance pattern draining toward its natural ostium irrespective of additional openings that may have been created into the sinuses.[1] This philosophy of opening the natural ostium of the diseased sinus was then popularized by Stammberger[2] and Kennedy.[3] ESS is now accepted as the surgical management of choice for chronic sinusitis. In addition, as our knowledge of the anatomy of the sinuses has improved, other ancillary techniques such as endoscopic lacrimal surgery[4] and orbital decompression[5] have been developed. The development of specialized instruments has facilitated the endoscopic management of benign endonasal tumors[6,7] and, more recently, the endoscopic management of malignant tumors[8] of the nose and sinuses. ESS, ancillary nasal and sinus procedures, and, more recently, endoscopic transnasal intracranial surgery require a broad range of specially designed endoscopic surgical instruments.

◆ Instruments

Disclaimer: Several instruments that are discussed in this book are manufactured and sold by Medtronic ENT. Those that are identified by an asterisk here and in subsequent chapters have been designed by the author; a royalty is received from the sale of these instruments. There are no undeclared financial incentives associated with any of the instruments discussed that do not bear the identifying asterisk.

A complete list of the ESS instruments used by the author is presented in **Table 1.1**. In this table and here, the manufacturer is named if the particular instrument is produced by only that company, but if the instrument is produced by several

companies then no manufacturer is named. The following instruments are the most important for basic sinus surgery:

- Small rotating backbiting forceps
- Sickle knife
- Small (2.5 mm) straight and 45-degree upturned Blakesley forceps
- Small (2.5 mm) straight and 45-degree upturned through-biting (cutting) Blakesley forceps
- Endoscopic scissors
- Double right-angled ball probe
- Forceps: 45- and 90-degree giraffe cup forceps, 45- and 90-degree through-biting giraffe forceps
- Hajek Koffler forward-biting punch
- Suction Freer elevator
- Curettes (straight, 45- and 90-degree curette)
- Malleable suction Freer elevator* (Medtronic ENT, Jacksonville, FL)
- Malleable suction curette* (Medtronic ENT)
- Malleable frontal sinus probe* (Medtronic ENT)

Powered Microdebriders

Powered microdebriders now form an essential part of the instrumentation required to perform ESS. These instruments allow the surgeon to remove blood from the operating field with the gate open and then the tissue can be cut with considerable precision by the rotating inner blade of the microdebrider. This precise cutting of mucosa minimizes the potential for stripping of the mucosa and helps to achieve maximum mucosal preservation which should improve postoperative healing and, consequently, the results of the surgery. These instruments are very effective at removing tissue and, if placed in the wrong area, such as the orbit, can create significant damage to the orbital contents in a very short space of time.[9,10] Due to its soft consistency, orbital fat can be sucked into the blade opening and cut by the rotating inner blade at a frightening rate. If the surgeon is unaware of having penetrated the orbital periosteum with the microde-

Table 1.1   Full List of Operating Instruments and Equipment*

General Instruments
Jacobson angled 7-inch needle holder
6-inch fine needle holder
Small Luc forceps
Angled Heyman turbinectomy scissors
Tilley Henkel forceps
Tilley packing forceps
Mosquito curved artery clips
Backhaus towel clips
Sponge holder
McIndoe forceps
Adson toothed OR Adson Brown forceps
Adson plain OR tungsten tip forceps
Suture scissors
Iris curved scissors
No. 7 scalpel blade handle
Freer dissector
Frazier 9-French gauge sucker and stilette
Frazier 10-French gauge sucker and stilette
Dental syringe
Heath mallet
Small Killian speculum
Medium Killian speculum
Large Killian speculum

Sinoscopy Instruments
Medium straight Blakesley forceps
Medium upturned Blakesley forceps
Blakesley forceps straight through cut
Blakesley forceps upturned through cut
Right ostrum punch downcut
Left ostrum punch downcut
Sinus short sucker
Sinus long sucker
Sickle knife
Freer dissector
Double-ended probe
Kuhn Bolger frontal ostium seeker
Kuhn Bolger frontal sinus curette, 55 degrees
Antrum curette
90-degree curette
Suction Freer and stilette
Rotating microbite backbiter
Hajek Kofler sphenoid punch upcut forward

Special Instruments
Sinoscopy scissors, straight
Sinoscopy scissors, curved left
Sinoscopy scissors, curved right
Kuhn Bolger giraffe forceps, horizontal
Kuhn Bolger giraffe forceps, vertical
Kuhn Bolger forceps, 60 degrees
Kuhn Bolger forceps, 90 degrees
Kuhn Bolger forceps, 90 degrees right angled
Kuhn Bolger forceps, 90 degrees left angled
Ligature clip carrier

Branded Instrument Sets
Wormald Sucker Bipolar* (Medtronic ENT)
  Wormald suction bipolar forceps, straight*
  Wormald suction bipolar forceps, upturned*
  Sterilization case
  Bipolar cable

Medtronic ENT Frontal Trephine Set
  Medtronic frontal trephine set
  Drill guide
  Drill pin
  Irrigation cannula (reusable; keep six in stock)
  Sterilizing tray

Wormald's Malleable Frontal Sinus Instruments*
(Medtronic ENT)
  Wormald malleable frontal sinus probe
  Wormald malleable frontal sinus sucker
  Wormald malleable elevator blunt
  Wormald malleable frontal sinus curette
  Sterilization tray

Wormald Dacryocystorhinostomy Set* (Medtronic ENT)
  Sickle knife
  Spear knife
  Lusk MicroBite forceps

Wormald MicroFrance Anterior Skull Base and Pituitary
Instrument Set* (Medtronic ENT)
  5-mm fine scissors: left, right, and straight
  5-mm fine scissors: up
  8-mm fine scissors: left, right, and straight
  8-mm fine scissors: up
  1-mm forceps straight and 45-degrees
  Malleable probe, straight
  Malleable probe, right angled hook
  Malleable suction dissector
  Malleable suction
  Malleable suction cage
  Malleable small and large 45-degree ring curettes
  Malleable small and large 90-degree ring curettes
  Bending tool

MicroFrance Wormald Medtronic Hemorrhage Control Set*
  Clamp, straight rotatable
  Clamp, curved small
  Clamp, curved long
  Clamp, 45-degress straight
  Clamp, 45-degress curved small
  Clamp, 45-degress curved long
  Clip, applying forceps rotatable straight
  Clip, applying forceps rotatable 45-degress
  Needle holder, rotatable

Camera System
STORZ IMAGE 1 digital camera
0-degree endoscope (4 × 11 mm Hopkins)
30-degree endoscope
45-degree endoscope
70-degree endoscope

Lens Washer
Medtronic EndoScrub II

Consumables
0-degree EndoScrub II sheath
30-degree EndoScrub sheath

Microdebrider
Medtronic IPC (Integrated Power Console)
M4 handpiece
Midas Rex stylus handpiece
Skull base burrs

Topical Solutions
Cocaine solution (10%, 2 mL)
Adrenaline (1:1000 × 1 mL)
Normal saline (0.9 × 3 mL)

*Instruments identified by an asterisk were designed by the author.

Fig. 1.1 (**A**) The blade is open and (**B**) tissue is sucked into the blade prior to rotation of the inner blade and severing of the tissue.

brider, significant damage can occur within a few seconds. There are numerous case reports in the literature in which powered microdebriders have caused inadvertent injury to the orbital contents and to the medial rectus muscle.[9,10]

The blade is used in oscillate mode for the majority of the surgery. Most of the instruments will have a default setting that will allow the blade to oscillate at 3000 or 5000 rpm. The foot pedal will also usually have a switch to allow the surgeon to select either variable or full speed when the pedal is depressed. Variable mode allows the surgeon to slow the speed whereas full speed mode will result in the blade turning at 3000 or 5000 rpm as soon as the pedal is depressed. It is important to understand that the speed at which the blade turns determines the amount of tissue that is cut. The higher the speed, the less time the port is open and the less tissue is able to be sucked into the blade before the turning blade cuts the tissue. Conversely, the slower the speed, the more tissue is sucked in and the more aggressively the blade cuts. **Figure 1.1A** shows the blade in open mode, and **Fig. 1.1B** shows tissue being sucked into the port of the blade before rotation of the blade cuts the tissue.

In forward and reverse mode the revolutions may vary from 3000 to 15,000 rpm and, consequently, the blade is open for only a very short period of time. Tissue cutting in this mode is thus severely limited. Forward mode is usually used for the various burr attachments that can be used in place of the blade. However, forward mode can also be used for very gently shaving bony septations on the lamina papyracea or skull base. This needs to be done with absolute knowledge of the anatomy and great care because inadvertent penetration of either structure can be disastrous. When this is done the septations are brushed with the rotating blade without any use of pressure.

Endoscopic High-Speed Drills

Medtronic ENT has a microdebrider base box that takes both a microdebrider handpiece with power range up to 12,000 rpm and all standard microdebrider blades and burrs.

In addition this base box also takes an electronic endoscopic high-speed drill with curved irrigated diamond and cutting burrs with power range up to 60,000 rpm. The surgeon can switch between the standard microdebrider and high-speed electric drill by simply touching the button on the foot pedal. This high-speed electric drill, although irrigated, does not have built-in suction like a normal microdebrider drill and therefore is most suitable in a two-surgeon setup where the second surgeon can provide suction during drilling. This drill will speed up the access during endoscopic skull base procedures where large amounts of bone need to be removed before the surgical site is reached.

Endoscope Cleaners

A large number of companies manufacture endoscope cleaners or scrubbers. These are designed to wash the lens of the endoscope should it become obscured with blood. If the surgical field is bloody, the endoscope cleaner keeps the scope lens clear of blood and allows the operation to proceed without the need to remove the endoscope from the nose and manually clean it. The endoscope cleaner speeds up the operation, thereby decreasing the surgeon's frustration level, and improves the safety of the surgery by maintaining visibility.

Cameras and Monitors

Surgery can be performed either through the eyepiece of the endoscope (traditional technique) or by connecting a video camera to the endoscope enabling the surgeon to operate off the monitor. The traditional technique (viewing down the endoscope) may give some surgeons a degree of orientation and depth perception. However, most surgeons today prefer to operate from the video monitor. A significant advantage of operating from the monitor is the ergonomic advantage this affords the surgeon as he or she can sit or stand next to the patient and not have to bend either their back or neck to obtain a view of the nasal cavity. This is especially valuable if the frontal recess is being operated on because the surgeon viewing the procedure through the eyepiece may have to almost have their head on the patient's chest to obtain an adequate view. In addition, if a large instrument such as the microdebrider is being used at the same time, this instrument may touch the surgeon's head when it is being manipulated into tight spaces. The monitor provides a large magnified image which can be advantageous for delicate work (e.g., optic nerve, skull base, and intracranial surgery) and it allows two surgeons to operate together (pituitary, infratemporal fossa, and intracranial surgery). Another major advantage of operating from the monitor is that it allows a senior surgeon to monitor the trainee's surgery and allows the trainee (and all in the operating room) to watch the senior surgeon operate. The nurse can anticipate the surgical instrument required for the next step and the anesthesiologist can monitor the operating field and undertake anesthetic interventions to improve the surgical field as required. If the surgeon is operating from the monitor, a high quality three-chip or digital camera is required with a powerful light source and medical grade monitor. Single-chip cameras generally do not cope well with blood in the surgical field and depth perception and tissue contrasts can be lost. If inferior cameras are used visibility and orientation become increasingly difficult for the surgeon and the risk of complications increases.

Fig. 1.2 Picture of the operating setup with the surgeon, the patient's head, and the video monitor all in a straight line. The scrub nurse stands opposite the surgeon which allows a view of the monitor and facilitates the handing of instruments to the surgeon.

◆ Position of the Patient and the Surgeon

The author's preference is to sit at the right-hand side of the patient. The surgeon may stand but if his/her elbow is not resting on the operating table, then the monitor image tends to move excessively, reflecting the instability of the hand holding the endoscope. The patient should be prone and the operating table tilted to 30 degrees anti-Trendelenburg. The patient's head should be in a neutral position (neither flexed nor extended). This allows the surgeon to operate in a plane parallel to the skull base, which diminishes the risk for skull base injury by decreasing the angle of approach. The video monitor should be positioned so that the surgeon, the patient's head, and the monitor are in a straight line (**Fig. 1.2**).

A thin arm board is placed next to the patient's head to widen the upper part of the operating table so that the surgeon can comfortably rest their elbow on the arm board. If this position is too low and extra height is needed, sterile drapes folded into a square are placed to build this up. The patient's head can also be turned toward the surgeon, thus decreasing the height at which the elbow needs to be supported. The scrub nurse should position their instrument table so that the far edge of the table is parallel with the head of the operating table. This allows the monitor stack to be placed in a straight line with the patient's head and surgeon (**Fig. 1.3A,B**).

A

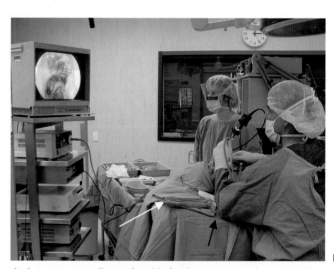

B

Fig. 1.3 The arm board is placed on the operating table (**A**, *white arrow*) to allow the surgeon to rest their elbow (**B**, *black arrow*) to stabilize the camera. This allows the surgeon's forearm and wrist to be straight, which is ergonomically comfortable for the surgeon. It also ensures that the monitor picture is stable (**B**). The height of the elbow can be adjusted with sterile towels (*white arrow*) as required.

Fig. 1.4 The scope is used to tent the nasal vestibule superiorly creating space below the endoscope (*white arrow*) through which the instrument is passed into the nose.

◆ Principles of Endoscope Placement and Instrument Placement during Endoscopic Sinus Surgery

With the surgeon's elbow resting on the added arm board, the endoscope is slid into the nose. The endoscope should then be pushed as far superiorly as possible. This should distort the nasal vestibule by placing the endoscope high in the nasal vestibule. This creates a space in the nasal vestibule below the endoscope through which all instruments are placed (**Fig. 1.4**).

The endoscope and the instruments should never cross during surgery. It is only very rarely when dissecting in the frontal sinus with a 70-degree endoscope that the endoscope needs to be placed below the instrument. When this is done the surgeon loses sight of the tip of the instrument and accurate and careful dissection is no longer possible. The 0-degree endoscope should be used whenever possible

and in the techniques described in the following chapters it is used unless otherwise stated. This makes the surgery as simple as possible and decreases the risk of unnecessary injury to the adjacent or surrounding mucosa during passage of the endoscope and instrument. It also limits the risk of disorientation that can occur when using angled endoscopes. If angled endoscopes are used, instruments need to be curved so that the tip of the instrument can be manipulated in the center of the endoscope view (see Chapter 7). The greater the angle of the endoscope, the longer the curve must be on the instrument. The greater the angle of the endoscope and curve of the instrument, the greater the degree of difficulty of dissection so it is best to use the angled endoscopes (especially the 70-degree endoscope) as infrequently as possible during surgery.

References

1. Messerklinger W. Endoscopy of the Nose. Munich: Urban and Scharzenberg; 1978: 52–54
2. Stammberger H. Endoscopic endonasal surgery—concepts in treatment of recurring rhinosinusitis. Part I. Anatomic and pathophysiologic considerations. Otolaryngol Head Neck Surg 1986;94(2):143–147
3. Kennedy DW. Functional endoscopic sinus surgery. Technique. Arch Otolaryngol 1985;111(10):643–649
4. Wee DTH, Carney AS, Thorpe M, Wormald PJ. Endoscopic orbital decompression for Graves' ophthalmopathy. J Laryngol Otol 2002;116(1):6–9
5. Wormald PJ. Powered endoscopic dacryocystorhinostomy. Laryngoscope 2002;112(1):69–72
6. Wormald PJ, Ooi E, van Hasselt CA, Nair S. Endoscopic removal of sinonasal inverted papilloma including endoscopic medial maxillectomy. Laryngoscope 2003;113(5):867–873
7. Wormald PJ, Van Hasselt A. Endoscopic removal of juvenile angiofibromas. Otolaryngol Head Neck Surg 2003;129(6):684–691
8. Knegt PP, Ah-See KW, Velden LA, Kerrebijn J. Adenocarcinoma of the ethmoidal sinus complex: surgical debulking and topical fluorouracil may be the optimal treatment. Arch Otolaryngol Head Neck Surg 2001;127(2):141–146
9. Graham SM, Nerad JA. Orbital complications in endoscopic sinus surgery using powered instrumentation. Laryngoscope 2003;113(5):874–878
10. Bhatti MT, Giannoni CM, Raynor E, Monshizadeh R, Levine LM. Ocular motility complications after endoscopic sinus surgery with powered cutting instruments. Otolaryngol Head Neck Surg 2001;125(5):501–509

2 The Surgical Field in Endoscopic Sinus Surgery

The presence of significant bleeding in the surgical field is a critical factor in the potential success or failure of endoscopic sinus surgery (ESS).[1-4] When significant bleeding is present, recognition of anatomical landmarks becomes difficult.[2-4] Bleeding obscures surgical planes and makes the identification of the drainage pathways of the sinuses difficult. Cell walls become difficult to distinguish from the lamina papyracea or skull base and the risk of causing complications increases.[3,4] If the patient has significant inflammation of the sinuses, from chronic infection or the presence of pus/fungal debris, increased vascularity will often contribute to more bleeding.[2,5] If the surgeon attempts to manipulate an instrument in the surgical field after the discernible anatomy is covered in blood, the risk of a complication increases. In addition, greater surgical trauma may occur, cells may be left behind and there is an increased likelihood of postoperative scarring and failure of the surgical procedure. It is therefore critical to optimize the surgical field and, in so doing, make the surgical dissection as easy as possible.[2-4]

Our department has a special interest in this aspect of ESS and has conducted several double blind randomized controlled studies in an attempt to establish which maneuvers to reduce bleeding are worthwhile. To date not all maneuvers have been scientifically evaluated but where there is evidence for a specific maneuver this will be presented. The first important issue to address is a grading system for bleeding in the surgical field. Boezaart and van der Merwe described and validated a grading system of five grades presented in **Table 2.1**.[3]

Although this grading system is valuable we have found that the majority of surgical fields are around grade 3 with some grade 2 and some grade 4.[2] Only on rare occasions are grade 1 and 5 fields encountered. This tends to compress the grading system and makes differentiation of more subtle changes difficult. Grade 3 may need to be further divided to allow variation within grade 3 to be discerned.[2] We have recently developed and validated an endoscopic sinus surgical field score which separates the middle grades and allows more accurate grading of the surgical field (**Table 2.2**).

◆ Local versus General Anesthetic

Local anesthetic has the advantage of not inducing generalized vasodilation. Increased circulating catecholamines may also improve the surgical field by continuing to act on the prearteriolar and precapillary sphincters. However, there are several limitations to local anesthetics.

- Patient anxiety and sudden patient movement during delicate surgery can be problematic.
- Surgery takes between 1 and 2 hours. Some patients (especially older patients) have difficulty remaining still for this length of time.
- Appropriate anesthesia needs to be achieved in all the sinuses and the nasal cavity.
- If the procedure is bloody the patient may have difficulty dealing with the volume of blood trickling into the pharynx. If the patient is sedated aspiration can occur.
- Water from the scope scrubber may add to the secretions in the pharynx that the patient needs to deal with.
- Teaching of residents can be more difficult when the patient is awake.

In our department local anesthetic is offered to patients having limited ESS confined to the middle meatus. We prefer general anesthesia for ESS that involves the frontal recess and/or posterior ethmoids and/or sphenoids.

◆ Standard Nasal Preparation for Endoscopic Sinus Surgery

Laryngeal Mask versus Endotracheal Intubation

It is our current practice to use laryngeal masks rather than endotracheal intubation for all our patients undergoing sinus surgery. The rationale for this is that it allows the patient to be kept under a lighter general anesthetic with less vasodilation and less intraoperative bleeding. In addition,

Table 2.1 Boezaart and van der Merwe Grading System for Bleeding During Endoscopic Sinus Surgery

Grades	Surgical Field
Grade 1	Cadaveric conditions with minimal suction required
Grade 2	Minimal bleeding with infrequent suction required
Grade 3	Brisk bleeding with frequent suction required
Grade 4	Bleeding covers surgical field after removal of suction before surgical instrument can perform maneuver
Grade 5	Uncontrolled bleeding; bleeding out of nostril on removal of suction

Source: Data from Boezaart AP, van der Merwe J, Coetzee A. Comparison of sodium nitroprusside- and esmolol-induced controlled hypotension for functional endoscopic sinus surgery. Can J Anaesth 1995;42:373–376.

the patient does not cough and strain on the endotracheal tube as they recover from the anesthetic thus avoiding the venous congestion and subsequent hemorrhage often associated with such straining. One of the potential downsides of a laryngeal mask is the possibility of contamination of the upper airway by blood. This is prevented by the placement of a small throat pack above the laryngeal mask in the back of the throat to catch any blood from the nasal cavity. Another possible downside is the potential difficulty with ventilation of the patient during surgery. Our standard protocol is total intravenous anesthesia (TIVA) with a laryngeal mask in a nonparalyzed patient. The remifentanil infusion (part of TIVA) suppresses spontaneous ventilation and allows the patients to be ventilated through the laryngeal mask. The lack of paralysis provides additional safety against intraoperative awareness because the patient should move if the level of anesthesia becomes too light.

Table 2.2 The Wormald Grading System for Bleeding During Endoscopic Sinus Surgery*

Grade	Surgical Field
0	No bleeding
1	1–2 points of ooze (no blood in the sphenoid)
2	3–4 points of ooze (no blood in the sphenoid)
3	5–6 points of ooze (slight blood accumulation in the sphenoid)
4	7–8 points of ooze (moderate blood accumulation of sphenoid; fills after 90 seconds)
5	9–10 points of ooze (sphenoid fills after 60 seconds)
6	> 10 points of ooze, obscuring surface (sphenoid fills between 40 and 60 seconds)
7	Mild bleeding/oozing from entire surgical surface with slow accumulation of blood in postnasal space (sphenoid fills by 40 seconds)
8	Moderate bleeding from entire surgical surface with moderate accumulation of blood in postnasal space (sphenoid fills by 30 seconds)
9	Moderately severe bleeding with rapid accumulation of blood in postnasal space (sphenoid fills by 20 seconds)
10	Severe bleeding with nasal cavity filling rapidly (sphenoid fills in < 10 seconds)

*Used when all sinuses have been opened.

Positioning the Patient

The positioning of the patient is described in Chapter 1. It is important to have the patient 30 to 40 degrees head up so that the venous return from the head and neck is facilitated. This puts the patient's head above the chest, which lowers the arterial pressure and prevents venous congestion, and thereby improves the surgical field.[6]

Topical Vasoconstriction

In a study recently published we showed that any packing material placed in the nasal cavity tends to cause damage to the nasal mucosa.[7] The more abrasive the packing, the worse the trauma.[6] Taking this into consideration, the least abrasive packing material is used, namely the neurosurgical Cottonoid patties (Codman, Raynham, MA). The anesthetist is consulted to ensure there is no contraindication to the use of cocaine. If there is a concern then 1% oxymetazoline is used in place of cocaine. In an adult patient a mixture of 2 mL of 10% cocaine, 1 mL of 1:1000 adrenaline, and 4 mL of saline is divided into two equal portions, with one portion used to soak six neuropatties. These six neuropatties are placed in the nose once the patient is anesthetized. The other half of the cocaine mixture and remaining four neuropatties are kept sterile on the instrument trolley for later use during surgery if required. Three neuropatties are placed on each side directly after intubation using a Freer elevator to manipulate them gently into place. The first neuropattie is placed in the sphenoethmoidal recess, the second under the middle turbinate, with the third being placed over the axilla of the middle turbinate (**Fig. 2.1**). If there is a concha bullosa or significantly lateralized middle turbinate, the neuropattie is placed along the inferior margin of the middle turbinate. No force is used to place the neuropatties in the middle meatus.

Fig. 2.1 Placement of the neuropatties in the left nasal cavity prior to surgery. A pattie is in the sphenoethmoidal recess (*1*), another is in the middle meatus (*2*), and another is in the region of the axillary flap (*3*).

As only half the solution is used at the beginning of surgery the total dose of cocaine that the patient is exposed to is ~100 mg. The toxic dose of cocaine is 3 mg per kg without the simultaneous use of adrenaline. It has also been shown that the presence of adrenaline inhibits mucosal absorption and that a proportion of the solution will remain in the neuropattie. This decreases the amount of cocaine that the patient is exposed to and the doses used are well below the toxic dose in adult patients. The dose needs to be appropriately adjusted in children.

Local Infiltration

A 2% solution of lidocaine ("lignocaine" in the UK and Australia) with either 1:80000 or 1:100000 adrenaline is administered with a dental syringe and needle. The injections are given after the patient has been draped and the camera and endoscope are available. Under endoscopic guidance the area above the middle turbinate is infiltrated. This is followed by infiltration into the anterior end of the middle turbinate. Note that the area anterior to the uncinate is not infiltrated as bleeding from an injection site can obscure the uncinate during its removal. In some patients, where there is expected increased likelihood of bleeding, a third injection is given into the back end of the middle turbinate in the region of the sphenopalatine artery. A spinal needle is used as the dental needle is usually not long enough to reach this area. **Figure 2.2** illustrates the routine infiltration points used.

Preoperative Antibiotics and Steroids

Inflammation increases the vascularity of tissues and, when surgery is conducted on highly inflamed tissues, increased bleeding results. Patients with acute sinusitis, who have an

Fig. 2.2 Injection sites in the right nasal cavity for local anesthetic prior to endoscopic sinus surgery. The needle is in the region of the axillary flap and the *white arrow* indicates the injection site on the anterior end of the middle turbinate.

infective complication requiring surgery, will often have a very bloody surgical field. It therefore stands to reason that using antibiotics in patients with a significant infection preoperatively should improve the surgical field. However, most of our patients undergoing ESS have had extended medical therapy which normally includes numerous courses of antibiotics and often systemic steroids, and therefore rarely have an acute infection present. The value of using antibiotics preoperatively in this elective patient group is unknown as there are no well-designed studies addressing this issue. The important questions that remain unanswered are the type of antibiotic, the length of time it should be used before surgery, and the patient group most likely to benefit from preoperative use. Currently I do not routinely place patients on antibiotics preoperatively.

It has been suggested that patients with significant nasal polyposis may benefit from a course of preoperative steroids.[8] The theory is that steroids should decrease the size of the polyps and the vascularity associated with these polyps. Although this argument seems logical, it is yet to be confirmed in properly designed and controlled studies. A recently published preliminary study evaluated the effect of preoperative steroids on the degree of bleeding during sinus surgery.[8] In this study prednisone 30 mg daily was given for 5 days preoperatively and the results showed a significant improvement in a visual analogue grading of the surgical field during surgery.[8] However, it remains unclear what doses of steroids should be given, for how long, and to which patient groups. Empiric treatment regimens range from 30[8] to 50 mg of prednisone daily for between 5 and 7 days preoperatively, and is usually only utilized in nasal polyposis patients.

◆ Additional Maneuvers for Optimizing the Surgical Field in Endoscopic Sinus Surgery

Suction Bipolar Cautery* of Isolated Bleeding Areas

It is common to see isolated bleeding vessels in the surgical field during ESS. These result from the transection of small blood vessels and may continue to ooze into the surgical field, significantly adding to the volume of blood which may obscure the surgical field.[4] In addition, such an ooze may obscure the end of the endoscope requiring either the endoscope scrubber to be used or the endoscope to be removed from the nose to be cleaned. If the axillary flap approach to the frontal recess is used (see Chapter 7), the cut mucosal edge may bleed and this can be controlled by the use of the suction bipolar cautery. Other common areas where bleeding is seen are the posterior region of the maxillary sinus, the sphenopalatine region of the lateral nasal wall, and from the anterior wall of the sphenoid below its ostium. The suction bipolar allows the bleeding vessels to be accurately identified and cauterized. Not having to remove the instrument from the nose after the suction clears the blood allows identification of the bleeding point, which is a significant advantage of this instrument (**Fig. 2.3**).

Fig. 2.3 (**A**) The suction bipolar is in the normal position. (**B**) The suction is extended beyond the bipolar paddles. When the manipulating lever (*black arrow* in **A**) is relaxed the suction retracts behind the bipolar paddles (**C**).

The Anatomy of the Greater Palatine Canal and Local Anesthetic Infiltration of the Pterygopalatine Fossa

Injection of local anesthetic into the pterygopalatine fossa does improve the surgical field.[9,10] The maxillary artery and its terminal branches make up the main blood supply of the nose. There are two approaches and the less reliable approach is direct infiltration into the region of the sphenopalatine foramen. The needle is introduced just under the posterior end of the middle turbinate. Sometimes the needle can be felt to slip into the sphenopalatine foramen but, in most cases, location of the foramen is difficult and the injection is given into the general region of the foramen. This should cause vasospasm of the vessels exiting the foramen. However, because the foramen is not easily located, the resulting vasoconstriction achieved may not be as great as injecting the pterygopalatine fossa through the greater palatine canal.

The second, more reliable approach is to inject the pterygopalatine fossa through the greater palatine foramen and canal. First the greater palatine foramen needs to be located on the hard palate (**Fig. 2.4**). The greater palatine foramen is located just anterior to the posterior edge of the hard palate opposite the second molar tooth.[11] It is usually halfway between the tooth and the midline of the hard palate. The

opening of the foramen into the canal is funnel-shaped and the canal is angled at ~45 degrees to the hard palate.

In a cadaver study performed in our department to evaluate the anatomy of the greater palatine canal, 20 cadaver heads underwent computed tomography (CT) scanning in the axial plane at 0.5 mm.[12] Parasagittal reconstructions were performed in the plane of the greater palatine canal. The length of the canal and depth of the soft tissue overlying the canal was measured. In addition, needles were bent at 10, 20, and 30 mm and inserted into the greater palatine canal prior to CT scanning to demonstrate the degree of penetration into the pterygopalatine fossa in four cadavers (**Fig. 2.5**).

This was done to ascertain the likelihood of damage to the contents of the fossa (branches of the maxillary nerve, maxillary artery, and pterygopalatine ganglion) and the orbit. Note that the bend in the needle stops at the soft tissue overlying the hard palate and that this soft tissue had a mean thickness of 6.9 mm (95% confidence interval [CI] = 6.2–7.6) (**Fig. 2.6**). The mean length of the greater palatine canal was 18.5 mm (95% CI = 17.9–19.1) and the mean height of the pterygopalatine fossa was 21.6 mm (95% CI = 20.7–22.5).[12] Therefore, to perform an effective infiltration of the pterygopalatine fossa, the needle should be bent at 25 mm from the tip at an angle of 45 degrees.[12] This will result in the tip of the needle just

Fig. 2.4 Blood staining can be seen from where the needle was introduced into the greater palatine canal (*black arrow*) of the left hard palate. The second molar tooth is marked with a *white arrow*.

Fig. 2.5 Cadaver with needle (*white arrow*) bent at 20 mm and inserted into the greater palatine canal after which the computed tomography scan was performed.

Fig. 2.6 The soft tissue measurement was from *A* to *B*, the greater palatine canal from *B* to *C*, and the height of the pterygopalatine fossa from *C* to *D*. The funnel-shaped opening of the greater palatine canal into the pterygopalatine fossa is indicated with a *white arrow*.

penetrating the pterygopalatine fossa without putting any of the contents of the fossa at risk.[12]

The greater palatine canal has an hourglass shape, dilating as it enters the pterygopalatine fossa. This funnel-shaped entrance into the greater palatine canal means that it can be difficult to determine exactly where the pterygopalatine fossa ends and the greater palatine canal begins (white arrow, **Fig. 2.6**).

The easiest way to locate the greater palatine foramen is by palpating the palate with the finger. This is performed by placing a tongue depressor in the mouth and holding down the tongue, then passing a finger and the endoscope into the mouth together. The finger first locates the posterior free edge of the hard palate and then slides anteriorly over this ridge onto the hard palate. The foramen should be felt as a depression directly anterior to the free edge about midway between the second molar tooth and the midline of the palate. Visualize the finger palpating the foramen on the monitor and identify the spot on the palate as the finger is withdrawn from the mouth. With the needle bent at 25 mm and at a 45-degree angle, insert the needle into the spot that you had visually marked on the palate. If the needle strikes bone then a small amount of lidocaine is infiltrated, the needle is withdrawn, and an adjacent spot it tried. The assumption is that the needle had just missed the foramen and that a slight adjustment needs to be made before the foramen is located. If repeated attempts to introduce the needle fail, then the landmarks for the foramen (the midpoint between the second molar tooth and midline of the palate) are reassessed and the finger and endoscope are replaced into the mouth and the foramen relocated. The needle is reintroduced until the foramen is located by the needle advancing into the greater palatine canal without any resistance up to the bend in the needle. After aspirating (to ensure that the needle is not in a blood vessel), the pterygopalatine fossa is infiltrated with 2 mL of 2% lidocaine and 1:80 000 adrenaline.

Our department has conducted a double blind randomized controlled trial in which the effects of local anesthetic

and adrenaline infiltration of the pterygopalatine fossa were assessed on the surgical field in 55 patients.[10] To be included in the study the patient required bilateral ESS with similar procedures having been performed bilaterally. A surgeon not involved in the surgery randomly infiltrated one fossa transorally so that the operating surgeon would not be aware of which side had been infiltrated. The surgeon then alternated the surgery on the patient and assessed the surgical field on each side. Statistical analysis showed that the side that had received the pterygopalatine fossa injection had significantly better surgical field (mean surgical grade of 2.59) than the control side (mean surgical grade of 2.99; $P < .01$).[10]

β-Blockers

Inhalational agents used during general anesthesia cause peripheral vasodilation by relaxing the prearteriolar muscle sphincters.[6] This significant peripheral vasodilation usually results in mild hypotension.[3,4,6] Peripheral vasodilation with paralysis of the arteriolar and precapillary sphincters may result in significant bleeding if surgery is performed when the tissues of the nose and sinuses are inflamed.[3,4,6] In an attempt to compensate for this reduced venous return and low cardiac output, reflexes increase the heart rate in an attempt to improve the cardiac output.[3,4,6] A seminal paper by Boesak and van der Merwe showed that vasodilation induced by sodium nitroprusside caused a significant worsening in the surgical field despite the lowered blood pressure.[3] What they also showed was that esmolol, a highly selective β1 β-blocker, improved the surgical field with a much smaller drop in blood pressure.[3] Esmolol is a short-acting cardioselective β adrenergic receptor-blocking drug that has a fast onset and short half-life. In contrast to a drug such as sodium nitroprusside, which while effectively lowering the blood pressure results in a compensatory increase in heart rate, esmolol is highly effective at depressing cardiac output and results in a slowing of the pulse rate despite a fall in blood pressure.[6] Esmolol is given by a constant IV infusion and has a very short half-life (around 3 minutes) so its effect can be closely controlled. Although this can be a very worthwhile maneuver, it is a very expensive drug and there is some resistance (based on cost) against using it as a regular or routine part of ESS anesthesia.

The expense of this drug stimulated our department to conduct a double blind placebo controlled prospective study in the effects of metoprolol taken orally 20 minutes before general anesthetic, as compared with a vitamin B placebo.[2] This study showed that patients who received the β-blocker (metoprolol) had a significantly lower pulse rate (mean of 59) than the placebo group (mean of 69). There was no significant difference in blood pressure or surgical fields in the two groups. However, what was interesting was the significant correlation between heart rate in the overall patient group with surgical grade.[2] Thus, irrespective of whether a β-blocker is given to the patient or not, if the heart rate of the patient can be kept below 60 beats per minute, the surgical field was usually good.[2] Therefore we recommend the use of a β-blocker (atenolol, metoprolol, or esmolol) as a worthwhile manipulation that can improve the surgical field in patients who have a pulse rate significantly above 60 beats per minute at induction of anesthesia and who do not have a contraindication (such as asthma). However, asthma is a common comorbidity in patients with chronic sinusitis and alternatives are needed. In this group of patients we use clonidine.

Clonidine

Clonidine is a centrally active α agonist that initially results in an elevation of blood pressure before depressing the cardiac output by inhibiting the central cardiac regulatory mechanism. It should be used with caution and should be given in small increments, as the effect is not easily reversible. It also results in mild postoperative sedation and its effects on the blood pressure are usually seen in the initial few hours after surgery. This is beneficial for the majority of patients as this mild hypotension allows the small blood vessels in the nose to coagulate with a reduced chance of postoperative epistaxis. There are no properly designed and controlled studies which quantify the effect of clonidine on the surgical field in ESS.

Total Intravenous Anesthesia and Inhalational Agents

As can be seen from the previous discussion, vasodilation is detrimental to the surgical field. General anesthesia results in vasodilation and the extent of the vasodilation is to a certain extent dependent on the type and quantity of inhalational agent used.[6] Halothane gives significant vasodilation and should not be used.[6] Isoflurane and sevoflurane produce less vasodilation but if they are used to deepen the level of anesthesia with the intention of lowering the blood pressure, significant vasodilation can occur.[6] TIVA is usually given by utilizing a constant infusion of propofol. Propofol induces anesthesia by enhancing the action of GABA neurotransmitter on the GABA receptor, which allows the chloride channels to be opened causing hyperpolarization and reduced excitability of the cell.[13] Propofol is short acting and needs to be administered as a constant infusion. Although it does depress the heart, this response is not dose-dependent and increasing the infusion rate of propofol will not result in an increasing suppression of pulse rate and cardiac output. It, however, does not affect the muscle tone of the prearteriolar and precapillary sphincters and does not cause vasodilation and increased bleeding. This allows inhalational agents to be avoided. If bleeding during ESS continues to be problematic despite the patient receiving TIVA, other drugs such as β-blockers or clonidine can be added. In a recent study in our department we performed a randomized controlled single blinded (to the surgeon) study using TIVA and isoflurane. This study showed that the surgical fields were better if TIVA was used.[14] All other factors were kept constant during the surgery. The pulse rate, when analyzed independently, again correlated to the surgical field thereby emphasizing the importance of the pulse rate on the surgical field. Some

anesthetists are uncomfortable using TIVA as it can be difficult to judge the depth of anesthesia so it is a good idea to discuss the merits of use of TIVA with the anesthetist before surgery.

◆ General Guidelines for the Maneuvers for Improving the Surgical Field

The ideal surgical field is grade 2 on the Boezaart scale and grades 1 to 4 on the Wormald scale. However, the majority of our patients fluctuate between grade 2 and 3 on the Boezaart scale. Operating in more bloody conditions can be aided by the use of suction dissection instruments* (see Chapter 1) such as the suction curette* and suction Freer.* These instruments allow the blood to be cleared from the surgical field during the dissection and obviate the need to change from a dissecting instrument to a suction to clear the surgical field.

Surgical Field Change from Boezaart Grade 3 to Grade 4 or 5

Please note that surgery should not be performed if the surgical field is grade 5.

- Check positioning of the patient
- Check that you have properly infiltrated the lateral wall of the nose with lidocaine and adrenaline
- Place neuropatties soaked with cocaine and adrenaline in the surgical field
- Check the patient's pulse rate and, if greater than 60, ask the anesthetist to adjust this to below 60 (using β-blockers if not contraindicated)
- If the patient is hypertensive ask the anesthetist to bring the mean blood pressure down to around a mean of 65 to 75 mmHg without increasing the inhalational agent (consider the use of a β-blocker or clonidine)

Recheck Your Surgical Field

- If there is a specific bleeder, cauterize it with the suction bipolar.*
- If the bleeding is emanating from the posterior region of the nasal cavity, consider replacing the neuropatties and performing a pterygopalatine fossa block.
- If bleeding is still not controlled or is coming from the anterior aspects of the nose, then consider asking the anesthetist to further lower the pulse rate with small incremental doses of clonidine. Remember to stay within the safe range of mean blood pressure (> 55 mmHg[6]) especially when considering the age of the patient and the previous mean blood pressure of the patient. If the patient was known to suffer from hypertension this figure should be higher.
- Consider changing the patient from inhalational anesthesia to TIVA.

References

1. Stankiewicz JA. Complications of endoscopic intranasal ethmoidectomy. Laryngoscope 1987;97(11):1270–1273

2. Nair S, Collins M, Hung P, Rees G, Close D, Wormald PJ. The effect of beta-blocker premedication on the surgical field during endoscopic sinus surgery. Laryngoscope 2004;114(6):1042–1046

3. Boezaart AP, van der Merwe J, Coetzee A. Comparison of sodium nitroprusside- and esmolol-induced controlled hypotension for functional endoscopic sinus surgery. Can J Anaesth 1995;42(5 Pt 1):373–376

4. Boezaart AP, van der Merwe J, Coetzee AR. Re: Moderate controlled hypotension with sodium nitroprusside does not improve surgical conditions or decrease blood loss in endoscopic sinus surgery. J Clin Anesth 2001;13(4):319–320

5. Mortimore S, Wormald PJ. Management of acute complicated sinusitis: a 5-year review. Otolaryngol Head Neck Surg 1999;121(5):639–642

6. van Aken H, Miller ED. Deliberate hypotension. In: Miller RD, ed. Anesthesia. Vol 2. New York: Churchill Livingstone; 1994: 1481–1503

7. Shaw CL, Dymock RB, Cowin A, Wormald PJ. Effect of packing on nasal mucosa of sheep. J Laryngol Otol 2000;114(7):506–509

8. Sieskiewicz A, Olszewska E, Rogowski M, Grycz E. Preoperative corticosteroid oral therapy and intraoperative bleeding during functional endoscopic sinus surgery in patients with severe nasal polyposis: a preliminary investigation. Ann Otol Rhinol Laryngol 2006;115(7):490–494

9. Wormald PJ, Wee DTH, van Hasselt CA. Endoscopic ligation of the sphenopalatine artery for refractory posterior epistaxis. Am J Rhinol 2000;14(4):261–264

10. Wormald PJ, Athanasiadis T, Rees G, Robinson S. An evaluation of effect of pterygopalatine fossa injection with local anesthetic and adrenalin in the control of nasal bleeding during endoscopic sinus surgery. Am J Rhinol 2005;19(3):288–292

11. Mercuri LG. Intraoral second division nerve block. Oral Surg Oral Med Oral Pathol 1979;47(2):109–113

12. Douglas R, Wormald PJ. Pterygopalatine fossa infiltration through the greater palatine foramen: where to bend the needle. Laryngoscope 2006;116(7):1255–1257

13. Sonner J, Zhang Y, Stabernack C, Abaigar W, Xing Y, Laster M. GABA$_A$ receptor blockade antagonizes the immobilizing action of propofol but not ketamine or isoflurane in a dose-related manner. Anesth Analg 2003;3:706–712

14. Wormald PJ, van Renen G, Perks J, Jones JA, Langton-Hewer CD. The effect of the total intravenous anesthesia compared with inhalational anesthesia on the surgical field during endoscopic sinus surgery. Am J Rhinol 2005;19(5):514–520

3 Imaging in Endoscopic Sinus Surgery

It is fortunate that the development of endoscopic surgery (ESS) has coincided with major advances in computed tomography (CT) scanning technology. Before CT scanning was available, the extent of sinus disease and the anatomy of the nose and sinuses were assessed on plain X-rays. Plain X-rays are no longer used in this role because they provide neither sufficient anatomical detail nor accurate information on the extent of nasal and sinus pathology. The CT scan has allowed the detailed anatomy of the sinuses to be evaluated and in this textbook CT scans are used extensively to reconstruct the anatomy of the sinuses thus enabling a surgical plan to be made before surgery begins. The surgical philosophy of this textbook is underpinned by the availability of high-quality CT scans in three planes.

◆ Computed Tomography Scans

The Value of Scans in Three Planes

CT scans are used as an aid for both the diagnosis of chronic sinusitis and for the planning of the surgery. However, there is a significant incidence of mucosal abnormalities seen in completely asymptomatic patients.[1] Thus it is important that the patient has undergone adequate medical treatment for the nasal and sinus condition before a CT scan of the sinuses is performed.[2] The coronal scan is the primary scan used to assess the anatomy of the sinuses.[3] These scans should be sufficiently close together so that an identified cell can be followed from one slice to the next. This allows a three-dimensional (3D) image of the anatomy to be reconstructed from the scans.[4–6] The axial scan is of particular value in determining the drainage pathway of the frontal sinus. This is important when deciding where the curette or probe is going to be slid during the dissection of the frontal recess. Our department recently published a study evaluating the value of the parasagittal scan in assessing the frontal recess and in the understanding and planning of the

surgery.[7] We found that the parasagittal scan significantly improved the surgeon's ability to assess the frontal recess and improved the understanding of the anatomy by a mean of 57% on a 10–point visual analogue scale. The parasagittal scan also altered the surgical plan for the patient in over 50% of patients studied. We therefore recommend that all patients undergoing ESS should have a high definition helical multislice CT scan of the sinuses with the scans presented in all three planes. An example of the quality of the CT scans that should be expected using this protocol is shown in **Fig. 3.1**.

Scanning Protocol

Good quality CT scans are critical to the ability of the surgeon to reconstruct the anatomy and drainage pathways of the sinuses. Ideally, images should be in the coronal, axial, and parasagittal plane and should be relatively close together so that a cell can be followed from one scan to the next. Our current CT scan imaging protocol on a multislice CT helical scanner requires scans to be performed in the axial plane at 0.5- to 1-mm intervals with coronal and parasagittal reconstruction. Images in all planes are printed for the surgeon. The windows of the scan are set at between 1500 and 2000 with a center of +100 to +300 for highest bony definition. If there is a suspicion of fungal sinus disease, the window settings are changed to soft tissue settings. This allows the opacified sinuses to be assessed for double densities that are often present in chronic fungal sinus disease.

Three-Dimensional Views and the Concept of Building Blocks

Some CT scanners have software where cursors can be moved through a series of scans in one plane while at the same time the views of where the cursor is in the other

Fig. 3.1 Computed tomography scans with slices in the coronal (**A**), axial (**B**), and parasagittal planes (**C**). The disease in the left frontal recess (*white arrow*) can be evaluated and the cellular structure better understood if all three planes are available.

planes are simultaneously displayed. Such software can be purchased independently if not available on the scanner (e.g., Voxar, Edinburgh, UK). For owners of Apple computers there are programs (OsiriX) that can be downloaded free from the Internet which accept DICOM images from CT scanners and will create images in all three planes with movable crosshairs. In addition, all computer-aided surgical (CAS) systems also have this facility. With these systems the CT scans can be scrolled in a particular plane and the other views change depending on where the cursor is placed on the scan being viewed. If either the software is available or an image guidance machine is going to be used for a particular patient, it is valuable to utilize this technology to try and get a better understanding of the 3D anatomy of the patient before the patient is operated on. An example of a cursor placed in a position in one plane and then displayed by the computer in the other planes is shown in **Fig. 3.2**.

A central theme throughout this book is the utilization of high quality CT scans in three different planes to build a 3D picture of the anatomy of the sinuses. In general the coronal scans are viewed first and cells identified and followed in an

attempt to build up a 3D picture of the anatomy. This is done in the frontal recess (see Chapter 6) and, after completion of the frontal recess, the process is repeated in the posterior ethmoids and sphenoid (Chapter 8). After the anatomy is reviewed on the coronal scans (**Fig. 3.2A**), the parasagittal scans are reviewed (**Fig. 3.2C**). This often helps with the anterior posterior placement of the cells. Finally, the axial view (**Fig. 3.2B**) is reviewed as this is often helpful for establishing the drainage pathway of the frontal sinus. The building block concept is based around using a single building block for each cell identified in the frontal recess and in the posterior ethmoids. Following placement or stacking of the building blocks, the drainage pathway of the frontal sinus is established. This is of vital importance as it allows curettes and probes to be passed along this drainage pathway and for the cells to be removed from the outflow tract of the frontal sinus and sphenoethmoidal drainage pathway (Chapter 6). The concept of 3D anatomical reconstruction by using building blocks to recreate the anatomical formation in the frontal recess and posterior ethmoids and then to surgically establish the drainage pathways is the central theme of this book.

Fig. 3.2 The cross-hairs are placed on one scan by the computer mouse. The position of the cross-hairs is seen in other planes.

◆ Magnetic Resonance Imaging Scans

Magnetic resonance imaging (MRI) scans are not routinely used for the assessment of patients undergoing ESS as they do not provide bony definition. In addition MRI scans are very sensitive to mucosal thickening of the nasal or sinus mucosa (especially of a vascular region such as the inferior turbinate). Normal mucosa may be enhanced and in some patients even appear pathological even though it is normal. The MRI scan, however, can be very useful in several situations. We routinely request a MRI scan in patients who had previously undergone an osteoplastic flap with obliteration who have ongoing symptoms.[8,9] In these patients it can differentiate sepsis or mucocele formation from those with healthy fat in their obliterated frontal sinuses. All patients who have an intranasal tumor are assessed with an MRI scan.[10] In these patients we are primarily interested in whether an opacified sinus is filled with tumor or retained mucus and whether a breach or invasion of the dura or orbital periosteum has occurred. An example of the usefulness of a MRI in surgical planning is shown in **Fig. 3.3A-D**. This patient had an adenocarcinoma with opacified frontal sinuses and right maxillary sinus on CT scanning. In the MRI it can clearly be seen that the left frontal sinus and right maxillary sinus are filled with mucus, not tumor.

Our protocol to assess these patients is to perform a T1-weighted fat saturation gadolinium-enhanced scan and a T2-weighted scan. The tumor enhances on the T1 gadolinium-enhanced scan but the fluid in the sinuses does not. If the T2-weighted scan is reviewed, fluid (mucus) usually enhances significantly. In the scans shown in **Fig. 3.3B,D**, the lamina papyracea and skull base are eroded. However, it appears that the orbital contents have been pushed laterally by the tumor rather than the tumor invading into the orbit. In this patient both orbits were preserved and there was a good surgical plane between the tumor and the orbital periosteum. The tumor also appears to push the dura superiorly rather than eroding through the dura. Again we were able to establish a good surgical plane between the tumor and the dura and achieve a complete macroscopic resection of the tumor without resection of the dura. The patient had postoperative radiotherapy and continues to be tumor free three years after the surgical procedure.

MRI scans are also useful in the assessment of complications of sinusitis particularly for orbital complications with subperiosteal abscess formation and intracranial

Fig. 3.3 Computed tomography (CT) scan and magnetic resonance imaging (MRI) scan of a patient with adenocarcinoma. CT scans (**A,C**) show opacification of the frontal sinuses (*broken white arrow* in **A**) and the right maxillary (*solid white arrow* in **C**). The T2-weighted MRI scans (**B,D**) show the left frontal sinus (*broken white arrow* in **B**) and that both maxillary sinuses (*solid white arrow* for right sinus) contain fluid and not tumor (right frontal unclear on this scan).

complications.[11] MRI scans are used as first-line assessment for pituitary tumors and for extended skull base lesions such as clival tumors.

◆ Angiography

Angiography is useful in patients who have a suspected vascular tumor and an attempt is to be made to remove this tumor endoscopically.[12] It is of great importance that the vascularity of the tumor be reduced as far as possible to facilitate endoscopic removal. Vascular tumors that have not been embolized can bleed so profusely during endoscopic resection that the procedure needs to be abandoned. Although several tumors can benefit from preoperative embolization, this intervention is of particular value in angiofibroma (**Fig. 3.4A-D**).[12]

◆ Dacryocystogram and Lacrimal Scintillography

A dacryocystogram (DCG) can be very useful for assessing the anatomy of the nasolacrimal system.[13,14] It is important to identify patients with a significant stricture of the common canaliculus as these patients are not suitable for dacryocystorhinostomy.[13,14] In some patients with significant epiphora a DCG reveals a free flow of dye from the canaliculus to the nose. A DCG is not a physiologic test as abnormally high pressures are generated in the nasolacrimal system during injection of the dye. In these patients lacrimal scintillography can be very useful as the placement of a radioisotope in the tear lake with subsequent detection of its passage into the nasolacrimal system and nose provides important information regarding the function of the system (**Fig. 3.5**). These tests are fully elaborated upon in Chapter 11.

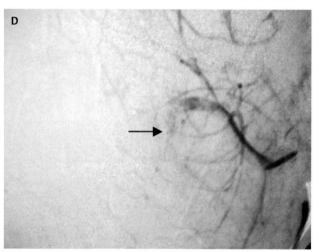

Fig. 3.4 The computed tomography scan (**A**) shows an angiofibroma (*white arrow*) filling the posterior nasal cavity with extension into the pterygopalatine and infratemporal fossas. The tumor (*white arrow*) extent is better seen on the magnetic resonance image (**B**). The digital subtraction angiogram (**C**) illustrates the intense vascularity of the tumor (*black arrow*) before embolization while the effectiveness of embolization is illustrated (**D**) where no tumor blush can be seen (*black arrow*).

Fig. 3.5 (**A**) The dacryocystogram: the right side is normal with the normal lacrimal sac (*black arrow*) and canaliculi clearly seen. On the left side the superior, inferior, and common canaliculi can be seen but dye does not penetrate the lacrimal sac (*white arrow*) and there is no filling of the lacrimal sac. This represents a common cannaliculus obstruction. (**B**) The corresponding lacrimal scintillogram. A normal scintillogram can be seen on the right. There is some isotope filling of the left lacrimal sac but no nasal penetration. This indicates probable kinking of the common canaliculus as it enters the sac.

References

1. Flinn J, Chapman ME, Wightman AJA, Maran AGD. A prospective analysis of incidental paranasal sinus abnormalities on CT head scans. Clin Otolaryngol Allied Sci 1994;19(4):287–289

2. Lusk RP, Muntz HR. Endoscopic sinus surgery in children with chronic sinusitis: a pilot study. Laryngoscope 1990;100(6):654–658

3. Kennedy DW, Zinreich SJ. The functional endoscopic approach to inflammatory sinus disease: current perspectives and technique modifications. Am J Rhinol 1988;2:89–96

4. Wormald PJ. The agger nasi cell: the key to understanding the anatomy of the frontal recess. Otolaryngol Head Neck Surg 2003;129(5):497–507

5. Wormald PJ. The axillary flap approach to the frontal recess. Laryngoscope 2002;112(3):494–499

6. Wormald PJ, Chan SZX. Surgical techniques for the removal of frontal recess cells obstructing the frontal ostium. Am J Rhinol 2003;17(4):221–226

7. Kew J, Rees G, Close D, Sdralis T, Sebben R, Wormald PJ. Multiplanar reconstructed CT images improves depiction and understanding of the anatomy of the frontal sinus and recess. Am J Rhinol 2002;16(2):119–123

8. Wormald PJ, Ooi E, van Hasselt CA, Nair S. Endoscopic removal of sinonasal inverted papilloma including endoscopic medial maxillectomy. Laryngoscope 2003;113(5):867–873

9. Wormald PJ. Salvage frontal sinus surgery: the endoscopic modified Lothrop procedure. Laryngoscope 2003;113(2):276–283

10. Wormald PJ, Ananda A, Nair S. The modified endoscopic Lothrop procedure in the treatment of complicated chronic frontal sinusitis. Clin Otolaryngol Allied Sci 2003;28(3):215–220

11. Mortimore S, Wormald PJ. Management of acute complicated sinusitis: a 5-year review. Otolaryngol Head Neck Surg 1999;121(5):639–642

12. Wormald PJ, Van Hasselt A. Endoscopic removal of juvenile angiofibromas. Otolaryngol Head Neck Surg 2003;129(6):684–691

13. Tsirbas A, Wormald PJ. Endonasal dacryocystorhinostomy with mucosal flaps. Am J Ophthalmol 2003;135(1):76–83

14. Wormald PJ. Powered endoscopic DCR. Laryngoscope 2002;112:69–72

4 Powered Inferior Turbinoplasty and Endoscopic Septoplasty

◆ Powered Endoscopic Inferior Turbinoplasty (Video 1)

Turbinectomy is seldom required in patients with chronic sinusitis because successful surgical management of the sinuses will in most cases result in normalization of the mucosa of the inferior turbinates. The inflammatory cytokines and cells contained within the mucus emanating from the diseased sinuses causes an inflammatory response from the mucosa of the inferior and middle turbinates. Once the sinuses are properly aerated and this inflammatory exudate resolves, the edema of the turbinate mucosa subsides. However, in patients with ostiomeatal complex disease or minimal maxillary mucosal thickening as their only computed tomography (CT) findings, who have nasal obstruction as their main nasal symptom, turbinoplasty with mini functional endoscopic sinus surgery (FESS) may be needed to resolve these patients' symptoms. In addition, there are some patients without sinus disease who have intractable inferior turbinate hypertrophy (nonresponsive to treatment), and in which turbinate reduction can improve the patient's nasal airway and quality of life. There have been many techniques described for inferior turbinate reduction and these include submucous turbinoplasty, partial turbinectomy, complete turbinectomy, and diathermy (usually performed in the submucosal plane).[1-5] Arguments against complete removal of the inferior turbinates cite the risk of the patient developing atrophic rhinitis, especially in hot and dry climates.[1] In addition, amputation of the turbinate flush with the lateral nasal wall will inevitably result in a significant bleed at the time of surgery as the branch of the sphenopalatine artery to the inferior turbinate is cut[6] (**Fig. 4.1**). This may require diathermy of the bleeder and this again increases the amount of necrotic tissue and results in significant postoperative crusting. Partial turbinectomy may also result in significant bleeding and require diathermy for control. Submucosal turbinoplasty and diathermy, although initially effective, does not appear to have the same long-term success as partial or complete turbinectomy.[1,7] In addition we are all aware of the patients who have undergone turbinectomy and have a capacious nasal airway but still have the sensation of nasal obstruction.[1] This may be due to the removal or destruction of airflow receptors on the medial and superior aspect of the inferior turbinate. However, this remains to be proven. The other significant problem patients suffer from after turbinectomy or diathermy (not submucous turbinoplasty) is crusting on the cut surface of turbinate.[6-8] This problem increases if diathermy has been used to control bleeding. These crusts can be uncomfortable and cause nasal obstruction. In addition, hemorrhage may occur when they either fall off or are removed.[1,3] In the group of patients undergoing submucosal diathermy and to a lesser extent submucosal turbinoplasty, they have significant postoperative swelling of the inferior turbinate which obliterates the nasal cavity and makes the first 3 weeks after surgery very uncomfortable for the patient who is usually unable to breathe through their nose.[7]

Powered inferior turbinoplasty was designed to preserve the medial wall of the inferior turbinate thereby preserving the airflow receptors. In addition the technique allows the inferior turbinate to be reduced in size by ~50% without leaving a raw surface for crusts to form in the postoperative period.

Surgical Technique (Video 1)

Under general or local anesthetic the anterior end of the inferior turbinate is infiltrated with lidocaine 2% and 1:80000 or 1:100000 adrenaline. A spinal needle attached to a 2-mL syringe is used to infiltrate along the posterior inferior border of the inferior turbinate. The turbinate is fractured medially allowing space for the endoscope (zero degree) and powered microdebrider to be placed. A 12-degree or straight blade is used in oscillate mode to remove the soft tissue from the lateral aspect of the vertical portion of the inferior turbinate (**Fig. 4.2**).

The debrider is then set on forward mode and the majority of the bone removed with the rotating blade. If the oscillate

Fig. 4.1 Cadaveric dissection of the right posterior lateral nasal wall demonstrating the inferior turbinate (*IT*) branch of the sphenopalatine artery (*SPA*). Note the relationship between the posterior attachment of the middle and inferior turbinates to the sphenopalatine foramen and palatine bone.

Fig. 4.2 Mucosa from the head of the inferior turbinate (*IT*) has been removed with the straight microdebrider demonstrating the underlying inferior turbinate bone. *MT*, middle turbinate.

mode is used for bone removal this may result in bone and portions of the medial surface of the turbinate being removed. If possible this should be avoided as the medial portion of the turbinate should be preserved so it can be rolled upon itself at the end of the procedure (**Fig. 4.3**). Any residual bony fragments are dissected free with a ball probe (**Fig. 4.4**). The inferior turbinate bone often thickens considerably as the dissection is continued anteriorly. It is often useful to use the pediatric backbiter to facilitate the dissection of this

bone. It is critical that this bone is removed as it is in this region that the nose is narrowest and where the greatest degree of benefit of the operation will be achieved.

Once all the lateral mucosa and bone has been removed the remaining mucosa is rolled upon itself covering the raw area. The Freer elevator is used to roll the mucosa and, if necessary, fracture the horizontal portion of the remaining inferior turbinate laterally. This reduces the size of the turbinate by ~50% (**Fig. 4.5**).

Fig. 4.3 (**A**) The inferior turbinate (*IT*) has been sufficiently mobilized to allow the microdebrider and endoscope to pass underneath it into the inferior meatus. The middle turbinate (*MT*) and septum (*S*) are seen. (**B**) The microdebrider blade is used to remove the tissue and some of the vertical bone from the lateral aspect of the inferior turbinate.

Fig. 4.4 The ball probe is used to remove the more posterior bony fragments and the backbiter used for the thicker more anterior bone.

Fig. 4.5 The medial mucosal flap (*black arrow*) is rotated on itself reforming the turbinate without any exposed mucosa. Note the turbinate is about half its original size.

The before and after pictures taken during surgery are presented in **Fig. 4.6**. It can clearly be seen that the size of the inferior turbinate is reduced by around 50%.

A rectangular sheet of Surgicel (Ethicon, Somerville, NJ) is placed over the rolled turbinate to keep it in place and prevent the mucosa from unrolling (**Fig. 4.7**). It also provides a degree of hemostasis. No other packing is placed in the nose.

Alternative Surgical Technique

This technique described by Dr. Ray Sacks follows the same principles as the technique described in the preceding paragraph but modifies the technique for removal of the vertical portion of the inferior turbinate bone. Infiltration of the inferior turbinate with local anesthetic remains unchanged.

However, to gain access to the inferior turbinate, the anterior head of the inferior turbinate is shaved (**Fig. 4.2**). This is done so that the endoscope and microdebrider blade can both be placed under the inferior turbinate without causing a fracture of the inferior turbinate bone. In addition, shaving the head of the turbinate exposes the vertical anterior end of the inferior turbinate bone. The removal of the lateral aspect of the inferior turbinate is performed as previously described without any attempt to remove the underlying turbinate bone. The bone is removed by creating a surgical plane between the exposed anterior end of the inferior turbinate bone and the medial vascular portion of the turbinate (**Fig. 4.8**). The malleable suction curette* (Medtronic ENT, Minneapolis, MN) is used as it provides both suction and has a relatively sharp anterior end which facilitates the dissection of the subperiosteal plane. After the bone has been dissected free

A   B

Fig. 4.6 The left inferior turbinate is seen (**A**). After inferior turbinoplasty the much smaller turbinate (**B**) is seen with the mucosal flap rolled on itself reforming the turbinate without exposed raw surfaces.

Fig. 4.7 A strip of Surgicel is placed over the rolled mucosal flap to keep it in place and prevent it from unrolling.

from the turbinate, the residual tissue is rolled on itself in the same manner as the previously described technique and supported with a strip of Surgicel.

Postoperative Care

The patient starts saline nasal douche within a few hours of the surgery. This is continued for a month postoperatively. After a day the patient is allowed to very gently blow their nose after saline wash. Systemic antibiotics are given for 5 days. The patient is reviewed after 2 weeks.

Results

To evaluate the effectiveness of this procedure, a prospective randomized comparative study was performed where

Fig. 4.8 The techniques are similar with the exception of the step in (**B**) where the vertical bone of the inferior turbinate is dissected with a suction curette* much in the same fashion as a septoplasty is performed.

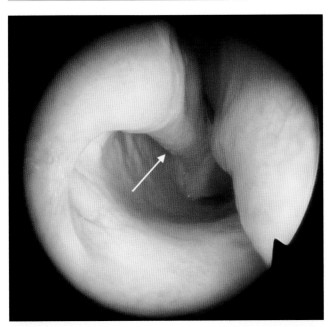

Fig. 4.9 This picture demonstrates the size of the turbinate after 1 year (*white arrow*).

patients were randomized to undergo powered inferior turbinectomy on one side and submucous diathermy on the other. Nineteen patients were assessed by a pre- and postoperative symptom score, endoscopic grading of turbinate hypertrophy, and acoustic rhinometry. The symptoms were scored individually for each side. This showed a significant improvement in symptoms of nasal patency on the powered turbinoplasty side in the immediate (first 3 weeks) postoperative period. The submucous diathermy side continued to have nasal obstruction during this period. Objectively there was also a statistically significant decrease in nasal crust formation at 3 weeks. After 3 weeks, objective nasal patency improved on the side that had undergone submucous diathermy but the difference in symptomatic and objective nasal patency was maintained on the powered turbinoplasty side at 1, 3, and 6 months but was not present at 1 year. There was no difference in postoperative hemorrhage rates. Long-term follow-up was performed at 5 years and this showed that turbinate hypertrophy had recurred on the submucous diathermy side but not on the powered turbinoplasty side when the nasal cavity was assessed endoscopically and with acoustic rhinometry.

Figure 4.9 shows a typical view of an inferior turbinate in a patient who had undergone powered inferior turbinectomy.

◆ Endoscopic Septoplasty (Video 2)

A significant percentage of patients have septal deviation which impedes adequate access to the middle meatus or to the axillary region of the middle turbinate. Following the surgical principle that exposure is one of the keys to successful surgery, we recommend having a fairly low threshold in straightening such a deflection and thereby improving the access to the middle meatus and to the frontal recess. As the surgeon has the

endoscopes all set up and ready to go, there seems little sense in using a headlight to perform an operation that is straightforward to perform with the endoscope. In addition, performing the surgery using the monitor allows all observers in the theater to view the surgery and has the significant advantage of allowing the surgeon to teach the operative steps to the junior resident. It is very difficult for the resident to follow the surgical steps if the surgeon performs the surgery utilizing the headlight and speculum. The key to successful endoscopic septoplasty is instrumentation. A suction Freer elevator helps to keep the surgical field clear of blood and it is extremely helpful to have an endoscope lens cleaner to remove any blood that may blur the end of the endoscope. If the septal deviation is to one side only then it is advisable to perform the ESS on the widely patent side and then perform the septoplasty with the incision on the side through which surgery had been performed. This decreases the likelihood of contaminating the endoscope as it is introduced through the nose.

Surgical Technique (Video 2)

The principle of endoscopic septoplasty is to preserve as much of the quadrilateral cartilage as possible. This is done by only elevating the mucosa off one side of the cartilage and leaving the other attached. In a large number of patients the septum is too long and dislocates off the maxillary crest creating an anterior septal spur. As the cartilaginous septum is often too long it bows and deviates aggravating the contralateral nasal obstruction. If there is a dislocation of the caudal end of the cartilaginous septum and the end of the septum protrudes into one of the nasal vestibules this should be addressed with a hemitransfixion incision rather than a Killian's incision. If the deviation starts in the region of the lower border of the upper lateral cartilage, then a Killian's incision is performed just beyond this landmark. The back of the scalpel is used to lift the presenting edge of the upper lateral cartilage. The vertical incision is started as high on the septum as possible, progressing to the floor of the nose, and curving posteriorly as it reaches the floor of the nose (**Fig. 4.10**). A suction Freer elevator is used to elevate the mucosal flap in the subperichondrial plane (**Fig. 4.10**).

The flap is raised in a posterior direction before the dissection proceeds to the floor of the nose. Once the floor is reached the flap is separated from the maxillary crest from posteriorly to anteriorly. If the cartilaginous septum is too long and is dislocated off the maxillary crest, a strip of cartilage needs to be removed from its lower insertion into the maxillary crest. The subperichondrial flap is brought down to the presenting edge of the spur but the flap is not raised over this deflection as it is likely to tear. Rather, using the sharp end of a regular Freer elevator, a horizontal incision is made above the spur through the cartilage from the bony cartilaginous junction ~2 to 3 mm above the maxillary crest up to the anterior Killian's incision (**Fig. 4.11**).

The subperichondrial flap is raised on the opposite side of this inferior segment down onto the maxillary crest. This segment of cartilage is then elevated out of the maxillary crest starting anteriorly and working under the cartilage in the groove of the crest. In this manner the mucosa over the anterior spur can often be preserved. If the maxillary crest

A   B

Fig. 4.10 **(A)** A Killian's incision has been performed just behind the leading edge of the upper lateral cartilage. **(B)** The mucoperichondrial flap has been raised with a suction Freer elevator and the deviation at the junction of the cartilaginous and bony septum is seen. Note the pearly white appearance of the cartilage indicating that the mucoperichondrium has been elevated in the correct plane.

is large or has a bony spur (**Fig. 4.12**), this can be trimmed back using a chisel. Usually only the half of the crest that is protruding into the nasal cavity is removed because damage to the nerves that supply the incisor teeth is more common if the whole maxillary crest is removed.

To manage the posterior bony septum, the bony and cartilaginous junction is disarticulated up to the roof of the nose (**Fig. 4.12**). The suction Freer is used to develop the subperichondrial flap on the other side of the bony septum. Bony deviations are removed with special attention given to the bony septum directly under the nasal bones which is often cancellous and quite thick. A great view of this is obtained with the endoscope and deviated bone is resected as this bone will often obstruct the view of the insertion of the middle turbinate onto the lateral nasal wall—the so-called axilla of the middle turbinate. No attempt is usually made

A

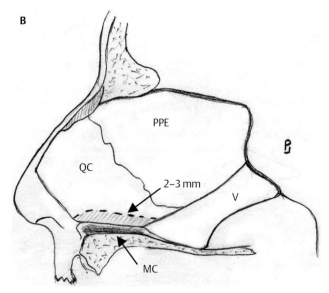

Fig. 4.11 **(A)** The horizontal incision 2 to 3 mm above the maxillary crest has been made. This cartilage is gently elevated out of the groove of the maxillary crest starting anteriorly and moving posteriorly.

(B) The quadrilateral cartilage (*QC*), perpendicular plate of the ethmoid (*PPE*), vomer (*V*), and maxillary crest are demonstrated. The 2 to 3 mm of cartilage to be excised above the maxillary crest is shaded.

Fig. 4.12 (**A**) The 2 to 3 mm strip of cartilage forming the lower border of the quadrilateral cartilage has been resected (*broken black arrow*). The maxillary crest is seen (*black arrow*) and the bony septum is indicated with a *white arrow*. (**B**) The cartilaginous septum has been dislocated from the posterior bony septum (*black arrow*). (**C**) The inferior bony septum has been resected (*white arrow*) and the thick upper bony septum remains (*black arrow*) and should be resected up to the roof of the nose.

to preserve bone in the posterior septum. The cartilaginous septum at this point has only had the lower 2 to 3 mm resected from it where it was dislocated from the maxillary crest. It still has the mucosal flap attached to one side and a subperichondrial flap raised on the opposite side. Superiorly the cartilaginous septum is attached to the undersurface of the upper lateral cartilages. The cartilage has a free lower and posterior margin and, if free of inherent bends or twists, should hang relatively straight.

Management of the remaining quadrilateral cartilage depends on the presence of any visible residual deviations within the cartilage. If there is a fracture line through the cartilage this can be excised and the remaining cartilage should then be straight. If, however, the cartilage has a bend or twist, the exposed surface is weakened with multiple incisions. The most difficult cartilaginous deviations are high anterior bends. This should be identified prior to surgery and the incision and flap elevation planned so that the concave surface of such a deviation is exposed during surgery. This allows multiple incisions and if necessary powered debridement with the microdebrider blade or septoplasty burr set on forward at a minimum of 12 000 rpm.

If no tear of either mucosal flap has occurred, the scalpel is used to make a posterior placed 2- to 3-cm horizontal incision on the floor of one of the mucosal flaps to ensure that no blood accumulated within the septum in the postoperative period.

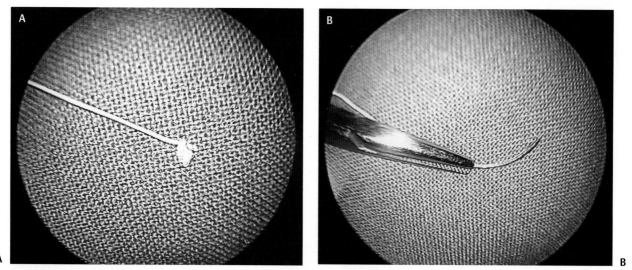

Fig. 4.13 (**A**) The knot at one end of the suture. (**B**) The shaft of the needle down the length of the needle-holding forceps.

Fig. 4.14 (**A**) The suture been passed through the septum from the left nasal cavity. (**B**) The quilting suture is seen in the left septum and (**C**) the suture catches a small bite of skin so it can be tied on itself in the right nasal vestibule.

After the ESS has been performed, a quilting suture is placed through the septum to hold the flaps together and to prevent hematoma formation. A 30 Vicryl suture (Ethicon) on a cutting needle is used. A standard needle holder holds the needle with the shaft of the needle positioned between the jaws of the needle holder (**Fig. 4.13**). A knot is made at the end of the suture and the needle is passed through the septum from one nasal cavity to the other (**Fig. 4.13**).

Counterpressure is often required with the endoscope to allow the needle to pass from one nasal cavity to the other. The stitch is pulled through the septum until the knot reaches the mucosa in the other nasal cavity and prevents further passage of the suture. The suture is then placed some distance from its exit point through the septum into the other nasal cavity. This results in a quilting suture which keeps the two mucosal flaps of the septum apposed. The suture is used to oppose the mucosal edges of the incision and then tied on itself through the vestibular skin (**Fig. 4.14**).

References

1. Clement WA, White PS. Trends in turbinate surgery literature: a 35-year review. Clin Otolaryngol Allied Sci 2001;26(2):124–128
2. Lippert BM, Werner JA. Long-term results after laser turbinectomy. Lasers Surg Med 1998;22(2):126–134
3. Warwick-Brown NP, Marks NJ. Turbinate surgery: how effective is it? A long-term assessment. ORL J Otorhinolaryngol Relat Spec 1987; 49(6):314–320
4. Gupta A, Mercurio E, Bielamowicz S. Endoscopic inferior turbinate reduction: an outcomes analysis. Laryngoscope 2001;111(11 Pt 1): 1957–1959
5. Kawai M, Kim Y, Okuyama T, Yoshida M. Modified method of submucosal turbinectomy: mucosal flap method. Acta Otolaryngol Suppl 1994; 511:228–232
6. Berenholz L, Kessler A, Sarfati S, Eviatar E, Segal S. Chronic sinusitis: a sequela of inferior turbinectomy. Am J Rhinol 1998;12(4):257–261
7. Elwany S, Harrison R. Inferior turbinectomy: comparison of four techniques. J Laryngol Otol 1990;104(3):206–209
8. Moore GF, Freeman TJ, Ogren FP, Yonkers AJ. Extended follow-up of total inferior turbinate resection for relief of chronic nasal obstruction. Laryngoscope 1985;95(9 Pt 1):1095–1099

5 Uncinectomy and Middle Meatal Antrostomy Including Canine Fossa Puncture/Trephine

Uncinectomy is the first step undertaken during endoscopic sinus surgery (ESS). If poorly performed it may result in failure of the ESS procedure[1–3] and may result in orbital or lacrimal complications.[4,5] It is important that the anatomy of the uncinate and ethmoidal infundibulum are properly understood. The uncinate is a sickle-shaped bone extending from the frontal recess superiorly and attaching to the inferior turbinate inferiorly. If the uncinate is viewed in the parasagittal plane, the upward extension of the uncinate into the frontal recess cannot be seen. The middle and horizontal portions of the uncinate form a sickle-shaped bone attaching to the lacrimal bone and the ethmoidal process of the inferior turbinate and lying below the bulla ethmoidalis (**Fig. 5.1**).

The middle third of the uncinate arises from the lacrimal bone and frontal process of the maxilla.[6] It projects posteriorly forming a gutter (the infundibulum) on its lateral aspect. It has a free edge which creates a space between this free edge and the bulla ethmoidalis.[6] This space is known as the hiatus semilunaris as it is crescent shaped (**Fig. 5.1**). **Figure 5.2** illustrates the orbital attachment of the uncinate process, the infundibulum, and the hiatus semilunaris. When viewed with an endoscope only the medially projecting middle portion of the uncinate can be visualized (**Fig. 5.3**).

The superior portion of the uncinate which extends into the frontal recess is considered in detail in Chapter 6. The attachment of the horizontal portion of the uncinate to the ethmoid process of the inferior turbinate is by a series of feet. This can clearly be seen in **Fig. 5.4** where the horizontal portion of the uncinate has been dissected free. Posteriorly it may have a free end or it may attach to the palatine bone.

◆ Uncinectomy

The Swing-Door Technique[4] (Videos 3, 4, and 5)

Removal of the Middle Part of the Uncinate

This technique was devised in an attempt to achieve a complete removal of the midsection of the uncinate process and in so doing expose the natural ostium of the maxillary sinus. If there is doubt about the position of the free edge of the uncinate, a ball-tipped right-angled probe can be used to palpate its free edge confirming its position (**Fig. 5.3**). The mid part of the uncinate is incised superiorly and inferiorly. The superior incision is performed with a sickle knife just under the axilla of the middle turbinate (**Fig. 5.5**). The tip of the sickle knife cuts the soft bone of the uncinate from its posterior free edge until the tip of the knife can be felt to strike the hard bone of the frontal process of the maxilla. In this area the uncinate attaches directly to the hard bone of the frontal process of the maxilla usually above the lacrimal bone (**Fig. 5.1**). It is highly unlikely that this incision will penetrate the lacrimal sac or lamina papyracea and expose orbital fat.

The pediatric backbiter is passed into the middle meatus and opened (**Fig. 5.6**). It is gently wriggled into the hiatus semilunaris so it engages the free edge of the uncinate process. It is easier to introduce the backbiter about midway up the middle portion of the uncinate before it is slid down the free edge until it comes to rest on the transition of the middle and horizontal parts of the uncinate. The uncinate is cut using sequential bites of the backbiter.[4] Usually (depending on the length of the uncinate and the size of the tooth of the backbiter) two to three bites are necessary. If the backbiter can still palpate residual uncinate, then a final bite is made. The backbiter should be turned upward to an angle of 45 degrees before this final bite is made. This brings the tooth of the backbiter medial to the nasolacrimal duct and protects it from injury. In patients with a lateralized uncinate, care needs to be taken that the tooth of the backbiter does not penetrate the lamina papyracea during positioning of the tooth on the uncinate. In these patients the proximity of the uncinate and lamina papyracea can result in the tooth penetrating the lamina papyracea as the tooth is opened and, while open, it is pulled anteriorly to engage the uncinate. To avoid this, the tooth is used to gently medialize the uncinate before the tooth is pulled anteriorly to engage the uncinate.

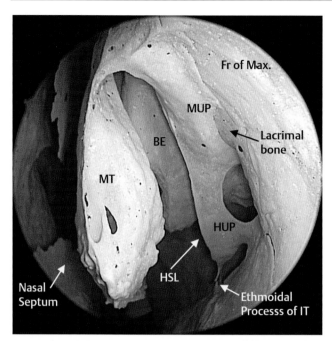

Fig. 5.1 Endoscopic image taken from a dry skull on the left side demonstrating the middle (*MUP*) and horizontal (*HUP*) portions of the uncinate attaching to the lacrimal bone and ethmoidal process of the inferior turbinate (*IT*). The uncinate lies beneath the bulla ethmoidalis, and the hiatus semilunaris (*HSL*) can be visualized between the free edge of the uncinate process and the bulla ethmoidalis (*BE*). *MT*, Middle turbinate; *Fr of Max*, frontal process of maxilla.

Fig. 5.2 This cadaver dissection specimen of the left nasal cavity is cut in the axial plane with the anterior aspect of the specimen on the right. The *black solid arrow* indicates the uncinate attachment, the *black arrow* the infundibulum, and the *broken white arrow* the hiatus semilunaris (entrance to the infundibulum).

Next a right-angled ball probe or curette is slid through the inferior incision behind the uncinate process fairly closely to the uncinate's insertion into the lateral nasal wall. The probe is pulled anteriorly and the uncinate is fractured at its insertion to the lateral nasal wall (**Fig. 5.7**).[4]

The posterior blade of a 45-degree upturned through-cutting Blakesley forceps is placed through the inferior cut in the uncinate and the forceps pushed against the lateral nasal wall bringing the forceps hard up against the frontal process of the maxilla. The middle section of the uncinate is then removed flush with the lateral nasal wall (**Fig. 5.8**).

In most circumstances the mid portion of the uncinate can be removed in one piece. In **Fig. 5.9** the superior, inferior, and anterior cuts as well as the free edge are labeled.

Several surgeons describe removal of the middle third of the uncinate with a microdebrider blade. This is NOT advocated as the lamina papyracea that lies directly behind the uncinate is the thinnest part of the medial orbital wall. Turning the microdebrider blade laterally and working onto the lamina with limited visualization of the lamina may end with inadvertent penetration of the lamina with the microdebrider with significant orbital complications.

Removal of the Horizontal Portion of the Uncinate (Videos 3, 4, and 5)

The zero-degree endoscope is changed for a 30-degree endoscope. This allows better visualization of the middle meatus and greater precision in the dissection. The next step is to dissect the horizontal portion of the uncinate bone out from between its two mucosal layers (**Fig. 5.10**).

The double right angled ball probe is used to elevate the mucosa off the medial aspect of the uncinate (**Fig. 5.10**). The bone is then fractured medially and the ball probe used to elevate the mucosa over the lateral aspect of the bone. Removal of this bone allows the mucosa covering the natural ostium to

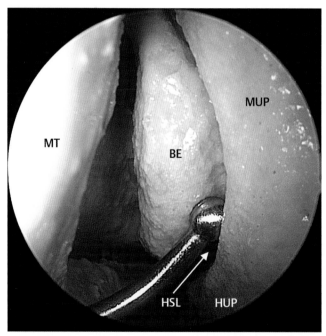

Fig. 5.3 This photo is taken in the left nasal cavity within the middle meatus. The middle (*MUP*) portion of the uncinate and horizontal (*HUP*) of the uncinate is visualized. The ball probe has been placed within the hiatus semilunaris (*HSL*), and lies between the free edge of the uncinate and the bulla ethmoidalis (*BE*).

Fig. 5.4 The uncinate bone is displayed in situ (right nasal cavity) with the medial mucosal flap dissected away from the bone in picture (**A**). (**B**) The horizontal portion of the uncinate has been removed from between the two layers of mucosa. (**C**) Feet-like process in a dry skull specimen. The feet-like attachments are indicated with *white arrows*. These feet attach to the ethmoidal process on the inferior turbinate (*IT*). *MT*, middle turbinate.

be delicately trimmed downward with the microdebrider exposing the natural maxillary ostium (**Fig. 5.11**). Note that the microdebrider blade here is positioned inferiorly so that it is working away from the orbit toward the nasal floor. Using the microdebrider allows these edges to be trimmed so that they lie directly opposed to each other without exposed bone separating these edges. This results in these mucosal edges healing by primary intention without scarring (**Fig. 5.11**).

If there is any doubt as to the location of the natural ostium, the right angled ball-probe or right-angled olive tip suction can be placed directly behind the cut edge of the middle portion of the uncinate in the ethmoidal infundibulum. The probe or suction is slid down this natural gutter as it must enter the natural ostium of the maxillary sinus. In this way the natural ostium of the maxillary sinus should always be able to be located.

Results with the Swing-Door Technique[4]

As part of the study comparing the swing-door and traditional techniques of uncinectomy, we examined the results of 636 consecutive swing-door uncinectomies. There were no orbital penetrations with fat exposure and all natural ostia of the maxillary sinuses were identified. However, there were four patients where the nasolacrimal duct was exposed and not opened and one patient in whom the nasolacrimal duct was opened. The important outcome was the ability of the surgeon to identify the natural ostium of the maxillary sinus in all 636 uncinectomies.

To compare the swing-door technique with the traditional technique of uncinectomy, a further 636 uncinectomies were performed using the traditional technique described later.[7] The traditional technique for uncinectomy starts

Fig. 5.5 Cadaver dissection on the left side. Superior incision of the middle portion of the uncinate process (*MUP*) is made with a sickle knife placed directly under the axilla of the middle turbinate (*MT*). *BE*, bulla ethmoidalis; *HUP*, horizontal portion of the uncinate; *HSL*, hiatus semilunaris.

Fig. 5.6 A pediatric backbiter is introduced and the lower cut is made. *BE*, bulla ethmoidalis; *MUP*, middle portion of the uncinate; *HUP*, horizontal portion of the uncinate; *MT*, middle turbinate.

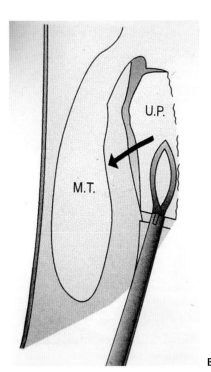

A

B

Fig. 5.7 **(A)** Insertion of a curette or ball probe behind the uncinate has allowed the middle portion of the uncinate (*MUP*) attachment to the lateral nasal wall to be fractured anteriorly in a swing-door technique for uncinectomy. **(B)** The 45-degree through-biting Blakesley used to cut the uncinate flush with the lateral nasal wall. *UP*, uncinate process; *MT*, middle turbinate; *BE*, bulla ethmoidalis; *Fr of Max*, frontal process of maxilla.

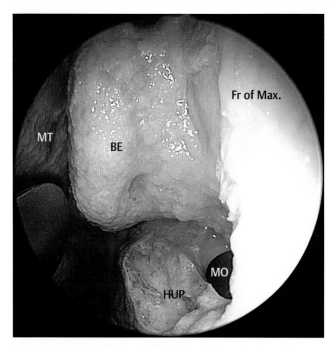

Fig. 5.8 Removal of the middle third of the uncinate process reveals the natural maxillary ostium (*MO*), with the remaining horizontal portion still in place. *Fr of Max*, frontal process of maxilla; *MT*, middle turbinate; *HUP*, horizontal portion of the uncinate; *BE*, bulla ethmoidalis.

Fig. 5.9 The middle section of the uncinate with superior (*white arrow*), inferior (*broken white arrow*), anterior cut edges (*black arrow*), and free edge (*broken black arrow*) labeled.

Fig. 5.10 A double right-angled ball probe dissecting the bone of the horizontal portion of the uncinate process (*HUP*). *MT*, middle turbinate; *MO*, maxillary ostium; *BE*, bulla ethmoidalis.

Fig. 5.11 Intraoperative picture of the right maxillary ostium (*black arrow*) after removal of the horizontal portion of the uncinate with apposition of the mucosal edges (*white arrow*). The final common drainage pathway is indicated by the broken white arrow.

with the identification of the uncinate's free edge. While the free edge is palpated, the surgeon attempts to gauge the site of the uncinate's insertion into the lateral wall of the nose. This decision is critical. If the surgeon starts too close to the uncinate insertion, the first incision may penetrate the lamina papyracea with a resultant prolapse of orbital fat. Surgeons tend to allow for such an error and tend to leave a few millimeters of uncinate behind incising distal to its insertion (**Fig. 5.12**).

If too much uncinate remains, the ostium may remain hidden behind this residual uncinate. In this situation the ostium should be sought behind the anteroinferior residual uncinate (**Fig. 5.13**).

In 636 consecutive traditional uncinectomies we were unable to locate the natural ostium of the maxillary sinus in 42. There were six cases of orbital fat exposure and no cases of nasolacrimal duct injury. In our hands the swing-door technique was more reliable to identify the natural ostium of the maxillary sinus and was less likely to result in penetration of the orbit.

Complications of Uncinectomy

The two areas at risk during uncinectomy are the orbit and the nasolacrimal duct.[4,5] To date penetration of the orbit has not occurred with the superior horizontal incision of the middle part of the uncinate. This is due to the insertion of this part of the uncinate on the thick bone of the frontal process of the maxilla (**Fig. 5.1**). The traditional technique of uncinectomy has a higher risk of orbital penetration. This is due to the knife penetrating the orbit during the anterior incision made into the uncinate at its insertion onto the lateral nasal wall.[4] This may result in the prolapse of orbital

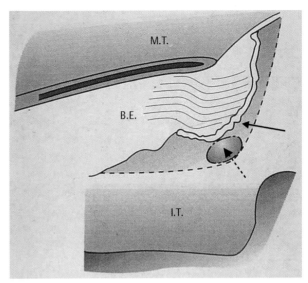

Fig. 5.13 After the uncinectomy has been performed, 2 to 3 mm of residual uncinate remains (*solid black arrow*). This obscures visualization of the natural ostium (*broken black arrow*) and may not be located by the surgeon. This may result in a posterior fontanelle ostium being created. *MT*, middle turbinate; *BE*, bull ethmoidalis; *IT*, inferior turbinate.

fat. Frequent palpation of the globe should be performed throughout the surgery. If inadvertent entry into the orbit or removal of the lamina papyracea has occurred, palpation of the globe will either cause a prolapse of orbital fat or cause the orbital periosteum to move. If orbital periosteum is exposed, care should be taken in this region during the rest of the surgery. If penetration of the orbit has occurred and orbital fat prolapse is seen, this should be left alone and not manipulated. The microdebrider should not be used in an area where orbital fat has prolapsed as it can be sucked very rapidly into the blade with rapid removal of fat and damage to the medial rectus muscle. Damage to the nasolacrimal duct is less likely with the traditional technique than the swing-door technique as there is less utilization of the backbiter and therefore less risk to the nasolacrimal duct. If the nasolacrimal duct is opened, any small bony pieces are removed and the opening left as it is. Normally no symptoms will result as the duct has not been obstructed. A crush injury of the duct has a worse prognosis as this may result in scar tissue formation within the duct with subsequent obstruction of the duct.

The surgeon should also be aware that collapse of the uncinate onto the lamina papyracea (so-called atelectatic uncinate) puts the orbit at greater risk of damage.[8] This occurs with complete opacification of the maxillary sinus with absorption of all gas within the sinus and resultant negative pressure sucking the uncinate laterally onto the lateral nasal wall. If this is long-standing, expansion of the orbit may occur with enophthalmos: the so-called silent sinus syndrome (**Fig. 5.14**). Anterior incisions into an atelectatic uncinate will result in a high incidence of orbital penetration and should not be used. The retrograde removal of the uncinate (swing-door technique) is preferred.

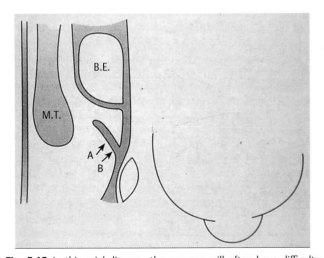

Fig. 5.12 In this axial diagram the surgeon will often have difficulty deciding exactly where the uncinate attaches to the lateral nasal wall and will usually make the incision into the uncinate as indicated by the *A arrow* as this gives a margin of safety when compared with the incision in the region of the *B arrow* which may traverse the lamina papyracea and expose orbital fat.

Fig. 5.14 Computed tomography scan of a patient with a right atelectatic uncinate (*white arrow*). The uncinate is plastered against the lamina papyracea over a considerable length.

◆ Posterior Fontanelle or Accessory Ostium

An accessory ostium is located within the posterior fontanelle of the maxillary sinus behind the natural ostium. Cadaveric studies have shown that 10% of the general population have an accessory ostium.[9] In addition, failure of the surgeon to locate the natural maxillary sinus ostium at surgery may result in the creation of a posterior fontanelle ostium. This is a common cause for ESS failure.[1-3] The presence of an accessory or posterior fontanelle ostium may result in the circular flow of mucus from the natural ostium of the maxillary sinus into the posterior fontanelle ostium with resultant recurrent chronic sinusitis symptoms (**Fig. 5.15**).

Patients who present with recurrent symptoms of sinusitis after ESS should have an endoscopic examination and, after

Fig. 5.15 Mucus draining from the natural ostium (*white arrow*) behind the uncinate process (*UP*) into an accessory ostium (*black arrow*).

appropriate medical treatment, a computed tomography (CT) scan. On clinical examination the presence of a posterior fontanelle and circular flow of mucus should be sought. This can often be seen on endoscopy with a 30-degree endoscope. In addition, the CT scans of the patient should be closely scrutinized for presence of a natural ostium and a posterior fontanelle ostium or accessory ostium (**Fig. 5.16**).

If a posterior fontanelle ostium or accessory ostium is identified, this should be surgically joined to the natural ostium to prevent ongoing circular flow of mucus. This can be done by inserting a backbiter into the accessory ostium and coming forward to the natural ostium. After creating this tissue edge, the microdebrider is used to trim away excessive tissue.

◆ Enlarging the Maxillary Ostium (Videos 6 and 7)

Currently there is debate as to whether enlarging the maxillary sinus ostium can be detrimental to the long-term health of the sinus.[10] The debate centers on the role of nitric oxide (NO) in the sinuses.[10] NO is produced by nitric oxide synthase (NOS) in the mucosa of the sinuses.[11,12] There are three types of NOS with type II thought to be most important in the production of NO in the sinuses.[11-14] Type II is found in various cells in the nasal mucosa and is induced by bacterial inflammation.[14-17] NO is believed to play an important role in the local innate defense of the nasal sinus mucosa by stimulating ciliary motility and by inhibiting infection by bacteria, viruses, and fungi.[17] In the early stages of the development of ESS, many surgeons advocated enlargement of the maxillary ostium toward the posterior fontanelle.[18-20] This results in a very large maxillary ostium. Recently there have been contrary opinions expressed where surgeons have argued that the proximity of the uncinate to the maxillary ostium results in a narrow transitional space that becomes easily obstructed and that removal of the uncinate alone is sufficient to restore the health of the maxillary sinuses.[21,22] Unfortunately there is little data published to support either argument. Kennedy et al.[18] described the natural size of the maxillary ostium to be 5 mm by 5 mm, which raises the possibility that significantly enlarging the ostium routinely may in some patients cause sufficient dilution of the sinus NO concentration to allow colonization of the sinus by bacteria with subsequent disease. Our department recently published a study where we measured the size of the maxillary sinus ostium and correlated this to the concentration of NO found in both in the maxillary sinus and nasal cavity.[10] There were 52 sinuses in the study with 22 sinuses having enlarged ostia and 30 sinuses having ostia less than 5×5 mm. This study showed that there was a significant decrease in NO concentration in sinuses and nasal cavities with large maxillary sinus ostia (greater than 5×5 mm). This does not mean that the study showed that a lower NO concentration predisposed patients to recurrent infections but only that a large maxillary ostium lowers the concentration of NO in the maxillary sinus and nasal cavity.[10] The association between large maxillary ostia and recurrent infections still needs to be formally studied. An example of a patient with recurrent maxillary sinus infection with a large maxillary antrostomy is presented in **Fig. 5.17**.

Fig. 5.16 The endoscopic picture and corresponding series of sequential coronal computed tomography (CT) scans reveal a partially obscured natural ostium (*white arrow* on photo and in CT scans **A** and **B**) and two accessory ostia (*black arrow* on scan **C**).

Fig. 5.17 Secretions filling a maxillary sinus with a large middle meatal antrostomy on the left side.

An additional consequence of removal of the posterior fontanelle during enlargement of the maxillary ostium may be dumping of secretions from the frontal sinuses and anterior ethmoids into the maxillary sinus. The natural drainage pathway of the frontal sinus and anterior ethmoids is above the natural ostium of the maxillary sinus along the base of the bulla ethmoidalis before crossing the posterior fontanelle and under the eustachian tube to the nasopharynx. In **Fig. 5.18** secretions can be seen coming from the frontal recess and anterior ethmoids across the natural ostium of the maxillary sinus.

Currently the decision as to whether the maxillary ostium is enlarged or not is dependent on the degree of disease within the maxillary sinus. If the maxillary sinus has minimal disease with only mucosal thickening present on the CT scan (**Fig. 5.19**) then only the uncinate is removed.

If the surgeon wishes to view the maxillary sinus then the ostium is enlarged until the dimensions are 10 mm by 10 mm. After removal of the horizontal bone of the uncinate, the mucosa is lowered onto the insertion of the inferior turbinate. In most cases this is sufficient to view the majority of the maxillary sinus with a 70-degree telescope. If there is submucosal abscess formation or polyps and mucus that

Fig. 5.19 Computed tomography scan of a patient with bilateral mucosal thickening in the maxillary sinus (*black arrow*) with an obstructed ostiomeatal complex (*white arrow*).

Fig. 5.18 Mucus (*black arrow*) from the left frontal and ethmoid sinuses moving over the left small maxillary ostium (*white arrow*).

need removal from the sinus, curved instruments and malleable suctions are used through this natural but enlarged ostium to achieve this. This sinus is still seen as having reversible mucosal disease or grade 2 maxillary sinus disease. If, however, the sinus has grade 3 disease where there is extensive polyp formation within the maxillary sinus or large amounts of thick and viscid secretions, particularly fungal mucin, a canine fossa trephine is performed and the maxillary ostium is opened into the posterior fontanelle and maximally enlarged with removal of the posterior fontanelle

(**Fig. 5.20**). In patients with Samter's triad and cystic fibrosis the ostium is always enlarged to its maximum size. This allows maximal penetration of nasal douching usually with topical medication into the maxillary sinus.

In **Fig. 5.21** a polyp pedicled on the roof of the maxillary sinus is seen. Polyps that are based on the posterior roof and posterior wall of the maxillary sinus can usually be removed through an enlarged maxillary ostium. If the majority of polyps or mucin remain after attempted removal through the large ostium, then a canine fossa trephine is performed as described later.

Fig. 5.20 A patient with a large right maxillary antrostomy (*white arrow*) after having extensive sinus disease.

◆ The Severely Diseased Maxillary Sinus

Grading

To date, when dealing with a severely disease maxillary sinus, emphasis has been placed on the creation of the maxillary antrostomy and ensuring that natural ostium is incorporated into any antrostomy created.[3,4] Although establishment of a patent maxillary ostium is a vitally important part of the management of the severely diseased maxillary sinus, management of the sinus and its contents should not be ignored.[3] The diagnosis of the severely diseased maxillary sinus should be suspected if the maxillary sinus is completely opacified on the CT scan.[18] **Figure 5.22** shows examples of severely diseased maxillary sinuses.

The diagnosis can only be confirmed, however, on endoscopy during surgery as the opacification may well be mucus which is easily cleared through the natural maxillary ostium. The first step at surgery is to perform an uncinectomy and middle meatal antrostomy. A 70-degree endoscope is used to visualize the natural ostium and contents of the maxillary sinus. The extent of disease affecting the maxillary sinus should be graded according to **Table 5.1**.

Grades 1 and 2 are reversible with adequate clearance of mucus and aeration of the maxillary sinus but grade 3 is

A   B

Fig. 5.21 (**A**) A large polyp on a twisted pedicle (*white arrow*) and (**B**) the maxillary sinus after removal of the polyp (*white arrow*).

Fig. 5.22 In both coronal computed tomography scans (**A**) and (**B**) there is complete opacification of the left maxillary sinus with double densities (*white arrow*) indicative of fungal sinusitis. (**B**) Previous surgery had cleared the ethmoid cavity on the left and this remains disease free.

Table 5.1 Grading and Management of the Diseased Maxillary Sinus

Grade	Endoscopic Findings	Suggested Surgery of Maxillary Ostium
1	Normal or slightly edematous mucosa (reversible disease)	Uncinectomy alone with visualization of the natural ostium
2	Edematous mucosa with small polyps (reversible disease) without significant eosinophilic mucus	Enlargement of the maxillary ostium to ~1 × 1 cm to allow suction clearance of maxillary, mucociliary clearance, and aeration
3	Extensive polyps and tenacious mucus (nonreversible disease)	Canine fossa puncture or trephine with complete clearance of polyps and mucus and creation of a large antrostomy

Fig. 5.23 The following pictures of the left maxillary sinus are taken after a maxillary antrostomy has been performed and illustrate the grades of disease. (**A**) Grade 1: the mucosa is cobblestoned in the floor of the antrum (*black arrow*) with edema of the residual sinus mucosa. (**B**) Grade 2: the polyps are seen in the floor and posterior wall of the maxillary sinus (*black arrows*) and could be left and should reverse with medical treatment provided there is no eosinophilic mucus around the polyps. If mucus was present a canine fossa trephine (CFT) should be performed. (**C**) Grade 3: the maxillary sinus is completely filled with polyps (*black arrows*) and eosinophilic mucus (*black arrow*) and should be managed with a CFT.

irreversibly diseased (**Fig. 5.23**) and therefore the polyps and especially the thick eosinophilic mucus should be cleared before adequate re-epithelialization and eventually re-ciliation will occur.

If standard ESS techniques and instruments are used, the polyps and mucus from the posterior region of the maxillary sinus can be removed with angled microdebrider blades and curved forceps.[18] However, due to the two fulcrums that microdebrider blades and instruments have when passed through the maxillary antrostomy or inferior meatal antrostomy, polyps in the anterior, inferior, and medial regions cannot be reached. The anterior fulcrum is the nasal vestibule and the posterior fulcrum is the antrostomy or inferior meatal antrostomy site. If the blade or instrument is passed through the anterior wall of the maxillary sinus it only has one fulcrum so a much greater degree of manipulation of the blade is possible (**Fig. 5.24**).

In current teaching the maxillary sinus is managed by creating a large antrostomy and then removing whatever can be removed through the maxillary antrostomy. Polyps and thick tenacious mucus in the anterior region or floor of the nose require removal (**Fig. 5.23C**). In patients with severe and aggressive sinus disease such as allergic fungal sinusitis, nonallergic eosinophilic fungal disease (**Fig. 5.23C**), and nonallergic nonfungal eosinophilic disease, leaving eosinophilic mucin in the maxillary sinus may contribute to a rapid recurrence of disease.[18,19] Whether this is due to a continuing exposure to fungus in the eosinophilic mucin or due to ongoing inflammation from the toxic substances within the mucin such as major basic protein and other substances released by the eosinophils is unclear. In other patient groups, such as Samter's triad and severe recurrent polyposis, it appears that if the maxillary sinus is left filled with polyps that these polyps do not resolve with only a maxillary antrostomy.

Is it Necessary to Remove Polyps and Thick Mucin from a Severely Diseased Maxillary Sinus?

We performed a study to establish whether this philosophy of clearing the polyps and mucus in a grade 3 maxillary

sinus improved patient outcome.[18] All patients who had undergone ESS in the department over the prior 3 years were identified and their CT scans reviewed. If there was complete opacification of the maxillary sinus or sinuses they were included in the study. The researcher at that stage was not aware what surgical procedures had been performed or what the current status of the patient sinuses were. This was therefore an unselected patient cohort. The surgical notes were reviewed and the patients were placed into two groups depending on whether the patient had undergone a large middle meatal antrostomy with clearance of all accessible polyps through the antrostomy or whether a canine fossa puncture/trephine (CFP/T) had been performed. If a trephine or puncture was performed our standard practice is to place a microdebrider blade through this puncture/trephine site and perform a complete clearance of polyps under visualization of a 70-degree endoscope placed at the middle meatal antrostomy (**Fig. 5.25**).

The polyps and thick mucin were removed from the sinus under direct visualization with the 70-degree endoscope. Care was taken not to strip the mucosa from the maxillary sinus. Only the polyp was taken while the base layer of mucosa underlying was preserved. This allowed rapid re-epithelialization after surgery and diminished crusting and secretion retention.

The patients in this study[18] underwent magnetic resonance imaging (MRI) scan at a mean time since surgery of 19.9 months. On the MRI scan the maxillary sinus was graded as normal, mucosal thickening < 4 mm, mucosal thickening > 4 mm but the sinus still aerated, or a completely opacified sinus (**Fig. 5.7**). This grading was confirmed on nasal endoscopy. In addition the patients were asked to grade their sinus symptoms on a visual analogue scale and to complete the Chronic Sinusitis Survey (CSS) quality of life questionnaire. In the CFP group the sinuses were normal in 62% of the patients compared with 12% in the patients that had undergone routine middle meatal antrostomy and as much maxillary sinus polyp resection that could be achieved through the natural ostium. The CSS symptom subscore and symptom score were statistically better in the CFP group indicating better symptom control in this group. If the overall disease burden

Fig. 5.24 (**A**) The microdebrider blade has been passed through an inferior meatal antrostomy. Note the anterior fulcrum (nasal vestibule, *broken white arrow*) and the posterior fulcrum (inferior meatal antrostomy, *white arrow*). The region of the maxillary sinus that can be cleared through this access is shaded. This shaded region is smaller with a middle meatal antrostomy. The single fulcrum of the canine fossa puncture is indicated (*white arrow*) (**B,C,D**), illustrating how the entire maxillary sinus can be accessed as the blade only has a single fulcrum.

A   B

Fig. 5.25 (**A**) The microdebrider blade has been passed through a canine fossa trephine site in the anterior face of the maxillary sinus (*black arrow*). (**B**) The polyps have been removed from the sinus without stripping the basement membrane from the sinus (note no exposed bone). The debrider blade can be seen entering the sinus through the anterior wall (*broken white arrow*).

was compared between the two groups using the Lund and Mackay score, it was found to be higher in the CFP group (Lund and Mackay = 10.3) as compared with the group undergoing standard ESS techniques.[6,8] In addition all the other sinuses were treated in exactly the same manner with complete removal of all polyps and mucin from these sinuses and exposure of the natural ostium of the sinuses. This study confirmed the clinical perception that complete clearance of the severely diseased maxillary sinus plays a major role in the control of the disease and decreases the overall incidence and severity of recurrence of the disease.[18]

◆ Old Technique of Canine Fossa Puncture (CFP)[21,22]

Technique

The old standard technique for canine fossa puncture was as follows[21]: the lip of the patient was elevated and the canine tooth identified (there are two front teeth either side of the midline before the canine tooth). The root of this tooth was traced with the finger under the lip until the canine fossa was palpated. One milliliter of 1:80 000 2% lidocaine and adrenaline is infiltrated in this region. A canine fossa trocar (Karl Storz, Tuttlingen, Germany) was placed in the fossa and directed posteriorly. The trocar was introduced with a rotating forward motion. When the bone was too thick, a couple of firm taps with the palm of the hand was usually sufficient to drive the trocar through the bone. However, in some patients in whom the bone was thicker, the trocar needed to be tapped with a mallet. After the tip of the trocar was felt to fully penetrate the sinus, it was withdrawn and the microdebrider blade was introduced through the mucosal and bony hole into the maxillary sinus. The blade was kept closed during introduction to prevent soft tissues from been sucked into the debrider during passage into the maxillary sinus. Once the blade was in the maxillary sinus, the 70-degree endoscope is introduced into the nasal cavity and the gate of the blade is opened. This helps remove most of the blood from within the sinus and allows the blade to be visualized within the sinus (**Fig. 5.25A**). This needs to be done before the blade is used to remove polyps. This visualization ensures that the blade is within the sinus and not in the orbit or soft tissues.

Complications[21]

The incidence of complications with the old CFP technique performed at the same time as ESS was 75%.[21] A telephonic survey revealed that the most common complications were cheek swelling, cheek pain, and facial pain. Most of these symptoms resolved within the first month after surgery. If the symptoms associated with the soft tissue dissection were removed, 28% of patients experienced a persistent significant complication of facial tingling, numbness, or continued pain. This incidence is similar to other studies where numbness of the upper lip and/or the upper teeth was seen in up to 38% of patients.[23] These persisting complications were thought to be a result of injury to branches of the infraorbital nerve. The infraorbital nerve divides before it exits the infraorbital foramen into the anterior superior alveolar nerve (ASAN) and the middle superior alveolar nerve (MSAN). These nerves traverse the anterior maxilla and supply sensation to the upper lip and teeth. Placement of the trocar through the anterior wall of the maxilla can injure these nerves and result in paresthesia and numbness of the upper lip and teeth. The risk of injury to this nerve increases if the trocar is placed too medially and cranially.[23] In most cases (91%) the paresthesia and numbness recovers within 12 months as the nerves either regrow or the area is reinnervated by nerves close by.[23] The area of numbness gradually shrinks, then disappears.

The Neural Anatomy of the Anterior Maxilla[23]

To determine the best way to avoid injury to these nerves, a cadaver based study was undertaken in our department on 20 cadavers.[23] The soft tissue overlying the maxillae was removed and the underlying pattern of the ASAN and MSAN determined. The ASAN and the MSAN both run in the bone of the anterior face of the maxilla. The infraorbital nerve divides prior to exiting the infraorbital foramen (IOF) within the maxillary sinuses. The ASAN usually enters the anterior face of the maxilla just below the IOF and then traverses across the anterior face of the maxillary sinus. There were six patterns of branching of the ASAN and MSAN (types 1 to 6). The most common pattern was a single trunk of the ASAN (75%) with no branches (30%, type 1) (**Fig. 5.26A**) followed by multiple branches (25%, type 2) (**Fig. 5.26B**), and a single branch (20%, type 3). Type 4 was a double trunk with no branches (10%) (**Fig. 5.26C**) and type 5 a double trunk with multiple branches (15%). The MSAN was present only as a single trunk with no branches (10%, type 6) and with multiple branches (13%) (type 7) (**Fig. 5.26D**).

Fig. 5.26 The most common nerve patterns are single trunk (75%) as seen in (**A**; type 1) and (**B**; type 2). (**C**) A double trunk is uncommon (10%; type 4). The middle superior alveolar nerve is seen in 23% of patients and may have no branches (10%) or multiple branches (13%; type 7) as seen in (**D**).

◆ New Technique of Canine Fossa Puncture or Trephine[23,24] (Videos 8 and 9)

Landmarks

To determine the region where neurologic injury would least likely occur, landmarks were determined on the cadavers as to the safest place to place the trephine.[24] The landmarks chosen were the intersection of the mid-pupillary line and a horizontal line drawn through the floor of the nose (**Fig. 5.27**). Canine fossa punctures were then performed on all 40 sides of the cadavers. In only 5 of the 40 punctures performed was there injury to one of the minor branches of the ASAN or MSAN confirming that these landmarks were the safest to perform a canine fossa puncture or trephine.

Rationale

One of the problems associated with canine fossa puncture is that the trocar is placed in a blinded manner. Although the soft tissue is dissected off the anterior face of the maxilla, the area through which the trocar is to placed is not visualized and the ASAN or the MSAN could be damaged. In addition placement of the trocar may cause fracture of the thin bone of the anterior wall of the maxilla around the puncture site. This is especially true if the trocar is not rotated with minimal pressure so that the edges of the trocar act as a drill as it penetrates the maxilla. If significant pressure is applied to the trocar a fracture of the surrounding bone will often occur. This enlarges the area of trauma and in so doing increases

Fig. 5.28 The maxillary trephination set* (Medtronic ENT) shows the endoscope sheath for holding the soft tissue away from the end of the endoscope (*white arrow*), the drill guide (*black arrow*), and the drill bit which fits into the end of the microdebrider.

the risk of possible associated neurologic injury. Also the currently available canine fossa trocar (Karl Storz) is 4 mm in diameter. When a 4-mm debrider blade is placed through this opening the fit is very snug and when the blade is manipulated within the maxillary sinus this may cause fracture of the surrounding maxillary bone, again increasing the potential risk of neurologic damage. To overcome these problems, an endoscope sheath* was developed with an extension to hold away the soft tissues (Medtronic ENT, Jacksonville, FL).

Technique[24] (Videos 8 and 9)

An ~6-mm incision is made in the gingivobuccal sulcus above and slightly lateral to the apex of the canine tooth. A suction Freer elevator is used to elevate the soft tissues off the anterior face of the maxilla in a sub-periosteal plane. Once this place is achieved the endoscope soft tissue sheath blade* (Medtronic ENT) is placed into the incision and the soft tissues held away from the bone allowing the surgical plane to be endoscopically visualized (**Fig. 5.28**).

Dissection is continued in a superior and superolateral direction, exposing the canine fossa and the region lateral to the fossa where the mid-pupillary line and line through the nasal floor intersect. If any nerve or branch of one of the nerves is seen (**Fig. 5.29**), further dissection is performed to create space so that the nerve can be avoided.

The canine fossa drill guide* (Medtronic ENT) is then placed on the anterior face of the maxilla at the intersection of the previously described lines. The canine fossa drill* (Medtronic ENT) is attached to the microdebrider handpiece and irrigation to the back of the drill guide. This allows irrigation of the burr during trephination. The drill should be used at 12 000 rpm for best results (lower revolutions may result in the burr sticking in the bone). A 5-mm diameter hole is neatly drilled through the anterior face of the maxilla (**Fig. 5.29B**). A Frasier suction is used to remove any bone dust from the

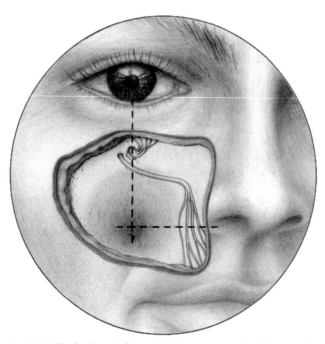

Fig. 5.27 The landmarks for canine fossa puncture/trephine are the intersection between a vertical line through the pupil and a horizontal line drawn through the floor of the nose.

Fig. 5.29 (**A**) The left anterior superior alveolar nerve (*white arrow*) is exposed and therefore can be avoided during placement of the canine fossa trephine (**B**).

hole and surrounding soft tissues and the 4-mm microdebrider blade is placed through the trephine into the maxillary sinus. Using a 70-degree endoscope placed transnasally at the maxillary antrostomy, the debrider blade can be opened and then visualized in the sinus. Activating the blade before it is visualized could result in damage if the blade had inadvertently been placed into the orbit or soft tissues (**Fig. 5.30**). The blade is then used to enlarge the maxillary sinus antrostomy. Any residual uncinate is removed and the posterior fontanelle is removed up to the posterior wall of the maxillary sinus. Polypoid tissue and residual uncinate are removed from the anterior lip of the antrostomy. The widest possible view is now able to be obtained through the antrostomy and the surgeon can remove the polyps and thick mucin from the maxillary sinus. Angled microdebrider blades are used for the lateral regions and anterior face of the maxillary sinus. The endoscope can also be placed through the trephine and the

interior of the maxillary sinus inspected to ensure complete removal of polyps and mucin. Note that only the polypoid tissue and mucin are removed. The basement membrane of the maxillary sinus is retained. This allows speedy re-epithelialization in the postoperative period with re-ciliation and restoration of the maxillary sinus function (**Fig. 5.25**).

Clinical Study of Complications[24]

To assess whether these new landmarks and technique reduced the incidence and severity of complications, a clinical study of 63 patients was performed.[24] Thirty-six patients had bilateral procedures resulting in 99 canine fossa punctures or trephines. Initial postoperative complication rate was reduced from 75 to 44% with only 3.3% of patients having a persisting neurologic complication after 6 months compared with 28.8% with the old CFP technique. In addition, the number of patients suffering from more than one side effect decreased from 70 to 31%. If the 99 sides were separated into patients who underwent canine fossa trephine ($n = 67$) as opposed to puncture ($n = 32$) with the new guidelines, a further reduction in complications is seen. In patients who had CFT and in whom the anterior face of the maxillary sinus was inspected for a visible ASAN or MSAN, the complication rate was 40%. This was significantly less than the 53% seen in patients who had a CFP and in whom the trocar was introduced in a blind manner. Also the CFT patients recovered from their symptoms faster with an 83.3% full recovery in 1 month compared with 62.5% full recovery in CFP patients. Although both techniques utilized the described landmarks to place the trephine/puncture, it is thought that the additional visualization provided by the trephine technique allowed the ASAN and its branches to be seen and avoided.[24] In addition the trephine technique creates a neat hole through which the debrider blade is passed while the puncture technique potentially creates fracture lines in the anterior face of the maxilla which may disrupt the nerves running in the bone and cause injury to these nerves.

Fig. 5.30 The microdebrider blade (*white arrow*) has been placed through a canine fossa trephine access port and can be seen emerging from among the massive polyposis filling the left maxillary sinus.

◆ Postoperative Care

Patients who have undergone either CFT or CFP are advised to rinse their mouth after eating with saline for the first few days until the gingivobuccal incision seals. This incision is usually not stitched. All patients are advised to perform saline douches starting the day after surgery and all patients receive 5 days of broad spectrum antibiotics. Toilet of the nasal cavity and maxillary sinuses is performed at 2 weeks.

Conclusion

The severely diseased maxillary sinus should be dealt with in the same way as any other severely diseased sinus by removal of all polyps and mucus or pus. A large middle meatal antrostomy combined with canine fossa trephine or puncture utilizing the landmarks described allows access to all regions of the maxillary sinus with the microdebrider blade. This in turn allows polyps and mucus to be removed with the retention of the basement membrane of the sinus and rapid postoperative healing with restoration of the function of the maxillary sinus.

◆ Key Points

Uncinectomy

Uncinectomy is the first and often the most important step of ESS.[1–4] If it is poorly performed there is a significant likelihood that the ESS will fail.[1–4] Critical evaluation of the CT scan before uncinectomy is important so that an atelectatic uncinate can be identified before surgery is undertaken. In our hands the swing-door technique of uncinectomy has few complications and a higher incidence of identification of the natural ostium.[4]

Enlargement of the Natural Maxillary Sinus Ostium

In revision ESS the surgeon should specifically look for a posterior fontanelle ostium during both the clinical examination and the CT evaluation. It is critical that the natural ostium of the maxillary sinus is identified and if there is a posterior fontanelle or accessory ostium that the two ostia are joined to form a single ostium. The natural ostium should be enlarged posteriorly if there is evidence of significant disease within the maxillary sinus that needs to be addressed through the natural ostium.

Canine Fossa Puncture/Trephine

A canine fossa puncture/trephine can be used to access anterior, medial, and inferior disease within the maxillary sinus.

The patient should always be warned about the possibility of lip and teeth numbness after the surgery with a small risk of permanent numbness.

References

1. Owen R, Kuhn F. The maxillary sinus ostium: demystifying the middle meatal antrostomy. Am J Rhinol 1995;9:313–320
2. Richtsmeier WJ. Top 10 reasons for endoscopic maxillary sinus surgery failure. Laryngoscope 2001;111(11 Pt 1):1952–1956
3. Parsons DS, Stivers FE, Talbot AR. The missed ostium sequence and the surgical approach to revision functional endoscopic sinus surgery. Otolaryngol Clin North Am 1996;29(1):169–183
4. Wormald PJ, McDonogh M. The "swing-door" technique for uncinectomy in endoscopic sinus surgery. J Laryngol Otol 1998;112:547–551
5. Levine HL. Functional endoscopic sinus surgery: evaluation, surgery, and follow-up of 250 patients. Laryngoscope 1990;100(1):79–84
6. Yoon JH, Kim KS, Jung DH, et al. Fontanelle and uncinate process in the lateral wall of the human nasal cavity. Laryngoscope 2000; 110(2 Pt 1):281–285
7. Stammberger H. Endoscopic endonasal surgery—concepts in treatment of recurring rhinosinusitis. Part I. Anatomic and pathophysiologic considerations. Otolaryngol Head Neck Surg 1986;94(2):143–147
8. Joe JK, Ho SY, Yanagisawa E. Documentation of variations in sinonasal anatomy by intraoperative nasal endoscopy. Laryngoscope 2000; 110(2 Pt 1):229–235
9. Jog M, McGarry GW. How frequent are accessory sinus ostia? J Laryngol Otol 2003;117(4):270–272
10. Kirihene RK, Rees G, Wormald PJ. The influence of the size of the maxillary sinus ostium on the nasal and sinus nitric oxide levels. Am J Rhinol 2002;16(5):261–264
11. Moncada S, Palmer RMJ, Higgs EA. Nitric oxide: physiology, pathophysiology, and pharmacology. Pharmacol Rev 1991;43(2):109–142
12. Nathan CF, Hibbs JB Jr. Role of nitric oxide synthesis in macrophage antimicrobial activity. Curr Opin Immunol 1991;3(1):65–70
13. Bentz BG, Simmons RL, Haines GK III, Radosevich JA. The yin and yang of nitric oxide: reflections on the physiology and pathophysiology of NO. Head Neck 2000;22(1):71–83
14. Nakane M, Schmidt HHHW, Pollock JS, Förstermann U, Murad F. Cloned human brain nitric oxide synthase is highly expressed in skeletal muscle. FEBS Lett 1993;316(2):175–180
15. Arnal J-F, Flores P, Rami J, et al. Nasal nitric oxide concentration in paranasal sinus inflammatory diseases. Eur Respir J 1999;13(2):307–312
16. Lundberg JON. Airborne nitric oxide: inflammatory marker and aerocrine messenger in man. Acta Physiol Scand Suppl 1996;633:1–27
17. Schlosser RJ, Spotnitz WD, Peters EJ, Fang K, Gaston B, Gross CW. Elevated nitric oxide metabolite levels in chronic sinusitis. Otolaryngol Head Neck Surg 2000;123(4):357–362
18. Sathananthar S, Nagaonkar S, Paleri V, Le T, Robinson S, Wormald PJ. Canine fossa puncture and clearance of the maxillary sinus for the severely diseased maxillary sinus. Laryngoscope 2005;115(6):1026–1029
19. Desrosiers M. Refractory chronic rhinosinusitis: pathophysiology and management of chronic rhinosinusitis persisting after endoscopic sinus surgery. Curr Allergy Asthma Rep 2004;4(3):200–207
20. Owen R, Kuhn F. The maxillary sinus ostium: demystifying the middle meatal antrostomy. Am J Rhinol 1995;9:313–320
21. Robinson SR, Baird R, Le T, Wormald PJ. The incidence of complications after canine fossa puncture performed during endoscopic sinus surgery. Am J Rhinol 2005;19(2):203–206
22. Bernal-Sprekelsen M, Kalweit H, Welkoborsky HJ. Discomforts after endoscopy of the maxillary sinus via canine fossa. Rhinology 1991; 29(1):69–75
23. Robinson SR, Wormald PJ. Patterns of innervation of the anterior maxilla: a cadaver study with relevance to canine fossa puncture of the maxillary sinus. Laryngoscope 2005;115(10):1785–1788
24. Singhal D, Douglas R, Robinson S, Wormald PJ. The incidence of complications using a modified technique of canine fossa puncture. Am J Rhinol 2007;21(3):316–319

6 Anatomy of the Frontal Recess and Frontal Sinus with Three-Dimensional Reconstruction

In recent years endoscopic sinus surgery (ESS) has become accepted as the treatment of choice for chronic sinusitis that is resistant to medical management.[1] As ESS has become more widely adopted so the understanding of the complex and varied anatomy of the sinuses has improved.[2,3] However, the frontal recess and frontal sinus remain a challenge for surgeons. The anatomy is complex, varied, and can be confusing.[4,5] To better understand the anatomy of the paranasal sinuses, it is important to be aware of the embryology of the turbinates and sinuses. There are six embryological lamellae, or "ridges," that form from the lateral nasal wall and give rise to important structures in the nose. Early in the fetal development these lamellae fuse to form four lamellae. Persistence of the fifth lamella will result in the presence of a supreme turbinate. This is rare and only present in 15% of the population. The first lamella forms the uncinate process, the second the bulla ethmoidalis, the third the middle turbinate, the fourth the superior turbinate, and the fifth (if present) the supreme turbinate (**Fig. 6.1**). The frontal, anterior ethmoid, and maxillary sinuses pneumatize from the furrow between the uncinate and bulla ethmoidalis. The posterior ethmoids pneumatize from the furrow between the middle and superior turbinates and the sphenoid sinus from the furrow above the superior turbinate.

The key to safe surgery in the frontal recess is a clear understanding of the anatomy. This chapter explains how two-dimensional (2D) computed tomography (CT) scans in coronal, parasagittal, and axial planes can be used to create a three-dimensional (3D) picture of the anatomy of the frontal recess. Such a 3D picture allows the surgeon to plan a surgical approach to the frontal recess so that each cell in the frontal recess can be entered in a predetermined sequential manner and then removed. This allows the surgeon to be able to turn to the CT scan at any point during the dissection and identify the cell that is currently being dissected. This mental picture gives the surgeon greater confidence that the complex anatomy of the frontal recess and frontal sinus is fully understood and removal of obstructing cells can be safely achieved. Insecurity during dissection in the frontal recess may result in either inadequate surgery with ESS failure or may increase the risk of injury to the skull base, orbit, and the anterior ethmoid artery.[4,6]

◆ Basic Anatomy of the Frontal Recess and Frontal Sinus

A common reason for ESS failure is inadequate removal of cells obstructing the outflow of the frontal sinus.[4,6] The location of the frontal recess creates anxiety for the surgeon as operating in this region places the lateral wall of the olfactory fossa (the thinnest part of the skull base), the anterior skull base (fovea ethmoidalis), the anterior ethmoidal artery, and the orbit at risk. The anterior wall of the frontal recess is formed by the thick bone of the frontal process of the maxilla, the so-called "beak" of the frontal process (**Fig. 6.2**). The size of this beak will vary according to the degree of pneumatization of the agger nasi cell. If there is a large agger nasi cell then the beak will be small. If, however, the agger nasi cell is absent or under-pneumatized, then the beak will extend significantly into the frontal recess and create a narrow frontal ostium as the beak approaches the forward projecting anterior skull base. Thus the anteroposterior distance from the skull base to the frontal beak is largely determined by the pneumatization of the agger nasi cell (**Fig. 6.3**).

The medial wall of the frontal recess is formed by the lateral wall of the olfactory fossa. The height of this wall is determined by the level of the cribriform plate. Keros[7] classified the depth of the olfactory fossa as a Keros type 1 (< 3 mm), type 2 (3–7 mm), and a type 3 (> 7 mm). Depending on the Keros type, a variable amount of the lateral wall of the olfactory fossa will be exposed during dissection in this region. The bone of the lateral wall of the olfactory fossa varies in thickness between 0.05 and 0.2 mm and provides little resistance to penetration.[8]

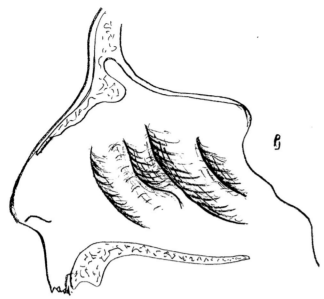

Fig. 6.1 This drawing demonstrates the four lateral lamellae and the corresponding structures into which they develop.

Fig. 6.2 Endoscopic image of dry skull demonstrating the dry bone anatomy of the frontal recess and frontal beak. Both frontal processes of the maxilla (*Fr of Max*) join in the midline to form the frontal beak. The olfactory fossa (*olf. fossa*) are bounded by the middle turbinates (*MT*) and the nasal septum, and roofed by the cribriform plate. The location of the agger nasi cell (*AN*) is shown, and the extent of pneumatization of this cell will determine the size of the frontal beak. *UP*, uncinate process.

The lateral wall of the frontal recess is formed by the lamina papyracea and the posterior wall by the upward continuation of the anterior face of the bulla ethmoidalis. On occasion this anterior wall of the bulla ethmoidalis may not reach the skull base and a suprabullar recess is formed (**Fig. 6.3**). The frontal recess is then continuous with this recess.

The roof of the frontal recess is formed by the fovea ethmoidalis. This bone is relatively thick and normally provides significant resistance to penetration. In a study conducted in our department we found that the right fovea ethmoidalis was higher than the left in 59% of patients.[9] It should also be

noted that the roof (fovea ethmoidalis) may slope, thereby placing the medial aspect of the roof at a lower level than the lateral aspect. The anterior ethmoidal artery and nerve runs across the fovea ethmoidalis at a 45-degree angle from lateral to medial (**Fig. 6.4**). In most instances it can be found behind the upward continuation of the bulla ethmoidalis.

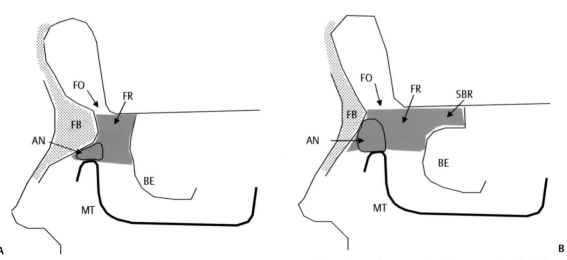

Fig. 6.3 (**A**) The effect of a small under-pneumatized agger nasi cell (*AN*). The frontal beak (*FB*) is large and the anteroposterior diameter of the frontal ostium (*FO*) small. The frontal recess (*FR*) is shaded and extends from the beak to the bulla lamella (*BE*). (**B**) The effect of a well pneumatized agger nasi cell (*AN*) cell with a small frontal beak (*FB*) and large frontal ostium. If the bulla lamella does not reach the skull base, a suprabullar recess (*SBR*) is formed. *MT*, middle turbinate.

Fig. 6.4 A cadaveric image taken of the left fovea ethmoidalis demonstrating the anterior ethmoidal artery (*AEA*) and nerve (*AEN*) leaving the orbit and travelling in a 45-degree angle from lateral to medial along the skull base. This artery can be seen giving off the anterior falcine artery (*AFA*) as it approaches the lateral wall of the olfactory fossa (*L. wall OF*). *M*, orbital wall, medial orb.

If the anterior ethmoidal artery is cut during surgery (this is only likely if it is on a mesentery) it may retract into the orbit and cause bleeding within the orbital tissues. This creates an increase in the intraorbital volume with resultant proptosis. Increasing pressure stretches the optic nerve and may result in decreased arterial blood flow to the retina and subsequent loss of vision.

◆ The Uncinate Process

The uncinate process, in the past, was thought to be the key to the frontal recess.[8] This text adopts an alternate approach and suggests that the agger nasi cell is the key that unlocks the frontal recess.[10,11] The agger nasi cell is present in more than 90% of patients.[12] As the agger nasi cell is the key, it is important to understand the interaction between the uncinate and the agger nasi cell. The interaction between the upward continuation of the uncinate and the agger nasi cell is often poorly understood. The attachment of the root of the uncinate into either the lamina papyracea, skull base, or middle turbinate have been well described (**Fig. 6.6**),[5,8,13] but how this upward continuation of the uncinate interacts with the agger nasi cell and anterior ethmoidal cells in the frontal recess is sometimes poorly understood.

However, when this is absent and a suprabullar recess is present, the anterior ethmoidal artery will be in the frontal recess. The anterior ethmoidal artery may lie in a mesentery suspended from the skull base in 14 to 43% of patients (in our study the incidence was 34%).[9] It is important that the CT scan is reviewed carefully before surgery to establish if the anterior ethmoidal artery is against the skull base or in a mesentery and if a suprabullar recess is present or not (**Fig. 6.5**).

Attachment of the Uncinate to the Lamina Papyracea

In most cases the uncinate/medial wall of agger nasi cell implants on the lamina papyracea. In a large proportion of these patients, this upward extension will give off a

Fig. 6.5 The right anterior ethmoidal artery is on a mesentery (*white arrow*). Note the pinching of the lamella papyracea as the artery exits the orbit.

Fig. 6.6 The classical description of the insertions of the uncinate process.[8] 1, insertion into the lamina papyracea; 2, insertion into the skull base; 3, insertion into middle turbinate.

A, B   C

Fig. 6.7 Intraoperative pictures in the right frontal recess illustrating (**A**) the upward continuation of the uncinate (*black arrow*) forming the medial wall of the agger nasi cell (*AN*). (**B**) The further removal of the medial wall/uncinate superiorly reveals the roof of the agger nasi cell (*AN*) and frontal ostium (*FS*). (**C**) A small residual part of the roof of the agger nasi cell remains. The frontal sinus ostium (*FS*) can be seen.

leaflet of bone to the bulla lamella forming a plate of bone that divides the frontal recess vertically from posterior to anterior[14,15] as it extends from the bulla ethmoidalis to the medial wall of the agger nasi cell and onto the frontal beak. In this situation the frontal sinus will drain medial to this plate (**Fig. 6.7**).

The relationship of a single large agger nasi cell to the frontal sinus ostium is better understood by viewing the coronal and parasagittal scans. This example shows the simplest anatomical configuration of the frontal recess. The next important step is to decide where the frontal sinus drains in relation to these cells.[16–18] This concept is illustrated in **Fig. 6.8**.

Attachment of the Uncinate to the Middle Turbinate

The second anatomical variation to consider is that of a larger agger nasi cell. A large cell may push the upward continuation

A, B   C

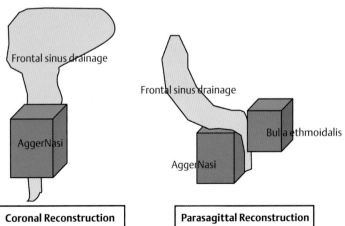

Coronal Reconstruction   **Parasagittal Reconstruction**

D   E

Fig. 6.8 Coronal and parasagittal scans illustrating a single agger nasi cell (*white arrow*) on the left side. Note that the three-dimensional building block reconstructions have been done in the anteroposterior (coronal) and parasagittal planes.

Fig. 6.9 A diagram illustrating how a single large agger nasi cell pushes the insertion of the uncinate onto the middle turbinate.

of the uncinate medially so that it attaches to the middle turbinate (**Fig. 6.9**).

This configuration alters the drainage of the frontal sinus as the agger nasi cell pushes the frontal drainage pathway posteriorly. Therefore, the surgeon can no longer access the frontal recess medial to the uncinate. Access is obtained by passing the curette along the frontal sinus drainage pathway behind the posterior wall of the agger nasi cell and fracturing the posterior wall and roof of the agger nasi cell forward to fully expose the frontal ostium.

The following series of CT scans and operative dissection pictures illustrates the upward continuation of the uncinate which forms the medial wall of the agger nasi cell and has been pushed by this cell to insert on the middle turbinate before progressing superiorly, forming the roof of the agger nasi and then implanting on the lamina papyracea (**Figs. 6.10** and **6.11**).

Attachment of the Uncinate to the Skull Base

The third scenario involves the further upward continuation of the uncinate onto the skull base. In a small percentage of patients the uncinate may have no relationship with the agger nasi cell. Usually in this configuration the uncinate will progress superiorly to implant on the skull base. The following series of CT scans and anatomical dissections illustrates this variation (**Fig. 6.12**).

The uncinate can be seen passing medial to the agger nasi cell and implanting at the junction of the middle turbinate and skull base. The broken line indicates the position of the parasagittal scan.

Alternatively the uncinate process may form the medial wall of a frontoethmoidal cell that is sitting above the agger nasi cell. This frontoethmoidal cell may push the upward continuation of the uncinate superiorly to attach onto the skull base (**Fig. 6.13**). The variations associated with the frontoethmoidal cells are considered later, in the discussion on the classification of the frontal ethmoidal cells. The following cadaver dissection and CT scan illustrate a cell on the right side pushing the insertion of the uncinate onto the skull base (**Fig. 6.13**).

The Agger Nasi Cell[10] (Video 10)

There are a large number of possible variations in the anatomy of the frontal recess. To gain a functional understanding of the anatomy of the frontal recess the simplest configurations should be understood first before more complex variations are tackled. The simplest anatomical configuration is the single agger nasi cell without frontal ethmoidal cells. The agger nasi cell is the most anterior ethmoidal cell and is present in 93% of people.[12] The agger nasi cell forms a bulge on the lateral nasal wall anterior to the middle turbinate (**Fig. 6.14**). If sequential coronal CT scans are evaluated in an anterior to posterior direction, the agger nasi cell can be seen before the middle turbinate comes into view (**Fig. 6.15**).[5,12]

Note that the uncinate only has a relationship with the posterior half of the agger nasi cell and not the anterior half which is why the uncinate cannot be seen on the coronal CT scans taken through the anterior half of the agger nasi cell, as seen in **Fig. 6.15**. This relationship can be viewed in **Figs. 6.16** and **6.17**.

The Transition from Frontal Sinus to Frontal Recess on the Coronal CT Scans

The surgeon reviewing a patient's CT scans before surgery needs to understand how the anterior coronal CT scan through the agger nasi cell relates to the frontal beak and

Fig. 6.10 The agger nasi cell is indicated by the *white arrow*. The *broken line* indicates the position of the parasagittal scan. The scans follow the sequence A, B, C, and D. The uncinate can be seen to be pushed medially by the agger nasi cell, touching the middle turbinate before it turns more posteriorly to form the posterior wall and roof of the agger nasi and implanting on the lamina papyracea.

Fig. 6.11 These left-sided operative pictures are taken of the patient in Fig. 6.10. The *black arrow* indicates the uncinate process which forms the medial wall of the agger nasi cell and attaches to the middle turbinate before progressing superiorly to form the roof of the agger nasi cell and implanting on the lamina papyracea.

Fig. 6.12 (**A–D**) On the right side (in CT scans **B**, **C**, and **D**) the *white arrow* indicates the agger nasi cell. The *black arrow* indicates the space anterior to the agger nasi cell in scans (**A**) and (**D**). The *solid white vertical line* in (**A**), (**B**), and (**C**) indicates the position of the parasagittal scan (**D**). The *broken white arrow* indicates the uncinate process separate from the agger nasi cell in scans (**B**) and (**C**). (**E–G**) These are the right-sided operative pictures of the CT scans shown in (**A–D**) and (**E**) corresponds to CT scan in (**A**) and shows the agger nasi cell intact (*white arrow*) and the *black arrow* indicating the uncinate process as it progresses upward to implant on the junction of the middle turbinate and the skull base. (**F**) The anterior face of the agger nasi cell opened with the uncinate process (*black arrow*) seen to be separate from the agger nasi cell. (**G**) The uncinate (*black arrow*) implanting onto the skull base. The *white arrow* indicates the remaining roof of the agger nasi cell.

A

B

Fig. 6.13 The CT scan is taken of the cadaver dissection specimen pictured along with it. On the right side, the uncinate process (*black arrow*) is pushed up toward the skull base and onto the middle turbinate by a small cell sitting above and medial to the agger nasi cell. On the left the

upward continuation of the uncinate can be seen forming the roof of the agger nasi cell (*white arrow*). Note the frontal sinus draining directly above the agger nasi cell.

frontal sinus and how to be able to tell on sequential coronal CT scans when the transition from frontal sinus to frontal recess occurs. **Figure 6.16** is a diagrammatic illustration of how a coronal CT scan through the anterior half of the agger nasi cell and through the frontal sinus can be identified on a coronal CT scan.

If line 1 is drawn in the coronal plane, the frontal beak can be seen as continuous ridge of bone with the frontal sinus above it (diagonally shaded area in **Figs. 6.16** and **6.17**). This line (line 1) is anterior to the uncinate and one can still see the continuous

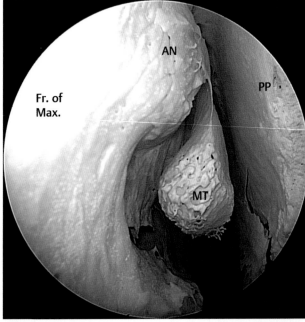

Fig. 6.14 Endoscopic image of a dry skull taken within the right nasal cavity. The bulge on the lateral nasal wall created by the agger nasi cell (*AN*) can clearly be seen above and anterior to the middle turbinate (*MT*). *Fr. of Max*, frontal process of maxilla; *PP*, perpendicular plate.

Fig. 6.15 CT scan illustrating agger nasi cells anterior to middle turbinate insertion (*white arrows*).

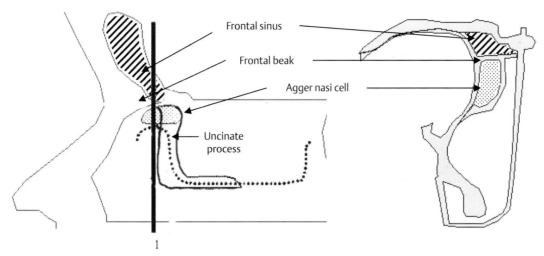

Fig. 6.16 An illustration of a parasagittal view of the agger nasi cell with line 1 representing a coronal cut through the anterior aspect of the agger nasi cell anterior to the middle turbinate. The diagonally striped shaded area represents the area of the frontal sinus above the frontal beak (*black arrow*).

ridge of bone of the beak (floor of the frontal sinus). This makes it simple to differentiate the frontal sinus (above the beak) from the frontal recess. Line 2 in **Fig. 6.17** shows a coronal cut through the uncinate process behind the beak. This illustrates the transition from the frontal sinus to the frontal recess with loss of the continuity of bone (illustrated as the "frontal beak" in **Fig. 6.16**) and by the presence of the uncinate. This coronal cut illustrates the posterior part of the agger nasi cell's relationship to the superior extension of the uncinate process. This part of the uncinate forms the medial and posterior medial wall of the agger nasi cell and represents the relationship between the anterior agger nasi cell (shaded with dots) and the frontal beak and the floor of the frontal sinus (diagonally shaded area).

The diagonally shaded area in **Figs. 6.16** and **6.17** is the frontal sinus above the frontal beak. The frontal beak forms the floor of the frontal sinus (**Fig. 6.2**). Frontal ethmoidal cells pushing into this shaded area are classified as Kuhn type 3

cells (**Table 6.1**).[14] From these diagrams it can be seen that most of the agger nasi cell is anterior to the uncinate but the posterior half of the agger nasi cell has an intimate relationship with the upward extension of the uncinate process (**Fig. 6.18**).[10]

Transition from Frontal Sinus to Frontal Recess on the Axial Scans

The surgeon should also be able to differentiate on the axial scans when transition occurs from the frontal sinus to the frontal recess. The frontal sinus scans should be viewed from the top down (cranial to caudal). The frontal sinus is relatively easy to identify because, as it narrows toward the frontal ostia, it forms a square (**Fig. 6.19**). At this level the posterior wall of the two frontal sinuses forms a straight line

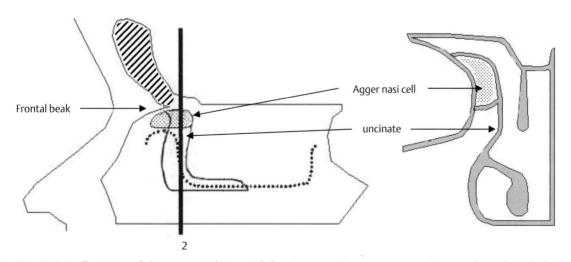

Fig. 6.17 An illustration of the parasagittal view with line 2 representing a more posterior coronal cut through the posterior aspect of the agger nasi cell.

Table 6.1   Kuhn Classification of Frontal Recess and Frontal Sinus Cells

Agger nasi cell	
Supraorbital ethmoid cells	
Frontal cells	
• Type 1	Single frontal recess cell above agger nasi cell
• Type 2	Tier of cells in frontal recess above agger nasi cell
• Type 3	Single massive cell pneumatizing cephalad into frontal sinus
• Type 4	Isolated cell in the frontal sinus
Frontal bulla cells	
Suprabullar cells	
Interfrontal sinus septal cell	

Source: Data from Kuhn FA. Chronic frontal sinusitis: the endoscopic frontal recess approach. Operative techniques. Otolaryngol Head Neck Surg 1996;7:222–229.

(**Fig. 6.19B**). As the skull base turns posteriorly these squares elongate posteriorly but still maintain a roughly rectangular shape. This is the transition stage from frontal sinus to frontal recess (**Fig. 6.19D,E**). As the posterior ends of these boxes become pointed the scans reach the frontal recess (**Fig. 6.19E**). **Figure 6.19A,B** shows the square formation of the frontal sinuses. The transition region is between **Fig. 6.19D** and **Fig. 6.19E**. Note how the bone of the anterior wall changes at each of these levels. At **Fig. 6.19A,B**, the bone of the anterior wall of the frontal sinus is even and relatively flat and not very thick. The anterior wall bone becomes much thicker as the upper region of the frontal beak is reached (**Fig. 6.19C**). At **Fig. 6.19D,E** the anterior wall is curved indicating that the nasion has been reached. In **Fig. 6.19D** the nasion is fully developed and the frontal beak bone is thick. Also note how the posterior wall has become pointed (**Fig. 6.19D,E**) as the axial cut goes into the frontal recess toward the anterior ethmoidal arteries. This artery is seen in its canal in **Fig. 6.19D** on the right side.

Frontal Ethmoidal Cells

Classification

A single agger nasi cell in the frontal recess is only one of the many anatomical variations. In 1995 Fred Kuhn classified the cells seen in the frontal recess and frontal sinus as presented in **Table 6.1**.[14]

This classification still forms the basis of our current classification although we have made significant modifications (**Table 6.2**). One of the important modifications is defining the types of cells that occur in the frontal recess and frontal sinus more precisely. The first cells to be considered are the frontal ethmoidal cells. For a cell to be called a frontal ethmoidal cell it needs to satisfy two criteria: first it must be an anterior ethmoidal cell and second it should be in close proximity to the frontal process of the maxilla. The frontal process of the maxilla is the bone forming the anterior wall of the frontal recess (**Figs. 6.2** and **6.20**).

This bone goes on to form the frontal beak. The frontal ethmoidal cells are further divided depending on how many there are and how far these cells extend into the frontal sinus through the frontal ostium.[16] Kuhn classified frontal ethmoidal cells into types 1 to 4.[14] However, we have modified this classification by clearly defining a frontal ethmoidal cell and by redefining the type 3 and 4 cells (**Table 6.2**).

◆ The Building Block Concept for the Reconstruction of the Anatomy of the Frontal Recess

To reconstruct the cells in the frontal recess in three dimensions, building blocks are arranged, one block for each cell.[10,18] This is done as an aid to the dissection of the frontal recess. When operating in this area the surgeon needs to know exactly which cell is being dissected and in what sequence each cell will be opened so that the frontal recess

A   B

Fig. 6.18 (**A**) Coronal CT scan anterior to uncinate with the floor of the frontal sinus ("beak") illustrated by *white arrow* on the left. (**B**) Coronal CT through the uncinate process (*white arrow*) with the uncinate forming medial wall and roof of agger nasi cell on the left.

Fig. 6.19 **(A)** to **(H)** are sequential axial CT scans. Approximate levels of cuts are demonstrated in parasagittal scan **(J)**. The transition from frontal sinus to frontal recess is between axial cuts **(D)** and **(E)**. Note the development of the nasion in **(E)** with thick bony beak visible. *White arrows* demonstrate the drainage pathway of the frontal sinus on the right side.

Table 6.2 Modified Classification of Frontal Recess and Frontal Sinus Cells*

Agger nasi cell	*Cell that is either anterior to the origin of the middle turbinate or sits directly above the most anterior insertion of the middle turbinate into the lateral nasal wall*
Frontal ethmoidal cells	*An anterior ethmoidal cell that needs to be in close proximity (touching) the frontal process of the maxilla*
• Type 1	Single frontal ethmoidal cell above agger nasi cell
• Type 2	Tier of frontal ethmoidal cells above agger nasi cell
• Type 3	Frontal ethmoidal cell that pneumatizes cephalad into the frontal sinus through the frontal ostium *but not extending beyond 50% of the vertical height of that frontal sinus on the CT scan that is evaluated (is usually found in the lateral region of the frontal ostium)*
• Type 4	*A frontal ethmoidal cell that extends more than 50% of the vertical height of the frontal sinus in the scan that it is evaluated; originally termed an isolated cell in the frontal sinus but, in our experience, isolated cells in the frontal sinus are extremely rare and seldom clinically important*
Frontal bulla cells	This is a cell that originates in the suprabullar region but pneumatizes along the skull base into the frontal sinus along the posterior wall of the frontal sinus
Suprabullar cells	These are suprabullar cells *(cells above the bulla ethmoidalis)* that do not enter the frontal sinus
Intersinus septal cell (also termed "interfrontal sinus septal cell" in Kuhn classification)	This cell is associated with the frontal sinus septum and compromises the frontal ostium by occupying part of the frontal ostium; *it is always medially based and opens into the frontal recess*

*Modifications from the original Kuhn classification are shown in *italic*.

Source: Data from Kuhn FA. Chronic frontal sinusitis: the endoscopic frontal recess approach. Operative techniques. Otolaryngol Head Neck Surg 1996;7:222–229.

Fig. 6.20 The region between the divergent *solid white arrows* is the frontal process of the maxilla. In this example we have a large agger nasi cell (*broken black arrow*) and a type 3 frontal ethmoidal cell (*broken white arrow*).

can be safely and competently cleared. To build a mental picture of the cells in the frontal recess, the coronal CT scans are viewed first. The first cell seen on the coronal CT that is anterior to and directly above the insertion of the middle turbinate is, in most cases, the agger nasi cell[10,18] (**Fig. 6.14**). This cell should now be identified on the parasagittal CT scan (**Fig. 6.21**). Make sure that you use all the information

available to you to confirm that the cell seen on the coronal is indeed the cell that you have identified on the parasagittal. Ask yourself if the cell has air or whether it is partially or completely opacified. Check on both the coronal and parasagittal scans that the cell that you have identified has the expected amount of opacification. A building block is now placed for this cell (**Fig. 6.21**).

The cell directly adjacent (above) to the agger cell is now identified (**Fig. 6.22**). This cell is followed in each sequential coronal scan and is again identified on the parasagittal by again using all the information available (**Fig. 6.22**). A building block is placed to represent this T1 cell. There are no other cells associated with the second cell in this example but, if there were, they would be identified in the same manner and a building block would be placed for each additional cell.

In most patients a suprabullar cell is present. This cell can be difficult to identify on the coronal scan if the septation between it and the frontal drainage pathway is not actively sought. This cell lies against the skull base so the skull base forms its roof (**Fig. 6.23**). It is often confused with the frontal sinus drainage pathway especially if it projects forward toward the frontal ostium. A building block should be placed for this cell and another for the bulla ethmoidalis which lies directly below this cell (**Fig. 6.23**). This sequential identification of each cell first on the coronal scan and then on the parasagittal scan allows the surgeon to begin to build up a 3D picture of the anatomy of the frontal recess.

A, B   C

D   E

Fig. 6.21 (**A**) The first cell just above the origin of the middle turbinate is marked with a *white arrow*. Follow this cell posteriorly (**B,C**; *white arrows*) then identify this cell on the parasagittal CT scan (**D**) (marked with *white arrow*). Place a building block for this cell in your three-dimensional reconstruction.

Fig. 6.22 The cell directly above the agger nasi cell is identified in the first coronal CT scan (**A**; marked with a *white arrow*) and followed in the subsequent coronal scans. This cell (type 1) is identified on the parasagittal scan and a building block placed for it directly above the agger nasi cell.

Fig. 6.23 The suprabullar cell is identified in (**D**; *white arrow*) and then identified on the parasagittal CT scan (**E**). A building block is placed to represent this cell. A building block is also placed for the small bulla ethmoidalis cell below the suprabullar cell.

Fig. 6.24 The axial CT scans (**F** to **I**) are added to the coronal and para-sagittal scans. The *black arrows* in (**F** to **I**) indicate the frontal sinus and its drainage pathway. (**I**) Note how this pathway gets compressed between the T1 cell and the suprabullar cell. The suprabullar cell is indicated with a *white arrow* in CT scans (**F–I**). This posterior and lateral drainage pathway has been added to the 3D reconstruction in this figure.

Drainage Pathways: A Critical Concept in Frontal Recess Dissection

However, it is not just the cellular construction and their relationship with one another that is important but also the drainage pathway of the frontal sinus around these cells.[16–18] It is critical to identify the drainage pathway of the frontal sinus on the CT scan and then to mentally place this pathway in the 3D reconstruction of the anatomy of the frontal recess. The axial CT scans of the frontal sinus and frontal recess are the most helpful in evaluating the drainage pathway. Sequential axial scans are viewed starting in the frontal sinus and progressively following the frontal sinus drainage pathway into the frontal recess. An example of this is presented in **Fig. 6.24**. The black arrows indicate the frontal sinus on the axial CT scans. As the axial scans are followed inferiorly, the T1 cell in the frontal recess comes into view (axial scan I in **Fig. 6.24**). Note the change in shape of the frontal sinus during the transition from the frontal sinus to the frontal recess and the thickening of the bone in the region of the nasion where the frontal beak is formed (**Fig. 6.24**).

During this transition the anterior wall (beak) also becomes more bowed in the region of the nasion (**Fig. 6.24**, axial scans H and I). This is the region of the frontal ostium. In this example the drainage pathway is pushed posteriorly between the suprabullar cell and the T1 cell. During the dissection of the frontal recess instruments (probes or curettes) are passed along this pathway and the identified cells fractured to clear the pathway.[16] Usually the pathway is medial or posterior to the cell(s) and the cell(s) can be fractured laterally or anteriorly quite safely. However, when the pathway is anterior, care needs to be taken when fracturing the cell wall posteriorly against the skull base. When the drainage pathway is lateral, the cell wall should be removed by a very gentle fracture if the bone is thin or by placing the instrument as far posterior to the cell wall as possible and fracturing the cell wall anteriorly. For removing residual bony fragments a through-cutting giraffe forceps can be used. Instruments should not be passed through the roof of a cell because, occasionally, the surgeon may be confident that he or she is in a cell with space between the roof of the cell and the skull base; but, if mistaken, and they are in the space above the cell, pushing the instrument through the "roof" of the cell will result in the instrument entering into anterior cranial fossa. If instruments are passed along pathways, and this can be done very gently without undue force or pressure, cell walls can be fractured safely clearing the drainage pathway of the frontal sinus without endangering the anterior cranial fossa or the orbit.[16–19]

◆ The Anatomical Variations of the Frontal Recess and Frontal Sinus

The Type 1 Cellular Configuration (Videos 11 to 14, 18, and 19)

A type 1 (T1) configuration is one frontal ethmoidal cell above the agger nasi cell (**Fig. 6.25**). This configuration of a single cell associated with the agger nasi cell is common but also may induce significant variability into the frontal recess. The 3D conceptualization of this arrangement is two building blocks sitting one on top of the other (**Fig. 6.25**). The lower building block is the agger nasi cell and the upper block represents the T1 cell.

The Type 2 Cellular Configuration

A type 2 (T2) configuration consists of two or more frontal ethmoidal cells in association with the agger nasi cell (**Fig. 6.26**). These cells are most commonly seen directly above the agger nasi cell and push the implantation of the uncinate higher on the lamina papyracea (**Fig. 6.26**).

The CT scan (**Fig. 6.26**) illustrates the T2 configuration on the right side with cell number 1 representing the agger nasi cell and cells 2 and 3 the frontal ethmoidal cells above it. Review of the parasagittal scan (not shown here) would confirm the position and placement of these cells. Note that the T2 frontal ethmoidal cells do not reach above the frontal beak and therefore do not migrate into the floor of the frontal sinus and removal of these cells does not involve the frontal ostium.[17] If **Fig. 6.16** is reviewed, the diagonally shaded area represents the inferior (floor) part of the frontal sinus.

A, B   C

Fig. 6.25 The cell numbered 1 is the agger nasi cell and the cell numbered 2 is the type 1 cell.

A, B

C

Fig. 6.26 The cell numbered 1 is the agger nasi cell, 2 and 3 are type 2 cells.

Type 3 Cellular Configuration[17] (Videos 15, 16, and 20)

Further pneumatization of these frontal ethmoidal cells into the floor (inferior part) of the frontal sinus above the frontal beak (into the diagonally shaded area in **Fig. 6.16**) are classified as type 3 (T3) cells (**Fig. 6.27**). If the section where the frontal sinus becomes the frontal recess is reviewed (**Figs. 6.16** and **6.17**), the transition from the frontal sinus to the frontal recess occurs when the continuous bony line that forms the floor of the frontal sinus disappears. For the cell to be pushing into the floor of the frontal sinus, the cell needs to be visualized above this bony line in the floor of the frontal sinus (**Figs. 6.16** and **6.17**). T3 cells are usually found in the lateral aspect of the frontal sinus ostium and push the drainage pathway medially and narrow (obstruct) the drainage pathway of the frontal sinus (white arrow, **Fig. 6.27**). The bony beak can be visualized forming the floor of the frontal sinus on the left side of **Fig. 6.27A** scan (broken white arrow).

The parasagittal scan (**Fig. 6.27B**) shows air in the roof of the T3 cell. In addition, on the parasagittal scan, a cell can be seen above the bulla (suprabullar cell) that almost touches the K3 cell as it pneumatizes forward. This creates a narrowing of the frontal outflow track.

Type 4 Cellular Configuration (Video 21)

The original definition of a type 4 (T4) cell was an isolated cell within the frontal sinus.[14] This is a very rare occurrence. Most cells that appear as isolated frontal sinus cells are frontal bulla cells that have pneumatized along the skull base into the frontal sinus and protrude from the posterior wall of the frontal sinus into the sinus. A T4 cell is a frontal ethmoidal cell that pneumatizes through the frontal ostium and extends more than 50% of the vertical height of the frontal sinus (**Fig. 6.28**).

Clinical Difference between T3 and T4 Cells

If we assume that with very few exceptions all apparent isolated frontal sinus cells originate in the frontal recess or from the bulla ethmoidalis/suprabullar cell, then what is the value in discriminating between T3 and T4 cells? In a recent article[17] we suggested that it is worthwhile to discriminate between very extensive pneumatization of a frontal ethmoidal or bulla frontalis cell and a cell which pushes only part way into the frontal sinus.[17] Most T3 cells

A, B

C

Fig. 6.27 **(A,B)** CT scans of a frontal ethmoidal cell (type 3 [T3]) on the right side pushing into the floor of the frontal sinus. The three-dimensional (3D) reconstruction illustrates the T3 cell pushing into the floor of the frontal sinus. The parasagittal scan is taken along the *white line* marked *. The frontal beak (floor of the frontal sinus) is the bony continuity marked by the *white broken arrow* in the coronal scan **(A)** and by the "beak" in the 3D reconstruction. The agger nasi cell is numbered 1.

Fig. 6.28 (**A,B**) In coronal CT scans the type 4 (T4) cell in the right frontal sinus is indicated with a *white arrow*. (**C**) In parasagittal CT scan the T4 cell can be seen pneumatizing from the frontal ethmoidal cell directly above the agger nasi cell. (**D**) A three-dimensional reconstruction of the cells.

that push into the floor of the frontal sinus can be removed from below through the frontal ostium. Cells that pneumatize extensively into the frontal sinus may require additional access (combined approach, endoscopic modified Lothrop/ frontal drillout, or osteoplastic flap)[14,17] for removal to be achieved. On review of the patients included in that study[17] we suggested it would be clinically relevant to create an artificial demarcation between T3 and T4 cells based on the height that the cell extends into the frontal sinus. If the cell extends further than 50% of the height of the frontal sinus on the coronal scans then the cell is a T4 cell (by our definition) rather than a T3 cell (**Fig. 6.29**). Such a T4 cell would usually not be able to be removed from below unless the frontal ostium was particularly large in its anteroposterior dimension.

Fig. 6.29 (**A**) is a drawing of a type 3 (T3) and type 4 (T4) cell illustrating that the T3 is less than 50% of the height of the frontal sinus on the coronal scan and that the T4 is greater than 50% of the frontal sinus. *FB,* frontal beak. (**B**) Coronal CT in which the T4 and T3 cells are illustrated. (**C**) Axial CT scan illustrates how these cells have migrated up the lateral walls of the frontal ostia into the frontal sinuses pushing the drainage pathways medially. (From Wormald PJ, Chan SZX. Surgical techniques for the removal of frontal recess cells obstructing the frontal ostium. Am J Rhinol 2003;17(4):221–226.)[17]

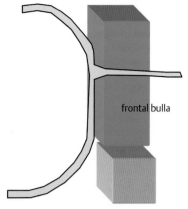

A, B   C

Fig. 6.30 In the coronal CT scan (**A**) the frontal bulla cell again appears as an isolated frontal sinus cell but again when the parasagittal scan is reviewed it can be clearly seen pneumatizing from the suprabullar region.

Further discussion on the selection and techniques used to remove T3 and T4 cells (and frontal bulla cells) is to be found in Chapter 7.

The posterior wall of the frontal sinus slopes and the definition of a T4 cell (> 50% of the height of the frontal sinus on the coronal CT scan under review) is used for the more anterior coronal CT scans as opposed to the CT scans performed in the region of the transition from the frontal sinus to the frontal recess.

Frontal Bulla Cells

Frontal bulla cells are cells that take origin in the suprabullar region and are therefore technically suprabullar cells. They become frontal bulla cells when they migrate through the frontal ostium into the frontal sinus. The skull base always forms the roof of these cells and they are seen on the parasagittal to hug the skull base as they migrate into the frontal sinus (**Fig. 6.30**). On the axial CT they can be clearly seen on the posterior wall of the frontal sinus. If these cells protrude off the skull base in an anterior manner, they will often appear as an isolated cell in the frontal sinus (**Fig. 6.30A**). The clinical importance of these cells is that they push the drainage pathway of the frontal sinus anteriorly and, to be removed, the curette or probe needs to be passed anterior to their wall and the cell wall carefully fractured in a posterior direction.

Intersinus Septal Cells (Video 17)

These are cells associated with the intersinus septum of the frontal sinus. This cell pneumatizes from the frontal recess through the frontal ostium and its medial wall is the intersinus septum of the frontal sinus. Intersinus septal cells (ISSCs) may vary in size but always push the frontal sinus drainage pathway laterally. If this cell is large it may significantly compromise the drainage of the frontal sinus (**Fig. 6.31**) and if the lateral wall of the cell is thick it may not be possible to fracture this wall and removal with

normal handheld instruments may not be possible. In these patients we do not advocate drilling this septum as the drill always creates significant mucosal trauma often leading to a scarred or stenosed frontal ostium as healing takes place (**Fig. 6.31**).

◆ Identifying the Frontal Sinus Drainage Pathways in the Different Anatomical Variations

Cellular Configurations and Associated Drainage Pathways

In the preceding pages the various cellular configurations are detailed. Although it is vital to determine the number of cells in the frontal recess and their relationship to the frontal ostium, it is equally important to understand how these cells interact with the drainage pathway of the frontal sinus.[16–18] One of the most difficult tasks is to determine with each cellular variation where the particular drainage pathway is. In the following examples the cellular configuration is first established and then for each configuration the drainage pathway is determined. Once the drainage pathway has been identified, the surgeon can work out where to slide the frontal sinus probe or curette so that the cells can each be removed sequentially, clearing the drainage pathway and exposing the frontal sinus ostium.

T1/T2 Variations

T1/T2 Configuration with a Posterior Drainage Pathway (Video 19)

To construct the 3D picture, the first step is to identify the agger nasi cell on the coronal CT scan (**Fig. 6.32A–C,** numbered 1 in CT) and to identify this cell in the parasagittal CT scan (numbered 1 on CT, **Fig. 6.32E**). The next cell seen in the coronal scans sits directly above this agger nasi cell and the

Fig. 6.31 (**A,B**) In the coronal CT scans and (**C**) the axial CT, the *black arrow* indicates the intersinus septal cell opening into the left frontal sinus and pushing the drainage pathway of the frontal sinus laterally (*white arrow*). (**D**) A intraoperative picture shows the large opening into the intersinus septal cell (*black arrow*) and the small lateral ostium of the frontal sinus (*white arrow*).

Fig. 6.32 The agger nasi cell (numbered 1) and type 1 cell (numbered 2) are first identified on the coronal scans (**A** to **D**) and then on the parasagittal CT scan. A building block is placed for each of these cells. The bulla ethmoidalis cell is seen on the parasagittal and a block placed for this cell.

Fig. 6.33 The coronal CT scans (**A,B**), parasagittal CT (**C**), and axial CT scans (**D–I**) are presented. The frontal sinus drainage pathway on each of the axial CT scans is illustrated on the accompanying drawing (*shaded area*) and this pathway can be followed from the frontal sinus into the frontal recess around the cells in the frontal recess.

T1 cell is numbered 2. This cell is also identified on the parasagittal CT. Building blocks are placed for both these cells (**Fig. 6.32**). The bulla ethmoidalis cell is noted on the parasagittal CT and a building block placed for this cell as well.

The next step is to work out how the frontal sinus drains around these cells. This is a crucial step as it will determine where the surgeon places instruments during the surgical dissection. Typically the surgeon will be faced with several potential drainage pathways once the agger nasi cell has been removed. When looking into the frontal recess, he or she needs to know if the pathway is posterior/medial/lateral or anterior as this will determine where the probe or curette is placed. Once this instrument is slid up the pathway the obstructing cells can be fractured and removed safely. Failure to correctly identify the frontal drainage pathway on the CT scan will cause indecision and may result in the probe being placed in the incorrect position and potentially, if force is used, may breach the skull base. In this example the T1/2 cell occupies the entire anterior region of the frontal recess and pushes the drainage pathway posteriorly. This can be clearly seen in the axial CT scans in the

accompanying **Fig. 6.33**. Drawings of the axial scans from the frontal sinus into the frontal recess are presented in conjunction with the axial CTs to help identify the drainage pathway and follow it from the frontal sinus into the frontal recess.

The first two steps were to construct a 3D picture and to place the drainage pathway in this 3D picture. The combined 3D reconstruction is presented in **Fig. 6.34**.

If the surgeon had created a 3D mental picture of the anatomy before the surgery, he or she would have visualized that after the agger nasi cell had been removed, that the T1 cell would be visible in the medial region of the frontal recess, and that the frontal sinus drainage pathway would be visible posterior to this cell.

T1/T2 Configuration with a Medial Drainage Pathway (Videos 11, 12, and 18)

This is one of the more common configurations where the T1/T2 cell sits directly above the agger nasi cell and pushes the

Fig. 6.34 Cell 1 is the agger nasi cell and cell 2 is the type 1 (T1) cell. Note the frontal sinus drainage pathway is posterior to the T1 cell (numbered 2) and anterior to the bulla ethmoidalis.

insertion of the middle turbinate comes into view. The agger cell (numbered 1) should also be identified on the parasagittal scan. On the coronal CT scan **Fig. 6.35C** a cell appears on the skull base (numbered 3). This is a suprabullar cell and is clearly seen on the parasagittal CT scan **Fig. 6.35E**. To create the 3D image a building block is placed for each one of these cells.

The next step is to identify the drainage pathway in this example. The series of axial CT scans are used and the frontal sinus identified. The frontal sinus is followed inferiorly into the frontal recess. Note how the first cell seen on the axial scans is the suprabullar cell (numbered 3) and that the drainage pathway is initially anterior to this cell (CT scan **Fig. 6.35H**) before it becomes medial to both this cell and the T1 cell (**Figs. 6.35I** and **6.36**).

To complete the 3D image the frontal sinus drainage pathway is drawn into the building block 3D picture (**Fig. 6.37**). This allows the surgeon to have a complete understanding of the anatomy of this frontal recess and to have a surgical plan to place the probe or curette and remove the frontal recess cells thereby clearing the frontal ostium.

drainage pathway of the frontal sinus in a medial direction. This is caused by the upward continuation of the uncinate process forming the medial wall of not only the agger cell but also of the T1/2 cell before finally implanting on the lamina papyracea. In this example the T1/2 cell is seen first and is identified on the parasagittal CT scan (**Fig. 6.35B–D**, cell numbered 2). The agger nasi cell is small and is seen in the CT scan **Fig. 6.35C** just as the

T1/T2 with an Anterior Drainage Pathway (Video 11)

If the T1/T2 cell expands so that it touches the suprabullar cell and the frontal process of the maxilla in the lateral region, it will push the drainage pathway of the frontal sinus anteromedially (**Fig. 6.38**). This T1/T2 configuration is illustrated by the following example on the left side. The

A, B

C

D, E

F

Fig. 6.35 On the right side of the coronal scans the type 1 (T1) cell (numbered 2) and agger nasi cell (numbered 1) are identified. These cells are then identified on the parasagittal CT scan (**E**). The suprabullar cell is seen in coronal CT (**C**) and on the parasagittal scan (**E**). A three-dimensional image is created with the building blocks.

Fig. 6.36 The axial CT scans are added so that the frontal sinus drainage pathway can be followed from the frontal sinus into the frontal recess. Note how the pathway passes initially anteriorly to the suprabullar cell (numbered 3) before passing medial to both the suprabullar cell and the type 1 cell (numbered 2).

Fig. 6.37 The three-dimensional picture of the cells in the frontal recess (1, agger nasi cell; 2, type 1 cell; 3, suprabullar cell) complete with the frontal sinus drainage pathway.

first cell identified in scan **Fig. 6.38B** is the agger nasi cell numbered 1. Directly above this cell is the frontal ethmoidal T1 numbered 2. A building block is placed for each of these cells. In the parasagittal scan **Fig. 6.38E** the suprabullar cell numbered 3 and bulla ethmoidalis numbered 4 can be seen. Building blocks are also placed for these cells.

It is important to be able to pick the drainage pathway of the frontal sinus around these cells. In this patient the frontal sinus drains anteromedial to the T1 cell as the T1 cell is attached to the anterior skull base and laterally to the frontal process of the maxilla (see **Fig. 6.39**). Again, if we follow the drainage pathway of the frontal sinus from the frontal sinus inferiorly into the frontal recess on the axial CT scans, the relationship between the pathway and the T1 cell is clearly seen (**Fig. 6.39**).

If we now add this drainage pathway to the 3D picture a clear understanding of the relationship of these frontal recess cells and the drainage pathway should be established (**Fig. 6.40**).

To add a clinical perspective, the following intraoperative pictures of this example are shown (**Fig. 6.41**). The surgeon should be able to visualize the configuration of the frontal recess cells and drainage pathway and should be able to picture this in his or her mind before surgery is commenced. When the surgeon looks up into the frontal recess, the T1/T2 cell should be seen anteriorly with the drainage pathway anteromedially.

Once the agger nasi cell is removed and the T1 cell identified, the surgeon should know where to look for the frontal sinus drainage pathway. In this patient, if attempts were made to push probes posterior to the cell, injury and penetration of the skull base would be possible. However, if the pathway is recognized, a small probe can be slid up between the T1 cell and the medial wall of the olfactory fossa and the cell fractured laterally thereby clearing the frontal recess. Review the Chapter 6 tutorials and online videos to see how this configuration was dissected and how it compares to your mental 3D reconstruction of the anatomy.

Fig. 6.38 The coronal CT scans (**A**) to (**D**) are viewed and each sequential cell identified and followed from anterior to posterior. A building block is placed for each cell. Additional cells can be seen in the parasagittal scan E which are not seen in the coronal scans as the coronal scans do not go far enough posteriorly. Building blocks are also placed for these cells.

A, B

C

D, E

F

G

H

Fig. 6.39 The following series of CT scans includes the axial scans (**E,F**) with associated drawings to illustrate how the type 1 cell pushes the frontal sinus drainage pathway anteromedially.

Fig. 6.40 This frontal sinus drainage pathway is placed in the three-dimensional picture. The type 1 cell (numbered 2) pushes the pathway anteromedially.

T1/2 with a Lateral Drainage Pathway

If a T1/2 cell abuts the insertion of the middle turbinate as it inserts to the skull base, the frontal sinus drainage pathway may be pushed laterally. This is relatively uncommon but is important to recognize when it occurs. It is more common for a medially based cell to be situated much higher and for it to be in contact with the frontal sinus septum and is termed an intersinus septal cell (see below). Recognition of a T1/2 cell situated medially in the frontal recess will allow the frontal sinus drainage pathway to be sought laterally and allow this cell to be safely removed and the frontal ostium to be fully exposed. The following example shows the medially placed T1 cell with the lateral drainage pathway (**Fig. 6.42**).

Now that the 3D reconstruction of the cells has been made, the drainage pathway of the frontal sinus into the frontal recess is established. This is done by following the frontal sinus inferiorly into the frontal recess. Note on **Fig. 6.43** the shaded region progressing from the frontal sinus lateral to the T1 cell and then medial to the agger nasi cell.

Fig. 6.41 **(A)** The frontal sinus drainage pathway is indicated with a *broken white arrow*. The anterior wall of the type 1 (T1) cell is indicated with a *solid black arrow* and the cell itself indicated with a *solid white arrow*. The suction curette is indicating the suprabullar cell.

(A) Taken prior to removal of the anterior wall of the cell and **(B)** after the wall has been removed the frontal ostium is seen (*broken white line*) with the insertion of the T1 cell indicated by the *solid black line* and cell by the *solid white line*.

Although the axial CT scans are our primary scan we use to follow the frontal sinus drainage pathway, it is also important to view the coronal CT scans as well. In this example the frontal drainage pathway can be clearly seen in the coronal CTs as well as the axials but what can also be seen from the coronal scans is how the frontal sinus drainage pathway swings below the T1 cells to move over the roof of the agger nasi cell to continue medial to this cell into the nasal cavity. This pathway can now be placed with the building blocks to form the 3D picture providing the surgeon with a clear understanding of the left frontal recess (**Fig. 6.44**).

If the surgeon had a clear 3D picture of the anatomy, then he or she would be able to visualize the T1 cell in the medial region of the frontal recess and the frontal sinus drainage pathway draining lateral to it. To aid the surgeon's conceptualization of this situation prior to any surgery being performed, the following clinical intraoperative pictures

Fig. 6.42 On the left side the agger nasi cell is numbered 1 and the type 1 cell numbered 2 on the coronal CT scans (**A–D**) and on the parasagittal CT scan (**E**). A building block is placed for each of these cells. A large bulla ethmoidalis extending to the skull base is seen behind these cells on the parasagittal CT (**E**) and a building block is also placed for this cell.

Fig. 6.43 When the axial CT scans (**E–H**) are reviewed, note with reference to the accompanying diagrams how the frontal sinus drainage pathway first is pushed anteriorly (**F**) then laterally (**G,H**).

Fig. 6.44 When both the coronal CT scans and axial CT scans are viewed together, note how the drainage frontal sinus pathway drains initially lateral to the type 1 cell before swinging medial to the agger nasi cell.

are provided (**Fig. 6.45**). Make sure that this is how you visualized the frontal recess after looking at the scans and if not re-do the scans until the clinical pictures are what you would expect to see.

T3/T4 and Intersinus Septal Cell Variations

T3/4 with a Medial Drainage Pathway (Videos 15, 16, and 20)

In most cases a T3 cell will enter the frontal ostium laterally pushing the frontal sinus drainage pathway medially (**Fig. 6.46**). In this example, on the right side, the T3 cell occupies most of the frontal ostium as it pushes through the ostium into the floor of the frontal sinus. The steps for creating a 3D image remain to identify each cell seen in each sequential coronal CT scan on the parasagittal scan. In this case the T3 cell is the first one identified, followed by a small agger nasi cell, and a small medial cell. The suprabullar cell also pushes forward onto the back wall of the T3 cell (**Fig. 6.46**).

Fig. 6.45 (**A**) The *white arrow* indicates the type 1 (T1) cell situated medially in the frontal recess whereas the *black arrow* indicates the frontal sinus drainage pathway. (**B**) The *white arrow* indicates the frontal ostium after the T1 cell has been removed.

The next step is to identify the drainage pathway of the frontal sinus. This is best appreciated in the axial CT scans and drawings. Note how the frontal drainage pathway is narrowed progressively as the T3 cell occupies more and more space and squeezes the frontal drainage pathway medially. The small medial cell (numbered 3) again pushes this pathway more anteromedially by occupying some of the medial drainage space (**Fig. 6.47**).

Once the frontal sinus drainage pathway around the cells has been established, this can be drawn on the 3D image, giving the surgeon a clear understanding of the anatomy of the frontal recess and allowing a surgical

Fig. 6.46 In the coronal CT (**A**), the type 3 cell is numbered 1 and can be clearly seen on the parasagittal scan (**E**). Note the small medial cell numbered 3 in CT scans (**C,D**).

Fig. 6.47 The coronal, parasagittal, and axial CT scans are presented with drawings of the medial frontal sinus drainage pathway on the right side of the patient. Note, on the axial CT scans (**E,F**), the small medial ethmoidal cell pushing into the drainage pathway from behind. This cell was numbered 3 in the previous figure.

plan to be developed for the frontal recess dissection (**Fig. 6.48**).

In some patients with very large T3 cells, only the medial wall that occupies the frontal ostium may need to be removed and the roof of the cell may be left if this no longer obstructs the frontal sinus drainage pathway. This is usually only done if there is technical difficulty in reaching the roof or dome of the cell or if the roof is too thick to fracture easily

with a probe or a curette. A T4 cell is a cell that usually enters the frontal sinus along the lateral wall of the frontal ostium pushing the drainage pathway medially. However, in the coronal plane, it can be seen that the cell extends more than 50% of the vertical height of the frontal sinus on the scan. The decision as to whether it would be possible to remove this is based on the anteroposterior dimension of the frontal ostium best evaluated on the parasagittal scan. In this case the

Fig. 6.48 The frontal sinus drainage pathway is medial to the type 3 cell (numbered 1) and lateral to the cell numbered 3.

frontal ostium is widely patent and the T4 cell was able to be removed from below. If this is not felt to be the case then a modified Lothrop/frontal drillout is performed for access and in all cases this provides more than adequate access to be able to remove T4 cells.

T3/4 with a Posterior Drainage Pathway

This situation occurs when a frontal ethmoidal cell pneumatizes through the frontal ostium and occupies the entire anterior region of the frontal ostium, pushing the frontal sinus drainage pathway posteriorly. In some instances this pathway can be very narrow and there may be significant risk when trying to manipulate a probe or curette through this narrow space due to the proximity of the skull base. In most patients this portion of the skull base (fovea ethmoidalis) is quite thick and there should be resistance to penetration. This should be checked on the CT scan prior to the probe being placed. In the following example the T3 cell almost reaches 50% of the vertical height of the frontal sinus on the coronal scan and therefore it is marginal if this cell should be termed a T3 or a T4 cell (**Fig. 6.49**). In addition this patient has undergone prior surgery and the agger nasi cell and bulla ethmoidalis have been removed.

Once the 3D picture has been created, the drainage pathway of the frontal sinus around these cells needs to be established. In the following **Fig. 6.50** the T3 cell can be seen occupying most of the frontal ostium and pushing the drainage pathway of the frontal sinus posteriorly but anterior to the residual suprabullar cell.

If the frontal sinus drainage pathway is now added to the 3D picture its posterior course can be clearly seen and understood (**Fig. 6.51**).

Fig. 6.49 The large type 3 cell (numbered 1) occupies almost the entire frontal recess (**A–D,** coronal CT scans). A small residual suprabullar cell (numbered 2) is seen just posterior to the type 1 cell on the skull base (**E,** parasagittal CT). A building block is placed for each of these cells to create the three-dimensional picture.

Fig. 6.50 Axial CT scans (**E,F**) and the accompanying drawings illustrate the frontal sinus drainage pathway (*shaded area*). Note how compressed this pathway becomes and how closely associated it is with the posterior wall of the frontal sinus and fovea ethmoidalis. Fortunately, in the patient, this region of the skull base has thick bone and the risk of skull base penetration while placing the probe or curette should be low. If the surgeon remains concerned, a frontal minitrephine can be placed. This is discussed in Chapter 7.

Fig. 6.51 The frontal sinus drainage pathway can be seen behind the type 3 cell and anterior to the residual suprabullar cell.

T3/4 and Intersinus Septal Cell with an Anterior Drainage Pathway (Video 17)

If the T3/4 cell is large and fills the frontal ostium it will push the drainage pathway either medially, posteriorly, or anteriorly. The direction it pushes the drainage pathway is primarily dependent on where the cell is based (anteriorly, laterally, or posteriorly) and what other cells are present in the frontal ostium/recess. If, for example, an ISSC is present this will further narrow the frontal sinus drainage pathway and this cell will tend to push the pathway laterally. In such a case the pathway will be squeezed between these two cells. An example of this anatomical variation is presented in **Fig. 6.52**. On CT scan **Fig. 6.52B** the T3 cell is numbered 1 and the intersinus septal cell is numbered 3. The T3 cell extends further through the frontal ostium than the ISSC and initially pushes the drainage pathway anteriorly. As the drainage pathway continues inferiorly the ISSC is encountered which squeezes the pathway between itself and the T3 cell. If a building block is placed for each of these cells seen and for the bulla ethmoidalis (cell number 5) and suprabullar cell (cell number 4), a 3D picture of this complex cellular configuration is established (**Fig. 6.52**).

To work out the frontal sinus drainage pathway, the axial scans are viewed from cranial to caudal (**Fig. 6.53**). As the frontal sinus is followed into the frontal recess its pathway is initially pushed anteriorly by the T3 cell—then, as the pathway reaches the ISSC, it is squeezed between the T3 cell and the ISSC (**Fig. 6.53**).

If the 3D image is reviewed, the frontal sinus drainage pathway can be placed among these cells. This allows the surgeon to decide exactly where the probe or curette should be placed so that it can be slid up the drainage pathway and the cells that are obstructing the frontal ostium can be removed (**Fig. 6.54**).

To further illustrate this complex anatomical arrangement of cells, the following intraoperative photos show the ISSC and T3 cell (**Fig. 6.55A**) and the curette in **Fig. 6.55B** illustrates where the drainage pathway would be sought after the CT scans had been thoroughly evaluated, the 3D reconstruction performed, and drainage pathway determined.

Fig. 6.52 In a CT scan (**A**), no cells are seen. (**B**) The T3 cell is seen and the beginning of the interseptal sinus cell (numbered 3). The agger nasi cell (numbered 2) is first seen on scan (**C**). (**E**) The suprabullar cell (numbered 4) and the bulla ethmoidalis (numbered 5) are also seen.

Fig. 6.53 To determine the frontal sinus drainage pathway the frontal sinus is followed from within the frontal sinus (**E**, axial CT) into the frontal recess (**G,H**). Note how the drainage pathway is first squeezed anteriorly by the T3 cell. Then the ISSC appears and compresses the pathway laterally, compressing it between itself and the T3 cell.

Fig. 6.54 Block 1 is the type 3 cell and block 3 is the interseptal sinus cell. Note how the drainage pathway is squeezed between these cells.

Figure 6.55C is the frontal ostium once these cells have been removed.

Frontal Bulla Cell with Anterior Drainage Pathway (Video 21)

This cell has been commonly confused with the T4 cell of the original Kuhn classification in which a T4 cell was defined as an isolated cell within the frontal sinus. In **Fig. 6.56**, the cell numbered 1 appears to be an isolated cell in the frontal sinus. However, when this cell is followed posteriorly and viewed on the parasagittal scan, it is quite clear that this is a frontal bulla cell that originated in the suprabullar space and pneumatizes forward along the skull base into the frontal sinus.

In **Fig. 6.57**, the frontal sinus drainage pathway can be followed from the frontal sinus into the frontal recess. Note how the sinus drains anterior to the frontal bulla cell and then medial to the agger nasi cell.

If the 3D picture is reviewed and the frontal sinus drainage pathway is placed, a true 3D image of both the anatomy and the pathway is formed. This allows planning of each step of the surgical resection of the frontal bulla cell (**Fig. 6.58**).

◆ Conclusion

The anatomy and common variations that occur in the frontal recess are poorly understood by a large number of endoscopic sinus surgeons. The agger nasi cell is proposed as the key to the understanding of this complex area. Fine cut coronal and parasagittal reconstructed CT scans aid the identification of each individual cell and allow the surgeon to formulate a clear and precise surgical plan. Axial scans are useful for the identification of the frontal sinus drainage pathway. Before surgery is performed in the frontal recess the surgeon needs to fully review all the CT scans in the three planes and assume that he or she is in a surgical simulator. The surgeon should be able to mentally create an image of the cellular structure in the frontal recess and then be able to place the frontal sinus drainage pathway in this 3D picture. The surgeon should then go through the surgical steps to be performed. For example: create an axillary flap, raise the flap, remove the anterior wall of the agger nasi cell, place the curette medial or behind the agger nasi cell, and remove this cell (medial wall and roof). Identify the residual cells and the frontal sinus drainage pathway around these cells. Place the suction curette along the frontal sinus drainage pathway without force and fracture the cell and remove the cell(s) exposing the frontal ostium. Such a surgical plan, formulated from a thorough understanding of the anatomy, allows a confident dissection of a complex and difficult area.

A, B   C

Fig. 6.55 **(A)** The interseptal sinus cell (ISSC) extending from the intersinus septum (region of the black arrow) laterally and the type 3 (T3) cell (*white arrow*). Note that the roof of the T3 cell is higher than that of the ISSC as could be seen in the CT scans. **(B)** The curette is placed into the drainage pathway and slid into the frontal sinus allowing both the ISSC and the T3 cell walls to be fractured and removed from the frontal ostium. **(C)** Shows the frontal ostium after removal of the ISSC and T3 cell walls. The *white arrow* indicates the frontal sinus and the *black arrow* the edge of the ISSC wall where it attaches to the intersinus septum.

Fig. 6.56 On the left side the cell numbered 1 is a frontal bulla cell. This can be followed in the sequential coronal CT scans (**A–D**) into the suprabullar space. The parasagittal CT scan (**E**) illustrates the origin of the cell. The cell numbered 2 is an agger nasi cell. A building block is placed for each cell seen to complete the three-dimensional conceptualization of the anatomy in this region.

Fig. 6.57 In the axial CT scans (**E–H**), note how on the left the suprabullar cell attaches to the posterior wall of the frontal sinus (skull base) as it creeps along the skull base into the frontal sinus. It pushes the frontal sinus drainage pathway anteriorly. This can be seen on the axial CT scan drawings where this pathway is shaded, allowing this drainage pathway to be clearly followed on the scans.

Fig. 6.58 The frontal sinus drainage pathway is initially pushed anteriorly to the bulla frontalis cell (*1*) before moving medial to the agger nasi cell (*2*).

Videos

The videos that accompany this book present a series of case studies in which the variations described above are illustrated. Each case is presented with a series of CT scans in the various planes. Attempt to draw the anatomy of the frontal recess using building blocks and establish a 3D picture including the frontal sinus drainage pathway. Then review the video of the surgical procedure so that you can see how the anatomy seen in the dissection relates to your 3D reconstruction. This illustrates the value of such a reconstruction before surgery is undertaken.

References

1. Kaliner MA, Osguthorpe JD, Fireman P, et al. Sinusitis: bench to bedside. Current findings, future directions. J Allergy Clin Immunol 1997;99 (6 Pt 3, Suppl)S829–S848

2. Davis WE, Templer J, Parsons DS. Anatomy of the paranasal sinuses. Otolaryngol Clin North Am 1996;29(1):57–74

3. Schaefer SD, Manning S, Close LG. Endoscopic paranasal sinus surgery: indications and considerations. Laryngoscope 1989;99(1):1–5

4. Kennedy DW, Senior BA. Endoscopic sinus surgery. A review. Otolaryngol Clin North Am 1997;30(3):313–330

5. Stammberger HR, Kennedy DW; The Anatomic Terminology Group. Paranasal sinuses:anatomic terminology and nomenclature. Ann Otol Rhinol Laryngol Suppl 1995;167(supplement 167):7–16

6. Thawley SE, Deddens AE. Transfrontal endoscopic management of frontal recess disease. Am J Rhinol 1995;9(6):307–311

7. Keros P. Über die praktische Bedeutung der Niveauunterschiede de Lamina cribrosa des Ethmoids. Laryngol Rhinol Otol (Stuttg) 1965;41: 808–813

8. Stammberger H, Hawke M, eds. Functional Endoscopic Sinus Surgery - The Messerklinger Technique. Philadelphia: B.C. Decker Publishers; 1991: 61–90

9. Floreani SR, Nair SB, Switajewski MC, Wormald PJ. Endoscopic anterior ethmoidal artery ligation: a cadaver study. Laryngoscope 2006;116(7): 1263–1267

10. Wormald PJ. The agger nasi cell: the key to understanding the anatomy of the frontal recess. Otolaryngol Head Neck Surg 2003;129(5):497–507

11. Kew J, Rees G, Close D, Sdralis T, Sebben R, Wormald PJ. Multiplanar reconstructed CT images improves depiction and understanding of the anatomy of the frontal sinus and recess. Am J Rhinol 2002;16(2):119–123

12. Bolger WE, Butzin CA, Parsons DS. Paranasal sinus bony anatomic variations and mucosal abnormalities: CT analysis for endoscopic sinus surgery. Laryngoscope 1991;101(1 Pt 1):56–64

13. Wake M, Takeno S, Hawke M. The uncinate process: a histological and morphological study. Laryngoscope 1994;104(3 Pt 1):364–369

14. Kuhn FA. Chronic frontal sinusitis: the endoscopic frontal recess approach. Operative techniques. Oper Tech Otolaryngol–Head Neck Surg 1996;7:222–229

15. Kim KS, Kim HU, Chung IH, Lee JG, Park IY, Yoon JH. Surgical anatomy of the nasofrontal duct: anatomical and computed tomographic analysis. Laryngoscope 2001;111(4 Pt 1):603–608

16. Wormald PJ. The axillary flap approach to the frontal recess. Laryngoscope 2002;112(3):494–499

17. Wormald PJ, Chan SZX. Surgical techniques for the removal of frontal recess cells obstructing the frontal ostium. Am J Rhinol 2003;17(4):221–226

18. Wormald PJ. Surgery of the frontal recess and frontal sinus. Rhinology 2005;43(2):82–85

19. Jacobs JB. 100 years of frontal sinus surgery. Laryngoscope 1997; 107(11 Pt 2):1–36

7 Surgical Approach to the Frontal Sinus and Frontal Recess

The frontal recess has always been considered to be the most difficult area to dissect.[1–4] This is largely due to its location behind the beak of the frontal bone.[5] There are three major philosophies regarding the management of disease of the frontal recess and sinus. The minimal invasive sinus technique (MIST) advocates management of the maxillary sinus and associated transitional spaces (hiatus semilunaris and ethmoidal infundibulum) without performing surgery in the frontal recess.[6–8] This philosophy states that treatment of the maxillary sinus and associated transitional spaces will result in clearance of the frontal recess and sinus disease. There are few published papers supporting this theory and all publications come from the same group of investigators.[6–8] Until there is substantial evidence that this approach works for a broad spectrum of frontal sinus and frontal recess disease, we do not advocate this approach. The second philosophy is that the frontal recess and frontal sinus should only be operated on if there are symptoms that can be directly ascribed to the frontal sinus such as frontal headache and pain. Although we agree that surgery on a diseased frontal sinus or recess that is symptomatic is appropriate, we disagree that this is the only indication for surgery in this region. Patients who present with nasal obstruction, postnasal drip, purulent rhinorrhea and anosmia, and who have radiological disease in the frontal sinus or recess need to have this region surgically addressed. These patients have their diseased maxillary sinuses, ethmoid, and sphenoid sinuses addressed and it makes no sense that just because they do not have localized frontal pain or tenderness, that the frontal sinus should not be addressed as well. It has been well recognized that retained or residual cells in the frontal recess/sinus is one of the most common causes of endoscopic sinus surgery (ESS) failure.[1,2]

In this chapter we present our graduated approach to surgery of the frontal recess and sinus. In the easy frontal recess and sinus, simple maneuvers in terms of endoscopy and surgical access (axillary flap) are advocated and are, in most cases, sufficient to allow clearance of the frontal recess and frontal ostium. In the difficult frontal recess or sinus, the additional technique of frontal sinus mini-trephination is presented. These difficult patients may also benefit from the surgeon having computer-aided surgical navigation available.

The mainstay of our surgical technique is the axillary flap technique. This technique has similarities to the frontal sinus rescue procedure described by Kuhn et al.[9] in that mucosal flaps are raised during the surgery on the frontal ostium. However, the major difference is that the frontal sinus rescue procedure is designed for the management of patients who have failed previous standard ESS and have a stenosed frontal ostium. The axillary flap technique is designed for all patients undergoing frontal recess or sinus procedure including previously operated patients. The central concept of the axillary flap procedure is removal of the anterior wall of the agger nasi cell. This is not new and was described by May and Schaitken[10] as part of their nasofrontal approach (NFA 1) to the frontal sinus. Schaefer and Close[11] have advocated a similar approach with removal of the bone above the insertion of the middle turbinate. The major difference between these approaches and the axillary flap approach is the elevation of a mucosal flap which can be replaced at the end of the procedure to cover the raw exposed bone that is seen after removal of the anterior wall of the agger nasi cell. This prevents granulation tissue from forming over the exposed bone with subsequent scarring and cicatrization of this area. Such scarring can pull the upper extension of the middle turbinate laterally and close off the anterior aspect of the frontal recess. This may in turn lead to blockage of the frontal outflow tract and result in recurrent frontal sinusitis.

May and Schaitkin advocated enlarging the frontal ostium in their NFA II and III approaches.[10] This is unnecessary and not advocated in the vast majority of patients as the removal of residual cells within the frontal recess with the exposure of the frontal ostium is usually sufficient to achieve resolution of frontal sinusitis. It is our philosophy that where patients have cells in the frontal recess or frontal ostium that obstruct the outflow of the frontal sinus, that these should be removed without enlarging the frontal ostium. Even very small frontal ostia can function well if their outflow pathway is not obstructed and the patient should be given the opportunity to see if the natural size of their frontal ostium is sufficient. In some patients, especially those with severe mucosal disease, this ostium may become edematous and obstruct and, if this causes symptoms, then enlargement of the ostium is indicated. However, this occurs in the minority of cases and it's not possible to predict which patients with a particular frontal ostium size will obstruct and become symptomatic. In most patients the only way to enlarge a frontal ostium is with a drill. Drilling in the frontal ostium without creation of the largest possible ostium is likely to result in an intense fibrous reaction from the exposed raw bone and in most cases will increase the likelihood of postoperative scarring and stenosis. As can be seen in Chapter 9, enlargement of the frontal ostium is usually done with a modified Lothrop procedure/Draf 3/frontal drillout and very rarely with a Draf type 2 (unilateral enlargement of the frontal ostium) procedure, due to the increased incidence of fibrosis and stenosis seen with unilateral drilling on the frontal ostium.[12] This is especially true for patients who have severe mucosal disease and in whom the inflammatory process continues in the postoperative period.[13]

◆ Which Patients Are Suitable for Frontal Recess and Frontal Sinus Surgery?

Our philosophy is that a patient who has undergone appropriate medical therapy (including systemic steroids) and is then found to have mucosal thickening in the frontal recess or sinus should have all cells cleared from the frontal recess and frontal ostium exposed (**Fig. 7.1**).[13–16] In patients

without significant disease of the frontal recess (**Fig. 7.1**), only the diseased sinuses are addressed and the frontal recess is left untouched. Partial surgery of the frontal recess is never indicated. If only the roof of the agger nasi cell is removed or one of the frontal ethmoidal cells is removed, scarring is likely to result. The cells in the frontal recess are usually in close approximation and partial clearance of cells will very likely result in adhesions forming between these closely approximated surfaces with obstruction of the drainage pathway of the frontal sinus. Our philosophy is an all or nothing approach. The frontal recess is either left entirely alone or all the cells are removed from the recess with visualization of the frontal ostium.

◆ Assessing the Frontal Recess and Frontal Sinus Prior to Surgery

In a patient who is to undergo frontal recess clearance and sinus surgery, the computed tomography (CT) scans need to be carefully assessed and the three-dimensional (3D) reconstruction of the anatomy performed (see Chapter 6). Once the surgeon has a clear understanding of the anatomy, a surgical plan should be formulated. An example of such a plan is presented in **Fig. 7.2**. In this patient, after uncinectomy and middle meatal antrostomy, an axillary flap is performed to expose the anterior face of the agger nasi cell. This is removed with the Hajek Koeffler punch (Karl Storz, Tuttlingen, Germany) and the agger nasi cell visualized. The malleable frontal sinus curette* (Medtronic ENT, Jacksonville, FL) is placed posteromedially to the agger nasi cell's posterior wall and roof, and the cell removed by fracturing it forward. The resultant debris is removed with a microdebrider. The residual roof of the agger nasi cell is cleared and

Fig. 7.1 In coronal CT (**A**) note the mucosal thickening in the left frontal sinus (*white arrow*) and recess with a normal right frontal sinus and recess. In coronal CT (**B**) note the mucosal thickening of the right maxillary sinus (*white arrow*). In this patient the left frontal recess would be

cleared of cells and the frontal ostium identified while on the right side no surgery would be performed in the frontal recess. Both maxillary sinuses would be surgically addressed.

Fig. 7.2 The T3 cell is numbered 1 in the coronal CT scans (**A–C**) and the parasagittal scan (**D**) and the agger nasi cell is numbered 2. In the axial CT scans (**E–G**), the T3 cell is numbered 1 with the frontal sinus drainage pathway medial to this cell (*white arrow*). (*continued*)

Fig. 7.2 *(continued)*

the type 3 (T3) cell visualized. After careful assessment of the axial scans we know that the frontal sinus drains medially around this cell and the suction curette is slid along this drainage pathway into the frontal sinus and the cell fractured laterally and removed. An angled microdebrider blade is used to clear debris, and small residual bony fragments are cleared with giraffe forceps and the malleable frontal sinus hooked probe* (Medtronic ENT). The frontal ostium is visualized but all mucosa around the frontal ostium is preserved.

Identifying the Easy from the Difficult Frontal Recess and Sinus

Surgeons should recognize potentially difficult frontal recesses by studying the CT scans at the time the patient is listed for surgery.[13–16] Recognition of potential difficulties can aid the surgeon when discussing the likelihood of success of the procedure and the probable need for further surgery such as enlargement of a very narrow frontal ostium. In addition, the likelihood of possible ancillary procedures, such as a mini-trephine of the frontal sinuses, can be assessed and discussed with the patient. The need for computer-aided surgical navigation is assessed at the same time. The surgeon should assess the degree of difficulty of the surgery and if the case is too difficult for their level of expertise, the patient should be referred to a specialist rhinologist. The following features should be sought on the CT scan.

Narrow versus Wide Anteroposterior Diameter of the Frontal Ostium

Patients who have a wide anteroposterior (AP) diameter will usually have a technically easier operation and will in most cases have a better prognosis for maintenance of health of the sinuses after surgery. This reflects the postoperative size of the frontal ostium that can be achieved without drilling on the ostium. **Figure 7.3** illustrates a patient with a wide AP

diameter compared with a patient with a narrow AP diameter. Note the space available to operate in the wide diameter patient.

Single Agger Nasi Cell or Simple T1/2 Configuration (Videos 10 to 14, 18, and 19)

Single agger nasi cell is the simplest configuration in the frontal recess and, after removal of this cell, the frontal ostium can be identified (**Fig. 7.4**). A simple cell configuration of one or two associated frontal ethmoidal cells is also relatively easy to deal with in the frontal recess.

Frontal Ethmoidal Type 3 and 4 Cells Obstructing the Frontal Sinus Ostium (Videos 15, 16, 20, and 21)

Even after an axillary flap approach these cells can be difficult to access and surgery often requires an angled endoscope thereby increasing the difficulty of the surgery. In addition a high T3 or type 4 (T4) cell can be confused with the frontal sinus and the CT scans should be reviewed to ensure that the drainage pathway of the frontal sinus is identified and instrumented. These cells need to be removed to allow adequate ventilation and drainage of the frontal sinus. An example of this is given in **Fig. 7.5**.

Small Frontal Sinus with Poorly Pneumatized Agger Nasi Cells and Small Frontal Ostium

This can be problematic if the frontal sinus is completely opacified and the surgeon wishes to ensure the pus or inspissated mucus is cleared from the sinus. Failure to clear thick mucus or pus from the frontal sinus may allow the inflammatory process to continue in the postoperative period in the region of the frontal ostium. This delays the healing process and can increase the risk of scarring and adhesions in the frontal region. An example of a small frontal sinus ostium is presented in **Fig. 7.6**.

Fig. 7.3 (A–C) The patient has a very narrow anteroposterior (AP) diameter. (**A**) The clue to the narrow AP diameter is the thick bone (*white arrow*) on either side of the frontal ostia, which is not present in equivalent coronal CT of the patient with a wide AP diameter (**D**). In the parasagittal scans (**B,E**) the difference between (**B**) a narrow AP and (**E**) a wide AP is apparent (*white arrows*). On the axial CT scans (**C,F**) the difference in the AP diameter is again apparent (*white arrows*).

Fig. 7.4 In coronal CT scan (**A**) the left frontal recess has a single agger nasi cell (*white arrow*). This can be clearly seen on the parasagittal scan (**B**, *white arrow*). This is the simplest configuration seen in the frontal recess.

Fig. 7.5 Bilateral type 3 cells are seen obstructing the frontal ostium. The parasagittal view is of the right side.

Fig. 7.6 This patient has a combination of an intersinus septal cell (*white arrow*) and a small frontal sinus on the right (*black arrow*) and on the left. The small drainage pathway of the frontal sinus on the right is marked with a *black arrow* (**B–D**). (*continued*)

Fig. 7.6 (*continued*)

New Bone Formation in the Region of the Frontal Ostium

New bone formation in the region of the frontal ostium and recess often indicates osteitis of the surrounding bone. If the new bone obstructs the frontal ostium, removal will often leave vascular and inflamed exposed bone, which will usually produce significant fibrosis and scar tissue. Re-stenosis and obstruction of the frontal ostium will often result. An example of the CT scan appearance of new bone formation is shown in **Fig. 7.7**. Cultures of removed bone should be performed and patients should then be started on appropriate antibiotics. Consideration should also be given to suppressing the inflammatory response during the healing period. This can be done by giving a 3-week course of oral steroids. Alternatively, or in combination with the oral steroids, the mini-trephine cannulas can be left in place for 3 to 4 days postoperatively and the frontal sinuses irrigated

with prednisolone drops after saline douching. This serves two purposes as it keeps the frontal ostium clear of blood clot (which can contribute to fibrosis and scarring) and the prednisolone diminishes the inflammatory response in the immediate postoperative period.

Previous Surgery with Scarring of the Frontal Recess

Previous surgery, especially amputation of the middle turbinate with lateralization of the remnant with associated scar tissue formation, can make exposure of the frontal ostium difficult. Diagnosis is made both on the CT scan appearance and on endoscopy. The CT scan can show residual cells and new bone formation and endoscopy can confirm the presence of scar tissue in the frontal recess. An example is shown in **Fig. 7.8**.

Extensive Disease in the Frontal Recess

Some patients may have extensive and severe disease in the frontal recess (**Fig. 7.9**). In this example the patient has allergic fungal sinusitis with expansion of the frontal recess and double densities visible on soft tissue settings (*white arrow*). The frontal recesses in this patient were filled with highly vascular polyps and inspissated fungal material. Not only were the normal anatomical landmarks distorted in this patient but there was extensive bleeding in the frontal recess as the polyps were removed. As previously stated such vascularity can significantly increase the degree of difficulty for the surgeon during removal of the polyps and cells, and during identification of the frontal ostium.

Resected Middle Turbinates and Patients with Few or No Operative Landmarks

Patients who have previously had resection of their middle turbinates can be difficult to manage as the absence of the

Fig. 7.7 New bone formation is seen in the right frontal recess (*white arrow*).

Fig. 7.8 The amputated right middle turbinate is marked with a *white solid arrow* in both the CT scan and on the endoscopy picture. The uncinate remains and abuts the retained anterior ethmoid cells obstructing the drainage of the frontal sinus. On the endoscopic view significant scarring is seen between the lateralized residual middle turbinate and lateral nasal wall (uncinate).

middle turbinate has removed the most important operative landmark (**Fig. 7.10**).

If there are polyps present, identification of the residual middle turbinate can be difficult (**Fig. 7.11**). The first step is to identify the maxillary ostium and to clear the maxillary sinus of polyps using the maxillary trephination procedure if necessary (Chapter 5). This will allow positive identification of the lamina papyracea, which is an important landmark in the further dissection of the frontal recess. The next step is to gently debride the polyps to reveal the underlying bony structures—the septum, olfactory recess, residual middle turbinate, and posterior bony choanae. If the anatomy is still unclear

then the polyps in the region of the posterior bony choanae and the anterior face of the sphenoid should be removed. The natural ostium of the sphenoid is usually ~12 mm above the bony posterior choanae. The microdebrider blade is 4 mm and this can be used to measure 12 mm from the posterior bony choanae. A useful additional landmark is the roof of the maxillary sinus which can be used as a guide to enter the sphenoid. Harvey et al.[17] have shown that a horizontal line taken from the maxillary sinus roof onto the anterior face of the sphenoid provides a safe point of entry into the sphenoid. Once the polyps in this region are cleared, the residual superior turbinate may come into view. If this has also been previously resected,

Fig. 7.9 Expansile disease of the frontal recess. Double densities marked with *white arrow*.

Fig. 7.10 (**A**) The *white arrow* indicates a residual T4 cell in the frontal sinus. (**B,C**) The *white arrow* indicates the previously resected middle turbinate. Note the absence of the inferior turbinate on the left side from previous surgery. (**D,F**) The *white arrow* indicates the anterior wall of the T4 cell. Note extensive polyps visible on all scans.

Fig. 7.11 Massive nasal polyps with no identifying landmarks visible.

Fig. 7.12 When a zero-degree endoscope is used, the instrument passed beneath the scope will be in the center of the field of view (**A**). If a 30-degree endoscope is used with a similar instrument passed below the scope, the instrument tip is on the extreme periphery of the visual field. If the tip of the instrument is brought into the center of the endoscope field of view the endoscope is pushed upward by the instrument and the area of dissection may no longer be visible. If a 45- or 70-degree endoscope is used, the instrument needs to be sufficiently angulated to be able to be placed in the center of the field of view of the endoscope (**C**).

then the polyps should be cleared from the skull base. The fovea ethmoidalis and olfactory fossa are normally in the same horizontal plane in this posterior region of the ethmoids and gentle removal of polyps (without bone removal) should safely expose the skull base and residual superior turbinate. The previously identified lamina papyracea is an important additional landmark. The next step is to identify the ostium of the sphenoid sinus (the method is described in Chapter 8) and enlarge the natural ostium of the sphenoid. This will allow the skull base to be positively identified and the dissection can then be brought along the skull base anteriorly. The surgeon needs to check the CT scan to identify the position of the anterior ethmoid artery and whether it is suspended within a mesentery or not. Using the lamina papyracea as the lateral landmark, the skull base as the superior landmark, and the beak of the frontal maxillary process as the anterior landmark, the frontal recess can be identified. In most patients a small stump of residual middle turbinate can be seen and an axillary flap is performed and the axilla opened with a Hajek Koffler punch. Now that all the landmarks for the frontal recess are established, the clearance of the frontal recess can continue according to the 3D reconstruction of the anatomy of that recess with localization of the frontal sinus drainage pathway and stepwise removal of each remaining cell in the frontal recess.

◆ Techniques for Managing the Frontal Recess and Frontal Sinus

1. Endoscopy
2. Surgical approach—the axillary flap
3. Frontal sinus mini-trephine
4. Computer-aided surgery (CAS, or image guidance surgery)

These techniques are used in a graduated approach. The combination of endoscopy utilizing the least angled endoscope

with the axillary flap technique is used for all frontal recess and sinus dissections. Frontal sinus mini-trephination and CAS are used in the more difficult frontal recess dissections.

Endoscopy

The classic description of the technique for dissection in the frontal recess and frontal sinus involves the use of 30-, 45-, and 70-degree endoscopes.[2–4] It is also recognized that the more angulated the endoscope the greater the degree of difficulty of the dissection because of surgeon disorientation and the manipulation of angled instruments. A recent paper[18] described increasing unwanted trauma within the nose and sinuses from the passage of angulated instruments during dissection.[18] **Figure 7.12** shows the increasing angulation of instruments required to keep the tip of the instrument in the center of the field of dissection with increasing angulation of the endoscope.

As illustrated in Chapter 1, the vast majority of surgery is conducted with the endoscope placed above the instrument. If the endoscope is placed below the instrument, the working tip of the instrument cannot be visualized (**Fig. 7.13**).

Fig. 7.13 If the instrument is positioned above the scope, the undersurface of the instrument is visualized (*block arrow*) and the working tip is not seen. This can be potentially dangerous if the working tip of the instrument is in a potentially vulnerable region of the frontal recess.

A 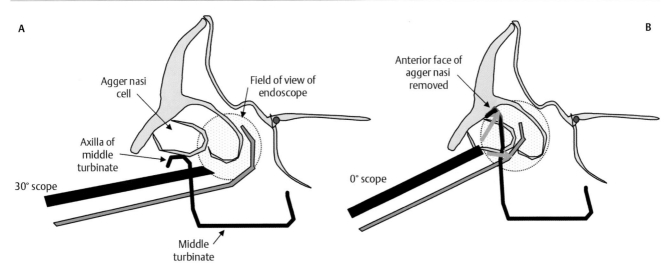 B

Fig. 7.14 **(A)** Illustrates the need to use an angled endoscope to view the frontal recess (visual field = *shaded circle*) with the axilla intact. After opening the anterior wall of the agger nasi cell **(B)**, a zero-degree endoscope can be used to view and operate in the frontal recess without having to use angled endoscopes and instruments.

The degree of difficulty is further increased if the surgical field is bloody. It can take longer for an angled endoscope (30- or 70-degree) and a curved instrument to be positioned in the frontal recess before surgical dissection can take place. If bleeding in the surgical field is profuse, the surgical field may be covered in blood before the dissection begins. This situation may lead to frustration for the surgeon at the slow progress of surgery and the surgeon may be tempted to proceed with dissection despite poor visibility. This can potentially lead to inadvertent injury to the skull base, lamina papyracea, or anterior ethmoidal artery. As with any surgical procedure the wider the exposure the easier the operation becomes. Most surgeons would recall a situation when they have needed the aid of a senior colleague during a procedure and that the first thing that the senior surgeon did was to widen the incisions to improve the surgical access. The axillary flap technique was designed to try to overcome some of the problems mentioned above by optimizing access to the frontal recess and allowing a large part of the dissection in the frontal sinus to be performed with a zero degree telescope (**Fig. 7.14**).[13–16]

Surgical Technique for the Axillary Flap

The first step in the axillary flap approach is to make an incision ~8 mm above the axilla of the middle turbinate and to bring this forward by ~8 mm.[15] The incision is turned vertically down to the level of the axilla. It is then carried back under the axilla onto the root of the middle turbinate (**Fig. 7.15**). A number 15 scalpel blade on a number 7 BP scalpel blade holder is used to make these incisions.

The full thickness mucosal flap is then raised with a suction Freer elevator. It is important to ensure that the tip of the suction Freer is on bone when the flap is being raised and that the flap extends behind the root of the middle turbinate (**Fig. 7.16A**). The flap is connected at its inferior edge to tissue under the axilla of the middle turbinate. This needs to be separated from the flap with a sickle knife or scalpel (see videos) before the flap is tucked between the middle turbinate and the septum (**Fig. 7.16B**). Failure to expose the vertical bone of the middle turbinate just below where it attaches to the lateral nasal wall will often result in this bridge of tissue remaining. If this bridge of tissue is pulled by an instrument or suction, then the flap will be pulled from between the turbinate and septum into the frontal recess. Here it may either be inadvertently removed by a microdebrider or instrument or irritate the surgeon by requiring it to be tucked away regularly before surgery can

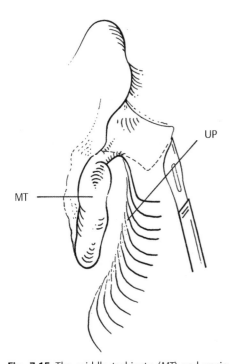

Fig. 7.15 The middle turbinate (*MT*) and uncinate process (*UP*) are marked in the left nasal cavity. The scalpel blade outlines the incisions for the axillary flap above the insertion of the middle turbinate on the left lateral nasal wall.

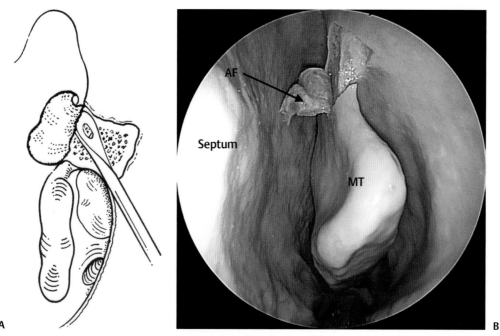

Fig. 7.16 (**A**) Suction Freer elevates the axillary flap. Identification of the root of the middle turbinate is necessary before the flap is tucked between the turbinate and septum. (**B**) Cadaveric image of a left-sided axillary flap. *AF*, axillary flap; *MT*, middle turbinate.

proceed. By exposing the vertical upper bony part of the middle turbinate, the surgeon ensures that the bridge of tissue is divided and, once the flap is tucked between the middle turbinate and septum, it should not be seen again until it is retrieved at the end of surgery to cover the raw bone of the newly created axilla.

A Hajek Koffler punch is used to remove the anterior wall of the agger nasi cell. The thickness of the bone depends on the extent of the pneumatization of the agger nasi cell. If it is well

pneumatized this bone is thin and easy to remove and should be removed to the edge of the mucosal incisions (**Fig. 7.17**). If the agger nasi cell is small or absent, the bone can be thick and may only be able to be partially removed. If there are polyps in the agger nasi cell, these are removed with the microdebrider so that the extent of the cell can be clearly seen.

Now that the agger nasi cell has been entered and positively identified, the surgeon should review the 3D reconstruction of the anatomy of the frontal recess that has previously been

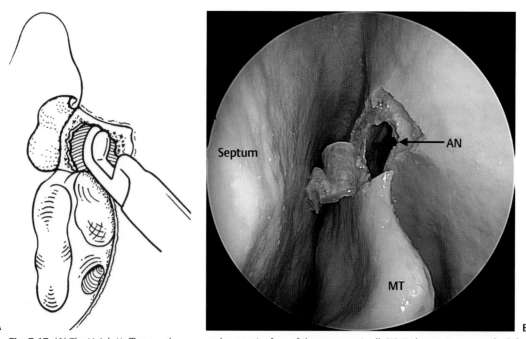

Fig. 7.17 (**A**) The Hajek-Koffler punch removes the anterior face of the agger nasi cell. (**B**) Cadaveric image on the left side showing the anterior face of the agger nasi cell (*AN*) removed. *MT*, middle turbinate.

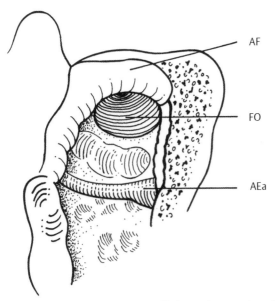

Fig. 7.18 The axillary flap (*AF*) is rolled over the raw edge of the newly formed axilla. The frontal ostium (*FO*) and anterior ethmoidal artery (*AEa*) are visible.

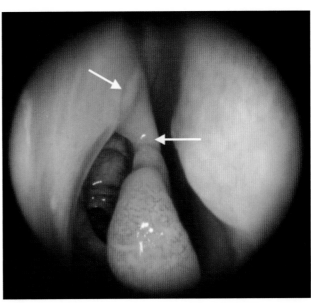

Fig. 7.19 Postoperative appearance of the right axillary flap. The *white arrows* mark the incision lines for the superior and inferior incisions.

performed (see Chapter 6). The location of the frontal drainage pathway should be sought with a probe or curette. The probe or curette should be gently slid up this drainage pathway and the obstructing cells removed by fracturing and removing the cells.

Once the frontal ostium has been visualized and is clear of any obstructing cells, the axillary flap is pulled forward and placed so that it partially rolls under the raw edge of bone of the residual anterior wall of the agger nasi cell (**Fig. 7.18**). This should provide cover for this area and prevent granulation tissue and subsequent adhesions from forming in this area.

Results of the Axillary Flap Technique[15]

In a recently published series[15] the axillary flap approach, in conjunction with the 3D building block concept, provided visualization of 96% of the frontal sinus ostia in 118 consecutive frontal recess procedures. The remaining frontal ostia were identified with the aid of the mini-trephine technique described below. Of the 118 cases, six had significant adhesions present which required outpatient treatment.[15] Therefore, the axillary flap approach does not increase the risk of adhesion formation in the middle meatus.[13–16] **Figure 7.19** shows the typical appearance of the region of the axillary flap after such an approach to the frontal recess.

Mini-Trephination of the Frontal Sinus (Videos 17 and 22)

The mini-trephine of the frontal sinuses is a very helpful technique when the drainage pathway of the frontal sinus is not easily seen. Placement of a cannula in the frontal sinus allows the sinus to be flushed with fluorescein-stained saline and

the pathway of this fluid in the frontal recess can be followed using a malleable frontal sinus probe* (Medtronic ENT). As the probe is passed up the fluorescein-stained pathway, the probe is used to gently widen this pathway until a curette can be placed along the pathway. The cells in the frontal recess can then be fractured (usually anteriorly or laterally) and removed to expose the frontal ostium (see video). In addition, the trephine can be used to ensure clearance of pus, mucus, or fungal material from the frontal sinus where the surgeon does not wish to place an instrument through the frontal ostium and risk damage to the mucosa of the frontal ostium. If a frontal sinus suction is nearly as large as the frontal ostium (often the case with a standard 3- or 4-mm olive tip suction), it may cause circumferential damage to the mucosa of the frontal ostium if it is forced through the ostium into the frontal sinus. This may in turn lead to stenosis or obstruction of the ostium. Clearance of the frontal sinus by irrigating through the mini-trephine cannula can avoid such injury. The mini-trephine cannula may be left in place for a variable period of time after the surgery so that the frontal sinus and frontal ostium can be flushed with saline. This flushing process can remove blood clots from the frontal ostium which in turn may help maintain its patency as it heals. If the mucosa is significantly inflamed or polypoid, steroid drops may be placed into the frontal sinus for the period of time after surgery before the cannulae are removed. This in turn may help reduce the inflammation and potentially the formation of early scar tissue in the frontal ostia.

Technique of Placing the Mini-Trephines

The CT scans should be reviewed to establish the presence and size of the frontal sinus. **Figure 7.20** shows absence of the right frontal sinus with a small left frontal sinus with a very narrow frontal ostium.

Fig. 7.20 The narrow left frontal ostium is indicated with a *black arrow*.

Note that the left frontal sinus does not extend above the eyebrow (bony rim of the orbit). The extent of superior pneumatization of the frontal sinus needs to be assessed on the CT scan before the mini-trephine is placed.

The landmark for placement of the skin incision is the medial aspect of the eyebrow. In most patients the eyebrow is on the superior orbital rim and one should follow this medially on the CT scan to ensure that there is sufficient pneumatization of the frontal sinus above the superior orbital rim. Placement of the mini-trephine too high can result in intracranial penetration by the drill. If the frontal sinus is sufficiently pneumatized on CT, the skin landmarks for placement of the skin incision are as follows: Draw an imaginary horizontal line from the middle of the medial end of the eyebrow to the medial end of the other eyebrow. Along this line pick the midpoint between the eyebrows and then estimate 1 cm from the midline along this imaginary line (**Fig. 7.21**).

Infiltrate with 1 to 2 mL of local anesthetic and adrenaline. A number 15 scalpel blade is used to make the stab incision through the skin onto bone. This incision can either be placed through a vertical frown line or, in the case of patients concerned about the possible aesthetic appearance of a scar, the incision can be placed through the medial hairs of the eyebrow. Although the latter two incisions may not be correctly placed between the medial aspect of the eyebrow and the midline, the skin of the frontal bone is mobile and, after placement of the mini-trephine guide, this guide can be shifted by moving the skin until it is correctly placed on the bone as described. If the bony trephine is placed too laterally it may either endanger the supratrochlear neurovascular bundle or be outside of the frontal sinus. The stab incision is gently dilated with a sharp-pointed scissors. A drill guide is placed through this incision by first laying the guide flat on the skin and then rotating it into the incision. This is done with the incision being held open by tension placed with fingers on either side of the wound (**Fig. 7.22**).

If the guide is pushed into the incision without opening the wound, a small ellipse of skin can be caught and removed as the guide is pushed into the wound. If the skin incision has been placed through the hairs of the eyebrow this point may be too lateral to perform the trephine. After placement of the drill guide, the skin is moved by pushing the guide to the point indicated by the previous guidelines before the bone is trephined. The guide has teeth on the surface that come in contact with the bone and these should be securely engaged onto the bone so that the guide does not move during

A

B

Fig. 7.21 **(A)** The black line marks the midline with the * marking the medial aspect of the eyebrow. The broken horizontal line joins the ends of the eyebrows. The needle with local anesthetic is placed through a skin crease midway between these points. After a stab incision, the wound is dilated with iris scissors **(B)**.

A

B

Fig. 7.22 **(A)** The guide is placed flat on the skin and rotated into the wound to avoid coring an ellipse of skin. **(B)** The drill is placed through the guide.

the trephination process. The drill bit should be removed almost as immediately as it touches the bone. It should be completely withdrawn from the guide and the tip irrigated with saline or water. Failure to do this results in significant heating of the drill tip and can lead to a burn of the bone and the skin around the trephine. On the skin this can result in a circular wound which leaves an unsightly scar and in the bone can predispose toward osteitis. The trephine burr is designed to extend 11 mm beyond the guide and should not be able to penetrate the posterior table of the frontal sinus. On rare occasions in patients with small (underpneumatized) frontal sinuses and a thick anterior table, the drill may not be long enough to penetrate the anterior table of the frontal sinus. Should this occur, the surgeon can move the trephine guide inferiorly (the bone of the anterior table tends to thin as one moves inferiorly) and reattempt frontal sinus trephination. The skin over the frontal sinus is mobile and easily moved by the guide. Do not attempt to move the trephine site superiorly as this can risk trephination of the intracranial cavity. The trephine is removed while the guide is held firmly in place. A wire stylet is placed through the guide into the trephine hole. The guide is removed and the frontal cannula is placed over the stylet into the frontal sinus (**Fig. 7.23**). The cannula is placed in a rotatory fashion and is not pushed too firmly into skin as the barrel widens and this can put pressure on the skin around the shaft of the cannula.

A syringe half-filled with saline and fluorescein (500 mL saline and 0.5 mL of 5% fluorescein) is placed on the cannula and aspiration attempted. Aspiration of clear fluid indicates intracranial penetration and the cannula should be immediately removed and the wound sutured. This concentration should not cause meningeal irritation if inadvertently injected into the intracranial space. Usually there is either air, mucus, pus, or blood withdrawn into the syringe. When the frontal ostium is completely blocked, only a vacuum will be created in the syringe. In this situation the frontal ostium is observed while gentle pressure is placed on the syringe. Pus or mucus followed by fluorescein-stained saline should be seen. This area of emergence of the fluorescein can then be probed to identify

A

B

C

Fig. 7.23 (A,B) The frontal cannula is slid over the stylet into the trephine hole and into the frontal sinus. **(C)** A syringe half filled with fluorescein-stained saline is attached to the cannula and the frontal sinus is aspirated before it is irrigated.

the drainage pathway of the frontal sinus. Before any significant pressure is placed on the syringe, check the CT scan to ensure that there are no dehiscences of the posterior table or floor of the frontal sinus. The saline and fluorescein mixture consists of 500 mL saline and 0.5 mL of 5% fluorescein.

Computer-Aided Surgery

CAS utilizes new technology where the patient has undergone either a CT or magnetic resonance imaging (MRI) scan (or both) prior to surgery. These images are downloaded onto a computer in the CAS machine and the images presented to the surgeon in three planes (coronal, axial, and parasagittal). This is similar to the standard CT scans performed on our patients. A software program that is free and can be downloaded from the Internet is OsiriX. It can only be used on an Apple Macintosh computer but reads all DICOM files so any CT scan copied onto a disk can be read in the same manner as is done on the CAS machines. Similar software programs are

available for PCs and usually come in the file set copied onto the disk by the radiology company providing the disk. The benefit of these software systems is that crosshairs can be placed on a cell and the crosshairs will appear in the same cell on the other two views (**Fig. 7.24**). The surgeon can identify a cell and see where that cell is in the other plane and, in the same way as described in Chapter 6, can build a 3D image of the anatomy of the patient. Surgical planning can also be effectively performed on the machine prior to surgery.

There are two systems: the first is an optical system where a camera tracks light emitting diodes (LEDs) on the patient (head frame) and the instruments. The second system is electromagnetic where the computer tracks movement of electromagnetic markers on the patient (head frame) and on instruments. Recent CAS machines are able to perform either the LED or electromagnetic tracking depending on the surgeon's preference. Both systems work well and have different advantages and disadvantages. To register the patient on the computer, landmarks are identified on the scans on the computer and then on the patient. The head frame monitors the

Fig. 7.24 In this patient with a large frontal sinus osteoma, computed-aided surgery was very helpful during endoscopic removal to identify and prevent injury to the skull base. The cross hairs indicate the roof of the frontal sinus after removal of the osteoma.

movement of the patient's head. The instruments are tracked either optically or electromagnetically. In patients without intranasal landmarks (absent middle turbinate etc.) these systems allow important structures such as the skull base, orbit, optic nerve, and carotid to be identified. In addition they allow residual cells within the frontal recess and sinus to be identified and removed. If a frontal sinus drainage pathway cannot be found, they can track an instrument tip so that the pathway can be identified and the instrument slid up the pathway and remaining cells removed from the frontal recess or sinus.

◆ Difficult Surgical Situations in Frontal Recess and Frontal Sinus During Surgery

Narrow Frontal Ostium with Obstructive Cells with Thick Bony Walls

This situation is not uncommon but results in a difficult intraoperative situation. In this particular example the patient

has a thick beak with a very underpneumatized agger nasi cell and an intersinus septal cell (ISSC) with thick bony walls that cannot be easily fractured with standard instruments to enlarge the frontal ostium (**Fig. 7.25**). The agger nasi cell is very small and narrow and the bulla ethmoidalis pushes forward into the frontal recess squashing the frontal sinus drainage pathway anterolaterally (best seen on the axial scans, **Fig. 7.25**). The beak of the frontal process is very thick and although there is an ISSC, the wall of this cell is formed by thick bone which separates this cell from the frontal drainage pathway. It would be impossible to enlarge the frontal sinus drainage pathway without resorting to a drill. As discussed previously, drilling in this situation is more likely to result in postoperative scarring and obstruction of the frontal ostium with iatrogenic long-term frontal sinusitis that can be difficult to manage. The intraoperative management of this patient should include complete clearance of the opacified maxillary sinus with a canine fossa trephine and creation of a large middle meatal antrostomy followed by an axillary flap with removal of as much of the axilla of the middle turbinate as possible. This will expose the small thin agger nasi cell. Because the bulla pneumatizes anteriorly this should be opened as well as the suprabullar cell allowing identification of the skull base and anterior ethmoidal artery which should be seen adjacent to where the posterior wall of this cell touches the skull base. The curette can now be slid up the frontal sinus drainage pathway

behind the agger nasi cell and this cell fractured forward and removed. Next the anterior wall of both the bulla and suprabullar cells should be removed up to the skull base. The intersinus septal cell will be seen with the frontal ostium pushed laterally. Because the frontal ostium is narrow

Fig. 7.25 The frontal ostium and frontal sinus drainage pathway are indicated with a white arrow on the left side (**C–G**). The small agger nasi cell can be seen (**C,D**, *black arrow*). The suprabullar cell (*broken white arrow*) can be seen (**E–H**). (*continued*)

Fig. 7.25 (*continued*)

and could not be enlarged, and due to the inflamed state of the mucosa around the frontal ostium, a frontal sinus mini-trephine was inserted and the frontal ostium irrigated for 3 days postoperatively with both saline flushes and prednisolone drops.

Postoperatively the frontal ostium was edematous for some months before settling down. The patient remains asymptomatic and the ostium healed (**Fig. 7.26**). This emphasizes the importance of removing the obstructive cells from the frontal recess (agger nasi, bulla, and suprabullar cells) and clearing the drainage pathway. I believe that any attempt to enlarge this ostium with a drill would not have had such a positive outcome.

That is not to say that all patients will respond in this manner and some patients may develop chronic edema with obstruction of a narrow ostium (**Fig. 7.27**). Such patients

should be treated with systemic and topical steroids, douches, and regular office toilet and, if the symptoms persist, revision surgery is indicated (usually an endoscopic modified Lothrop procedure/Draf 3/frontal drillout as described in Chapter 9).

Large Frontal Bulla Cell or T4 Cell Obstructing the Frontal Ostium (Video 21)

In some patients there are cells that extend significantly into the frontal sinus through the frontal ostium and, in so doing, compromise the ostium and the drainage and ventilation of the frontal sinus. These cells can be very difficult

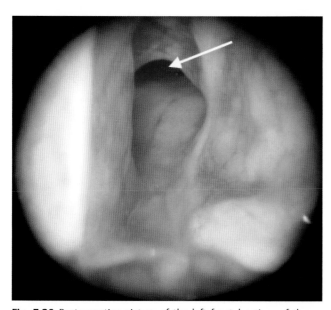

Fig. 7.26 Postoperative picture of the left frontal ostium of the patient presented in **Fig. 7.25**. Note the healthy left frontal ostium (*white arrow*).

Fig. 7.27 A patient who had a very narrow left frontal ostium with edema obstructing the ostium (*white arrow*). A thin suction could still be passed through this ostium but, despite ongoing medical treatment, the edema in this region has remained. If the patient remains symptomatic further surgery is indicated.

to manage and the approach depends on the size of the frontal ostium. If the patient has extensively pneumatized sinuses then there is a reasonable chance the anteroposterior (AP) distance of the frontal ostium may be quite large as is the case in this example (**Fig. 7.28**). Also note in this example that the anterior ethmoidal artery is on a mesentery (**Fig. 7.28**). This commonly occurs when there is extensive pneumatization and, in these cases, this region should be carefully scrutinized during surgery to avoid injury to this artery. In this case the large frontal bulla cell is originating from the suprabullar region and hugging the skull base into the frontal sinus and progressing almost to reach the roof of the frontal sinus. If the AP distance is large, then the cell can be reached through the natural frontal ostium and removed. In this case it was possible to remove the entire cell from below without enlarging the frontal ostium. However, if the AP distance was small then the cell would need ancillary measures for removal. In our department this would usually be an endoscopic modified Lothrop/Draf 3 procedure but removal may also be performed by a combined approach (trephine into the frontal sinus through the eyebrow big enough to admit either an endoscope or an instrument). The instrument is introduced through the frontal sinus trephine and viewed through the frontal ostium or vice versa. Alternatively, an osteoplastic flap into frontal sinuses can be performed and the cell removed under direct visualization.

The intraoperative picture is seen in **Fig. 7.29** where the base of the frontal bulla cell can be seen on the posterior table of the frontal sinus through the natural ostium (**Fig. 7.28**).

Fig. 7.28 The frontal bulla cell is numbered 1 and the roof of the agger nasi cell is numbered 2. (*continued*)

Fig. 7.28 (*continued*) Note the large anteroposterior distance in the axial scans (**E–G**) and marked as the distance between the *parallel black arrows* on the axial scan (**G**) and the parasagittal scan (**H**). (**D**) Note the broken *white arrow* indicating the anterior ethmoidal artery on a mesentery and at risk of damage during surgery.

Fig. 7.29 The left frontal ostium from the patient presented in **Fig. 7.28**. Note the attachment of the suprabullar cell (T4) to the posterior wall of the frontal sinus indicated by the *short white arrows*. The anterior ethmoidal artery in its mesentery is indicated by the *black arrow*. Note the wide anteroposterior distance of the frontal ostium.

◆ Postoperative Frontal Sinus Irrigation Regimens

The frontal sinus cannulae are left in place during the following scenarios: if there has been inadvertent trauma to the frontal ostium mucosa, if the natural frontal sinus ostium is very narrow (< 3 mm), if there was evidence of osteitis with new bone formation in the frontal recess or ostium, or if there was extensive polyposis resulting in significant traumatized mucosa after the polyp removal. The frontal cannulae are flushed with 5 mL of normal saline every 2 hours starting immediately after surgery. If prednisolone drops are to be used, 0.5 to 1 mL is instilled with a syringe into the frontal sinus after every second douche. No nasal packing is used as this has not been found to reduce adhesion formation or to promote healing.[19]

Postoperative Care and Debridement

All patients are placed on a 10-day course of broad spectrum antibiotics and requested to flush their nose and sinuses four to six times a day with saline after surgery. If significant polyps were found during surgery, patients are placed on a 3-week reducing course of oral prednisolone. Patients are reviewed in the office between 10 and 14 days after surgery. At this visit all residual blood clots are removed and the sinus ostia inspected. A thin curved suction is passed through the frontal sinus ostia and any secretions removed from the frontal sinus. All other sinus ostia are similarly checked. Any adhesions are divided. If these are significant, an early return visit is scheduled but if all appears to be healing well the patient is reviewed 4 to 6 weeks later.

References

1. Levine HL. Endoscopic sinus surgery: reasons for failure. Oper Tech Otolaryngol—Head Neck Surg 1995;6:176–179

2. Kennedy DW, Senior BA. Endoscopic sinus surgery. A review. Otolaryngol Clin North Am 1997;30(3):313–330

3. Stammberger H, Kopp W, Dekornfeld TJ, Hawke M. Functional Endoscopic Sinus Surgery - The Messerklinger Technique. Special Endoscopic Anatomy. Philadelphia: B.C. Decker Publishers; 1991: 61–90

4. Stammberger H, Posawetz W. Functional endoscopic sinus surgery. Concept, indications and results of the Messerklinger technique. Eur Arch Otorhinolaryngol 1990;247(2):63–76

5. Thawley SE, Deddens AE. Transfrontal endoscopic management of frontal recess disease. Am J Rhinol 1995;9(6):307–311

6. Setliff RC III. Minimally invasive sinus surgery: the rationale and the technique. Otolaryngol Clin North Am 1996;29(1):115–124

7. Catalano PJ, Setcliffe RC III, Catalano LA. Minimally invasive sinus surgery in the geriatric patient. Oper Tech Otolaryngol—Head Neck Surg 2001;12:85–90

8. Catalano PJ, Roffman E. Outcome in patients with chronic sinusitis after the minimally invasive sinus technique. Am J Rhinol 2003;17(1):17–22

9. Kuhn FA, Javer AR, Nagpal K, Citardi MJ. The frontal sinus rescue procedure: early experience and three-year follow-up. Am J Rhinol 2000;14(4):211–216

10. May M, Schaitkin B. Frontal sinus surgery: endonasal drainage instead of an external osteoplastic approach. Oper Tech Otolaryngol—Head Neck Surg 1995;6:184–192

11. Schaefer SD, Close LG. Endoscopic management of frontal sinus disease. Laryngoscope 1990;100(2 Pt 1):155–160

12. Kuhn FA. Chronic frontal sinusitis: the endoscopic frontal recess approach. Operative techniques. Otolaryngol Head Neck Surg 1996;7:222–229

13. Wormald PJ. Three dimensional building block approach to understanding the anatomy of the frontal recess and frontal sinus. Oper Tech Otolaryngol Head Neck Surg 2006;17:2–5

14. Wormald PJ. Surgery of the frontal recess and frontal sinus. Rhinology 2005;43(2):82–85

15. Wormald PJ. The axillary flap approach to the frontal recess. Laryngoscope 2002;112(3):494–499

16. Wormald PJ. The agger nasi cell: the key to understanding the anatomy of the frontal recess. Otolaryngol Head Neck Surg 2003;129(5):497–507

17. Harvey RJ, Shelton W, Timperley D, et al. Using fixed anatomical landmarks in endoscopic skull base surgery. Am J Rhinol Allergy 2010; 24(4):301–305

18. Kang SK, White PS, Lee MS, Ram B, Ogston S. A randomized control trial of surgical task performance in frontal recess surgery: zero degree versus angled telescopes. Am J Rhinol 2002;16(1):33–36

19. Wormald PJ, Boustred N, Le T, Hawke L, Sacks R. A prospective single blind randomized controlled study of use of Hyaluronic acid nasal packs (Merogel) in patients after endoscopic sinus surgery. Am J Rhinol 2006;20:145–149

8 Three-Dimensional Reconstruction and Surgery of the Bulla Ethmoidalis, Middle Turbinate, Posterior Ethmoids, and Sphenoid

Reviewing the embryology of the sinuses, the middle turbinate forms from the third lamella and the superior turbinate from the fourth lamella. The ground lamella of the middle turbinate divides the ethmoid sinuses into anterior ethmoid sinuses (anterior to the ground lamella) and posterior ethmoid sinuses (posterior to the ground lamella). Anterior ethmoid sinuses are further subdivided into those associated with the frontal process of the maxilla—the frontal ethmoidal cells, and cells associated with the bulla ethmoidalis. The bulla ethmoidalis forms from the second embryological lamella. It is a large ethmoid air cell directly anterior to the middle turbinate lamella. Cells directly above the bulla ethmoidalis are referred to as suprabullar cells. Posterior ethmoidal cells are found behind the middle turbinate ground lamella and anterior to the lamella of the superior turbinate.

◆ Surgery of the Bulla Ethmoidalis and Suprabullar Cells (Anterior Ethmoidectomy)

The bulla ethmoidalis is either a single cell or group of cells which are visible directly behind the free edge of the middle and horizontal portions of uncinate process. The gap between the anterior face of the bulla ethmoidalis and the free edge of the uncinate process is known as the hiatus semilunaris which is the entrance to the ethmoidal infundibulum. When the anterior face of the bulla ethmoidalis extends to the skull base it usually forms the posterior limit of the frontal recess. However, when its anterior lamella fails to reach the skull base, a suprabullar recess is created. The bulla ethmoidalis will usually have a posterior wall which is separate from the vertical portion of the ground lamella. The space between its posterior wall and the ground lamella is known as the retrobullar recess. A suprabullar recess can also form from the retrobullar recess as it pneumatizes over the top of the bulla. The bulla ethmoidalis like all sinuses drains via a

natural ostium. This can usually be found on its posteromedial aspect in the retrobullar recess.

To find the natural ostium a double right-angled probe is passed medial to the bulla between the bulla and the middle turbinate. The tip of the probe is gently rotated laterally until it falls into the natural ostium (**Fig. 8.1**). As the probe is pulled forward, the medial and anterior walls are fractured. This fracture should be in continuity with the natural ostium.

To open the bulla ethmoidalis the microdebrider is placed in this fractured area and the medial wall and anterior wall of the bulla removed. This allows the natural ostium to be enlarged and to be a part of the opening created into the bulla. This follows the general philosophy of endoscopic sinus surgery (ESS) of including the natural ostium in any opening made into a sinus. If only a mini-ESS has been performed (uncinectomy and opening of the bulla), then 3 or 4 mm of the anterior and inferior edge of the bulla is retained. This 3 to 4 mm of the anterior face of the bulla forms the posterosuperior part of the final common drainage pathway (see Chapter 5). This region is termed the "final common drainage pathway" as mucus from the frontal and anterior ethmoid cells and maxillary sinus is cleared to the nasopharynx along this pathway (**Fig. 8.2**).

If a posterior ethmoidectomy is to be performed in addition to opening the bulla, none of its anterior wall is retained. Removing the bulla in its entirety gives improved access to the posterior ethmoid complex.

The Three-Dimensional Reconstruction of the Posterior Ethmoids

As described in Chapter 6, three-dimensional (3D) anatomical reconstruction and planning of each surgical step is performed prior to dissection of the posterior ethmoids and sphenoid. In a similar manner as the agger nasi cell is used as the cornerstone of the dissection of the frontal recess dissection, a cell or space in the posterior ethmoids needs to be identified that can be accurately correlated to the computed

A   B

Fig. 8.1 **(A)** The ball-probe (*black arrow*) is slid medial to the anterior face of the bulla ethmoidalis (*BE*). **(B)** The anterior face of the bulla is fractured creating an edge for the microdebrider. The maxillary sinus ostium is marked by a *white arrow*.

tomography (CT) scan. The space used in the 3D reconstruction of the posterior ethmoids is the superior meatus. To be able to accurately identify the superior meatus on sequential CT scans, the transition from the anterior to the posterior ethmoids must be established on the CT scans. If the coronal CT scans are evaluated, the first landmark that is sought is the superior turbinate. Each sequential coronal CT is evaluated until the superior turbinate is identified (**Fig. 8.3**).

Once the transition between the anterior and posterior ethmoids is established on the CT scans, the superior meatus (SM) should be sought. This is clearly marked in **Fig. 8.3C,D**. This space is directly above the horizontal part of the ground

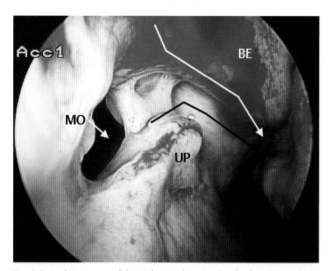

Fig. 8.2 In this picture of the right nasal cavity, the final common drainage pathway is indicated by the *black arrow*. This also indicates the drainage pathway of the maxillary sinus. The *white arrow* indicates the drainage pathway of the frontal and anterior ethmoidal cells along the anterior face of the bulla ethmoidalis (*BE*). This portion of the BE forms the posterosuperior part of the final common drainage pathway. The residual portion of the uncinate process (*UP*) after uncinectomy and the natural ostium of the maxillary sinus (*MO*) are marked.

lamella and should be easily located on all CT scans. The ability of the surgeon to locate this space on both the CT scan and the patient is critical as it provides the starting point of the surgery. Once penetration of the posterior ethmoids has taken place through the ground lamella, the superior meatus and superior turbinate are identified (**Fig. 8.1**). The surgeon now has a landmark in the dissection that can be clearly placed on the CT scan. Each sequential cell in the posterior ethmoids is identified and, using the building block principle, a 3D picture of the posterior ethmoids can be constructed. However, before a complete understanding of the anatomy of the posterior ethmoids is possible, a clear understanding of the transition between posterior ethmoids and sphenoid is necessary. This follows the theme of understanding the transition between the frontal sinus and anterior ethmoids, between the anterior and posterior ethmoids, and finally between the posterior ethmoids and sphenoid. The key to determining the transition from the posterior ethmoids to the sphenoid is identifying the first coronal CT scan in which the solid posterior bony choanae can be seen (**Fig. 8.4**).

In addition to the coronal CT scans, the parasagittal scan is helpful (**Fig. 8.5**). This scan is very useful in helping to place the cells either one on top of the other or anterior or posterior to the other cells of the posterior ethmoids. Cell number 3 is placed lateral to the parasagittal reconstruction and cannot be seen on scan **Fig. 8.5C**. Each configuration of the posterior ethmoids is different and each side of every patient needs to be independently assessed and the 3D picture built.

Figure 8.5 scans and diagram illustrate the building block 3D reconstruction of the posterior ethmoids. Although not all the posterior ethmoid and sphenoid scans can be shown, refer back to **Figs. 8.3** and **8.4** for additional CTs of the same patient if further clarification of the cells and reconstruction is needed. Note that once the superior meatus has been clearly identified in **Fig. 8.5A** scan, there is a single posterior ethmoid cell. This should be confirmed on both the parasagittal and coronal CT (**Fig. 8.5E-G**). Also note that the first CT on which the posterior bony choanae can be seen is **Fig. 8.5C**

Fig. 8.3 The following six sequential CT scans are marked (**A–F**) and show the transition of the anterior to the posterior ethmoids. (**A**) The series starts at the anterior ethmoidal artery marked with a *solid white arrow*. (**B**) The superior turbinate is visible and this scan marks the transition from the anterior to posterior ethmoids. The *broken arrow* marks the beginning of the superior meatus. (**C**) The *broken arrow* again marks the superior meatus with the horizontal part of the ground lamella directly beneath the superior meatus (*black arrow*). (**D**) The *solid white arrow* marks the single large posterior ethmoid cell with the superior meatus (*broken arrow*) and horizontal ground lamella (*black arrow*) visible. (**F**) The single posterior ethmoid cell and the solid bone of the posterior choanae beginning to form (*broken white arrow*). This marks the beginning of the sphenoid sinuses.

Fig. 8.4 (**A,B**) The superior meatus (*solid white arrow*) without any posterior bony choanae. (**C**) The solid bony choanae are first seen (*broken white arrow*) indicating the transition from the posterior ethmoids to the sphenoid. In most patients the cell directly above the solid bone of the choana is the sphenoid sinus. (**D**) A horizontal septation is seen (*solid white arrow*). This septation separates the sphenoid (always directly above the bony choanae) and the ethmoid cell pneumatizing over the top of the sphenoid.

Fig. 8.5 A series of coronal CT scans (**A–D**) followed by an axial CT scan (**E**) and two parasagittal CT scans (**F,G**). (**F**) Scan is close is to the midline; (**G**) more lateral. Cells are numbered on the CT scan and in the three-dimensional reconstruction with cell 1 the single posterior ethmoid and cell 2 the sphenoid sinus. *MT*, middle turbinate; *ST*, superior turbinate; *SM*, superior meatus.

and there is a horizontal septation seen in that scan (between cells 1 and 2). Note on the two parasagittal scans (**Fig. 8.5F,G**) that the anterior face of the sphenoid is angled posteriorly allowing this wall to be cut by the CT giving the horizontal septation. On the left this is not carried significantly over the sphenoid and the optic nerve is not seen in cell 1 and therefore this does not represent an Onodi (sphenoethmoidal cell). The right side will be discussed later in this chapter. The 3D reconstruction demonstrates this slight posterior angulation of the anterior face of the sphenoid and also gives the surgeon a clear indication of exactly what to expect once the surgeon has entered the superior meatus and clearly identified this space and the anterior end of the superior turbinate.

Surgical Plan for the Posterior Ethmoids (Videos 23 to 27)

Once a 3D reconstruction of the posterior ethmoids has been performed, a surgical plan is formulated as to how the

dissection will be performed in the posterior ethmoids. The first step is to enter the superior meatus through the ground lamella in a region that can be easily identified on the CT scans. To achieve this, the transition from the posterior horizontal ground lamella to the vertical ground lamella needs to be identified. To positively identify the horizontal ground lamella, slide the endoscope under the middle turbinate toward the back end of the middle turbinate. As the posterior end of the middle turbinate is approached, the horizontal portion of the ground lamella is directly above the endoscope. The endoscope is brought anteriorly following the horizontal ground lamella until it tuns vertically. At the point where it turns vertically, in the area directly adjacent to the middle turbinate, the microdebrider or straight Blakesley is pushed through the ground lamella (**Fig. 8.6**).

This access area is widened horizontally until the superior meatus and anterior edge of the superior turbinate are identified with certainty (**Fig. 8.7**).

The surgeon can now place the point of dissection on the CT scans and knows how many and in what order the

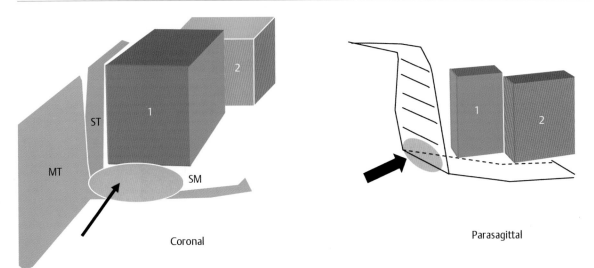

Fig. 8.6 The posterior ethmoids are entered at the junction of the horizontal and vertical portions of the ground lamella directly adjacent to the middle turbinate (as indicated by the *black arrow*). *MT*, middle turbinate; *ST*, superior turbinate; *SM*, superior meatus.

remaining cells are placed. These can then be sequentially entered and a complete dissection of the posterior ethmoids achieved. This low and medial entry into the posterior ethmoids minimizes the potential risk of damage to the skull base which may occur if entry is made higher on the vertical portion of the ground lamella.[1]

The Middle Turbinate

In most patients the middle turbinate is preserved. It is important that during the surgery that the middle turbinate is not destabilized. The most common cause for destabilization of the middle turbinate is fracturing its anterior vertical insertion from the skull base. The axillary flap is designed to preserve this insertion but does remove some

support from the anterior insertion of the middle turbinate. The horizontal portion of the ground lamella should also be preserved to give posterior stability to the middle turbinate. However, excessive manipulation of the middle turbinate can fracture the turbinate's insertion on the skull base and result in it becoming floppy. The maneuver that should be avoided is placing the endoscope and instruments medial to the middle turbinate. The combination of a 4-mm endoscope and a 4-mm instrument will usually be enough to fracture the middle turbinate. Therefore the techniques of posterior ethmoidectomy and sphenoidotomy are described through the middle meatus medial to the superior turbinate rather than medial to the middle turbinate. Despite all attempts to preserve the middle turbinate, there are some situations where partial or total resection of the middle turbinate is necessary.

Fig. 8.7 (**A**) Intraoperative picture illustrates the opening of the superior meatus on the left side (*broken white arrow*). The superior turbinate can be clearly seen (*solid white arrow*) and the partially opened posterior ethmoid (*PE*) cells are seen. (**B**) Cadaveric image on the left side. Penetration through horizontal ground lamella will immediately enter the superior meatus enabling a direct view of the superior turbinate.

A   B

Fig. 8.8 **(A)** The concha bullosa is seen. Note the breadth of the middle turbinate (*white arrow*). **(B)** The scalpel has been used to vertically incise (*white arrow*) the concha separating the medial and lateral lamella.

Concha Bullosa (Videos 6 and 7)

Patients with a concha bullosa need to have the lateral lamella of the middle turbinate removed to improve access to the middle meatus and, because this cell is often involved in the disease process, to clear the disease. To minimize damage to the lateral mucosa of the medial lamella, a scalpel is used to incise the anterior face of the concha bullosa vertically (**Fig. 8.8**).

A pair of 5-mm endoscopic scissors* (Medtronic ENT, Jacksonville, FL) are used to continue the incision along the inferior margin of the middle turbinate to the lateral insertion of the turbinate on the lateral nasal wall. The scissors are used to continue the superior incision posterior as high as possible on the turbinate but progressively moving inferiorly as the posterior region of the turbinate is approached. Once the lateral lamella of the turbinate has been resected it is removed. The residual upward continuation of the lateral lamella of the middle turbinate needs to be removed as part of the frontal recess and bulla ethmoidalis dissection. Failure to remove this upward continuation can result in residual disease in the medial compartment of the anterior ethmoids (**Fig. 8.9**).

Revision Surgery with Extensive Nasal Polyposis

The most common indication for middle turbinate resection is revision surgery with extensive polyposis. In patients who have previously undergone posterior ethmoidectomy, contracture of the horizontal part of the ground lamella may drag the middle turbinate laterally narrowing the ethmoidal space. This results in under ventilation of the posterior ethmoid region and could precipitate secretion retention in the posterior ethmoids and sphenoid and polyp formation.[2,3] In patients with massive polyposis often from Samter's triad (aspirin sensitivity, asthma, and polyps) or

fungal sinusitis, increased aeration of the posterior ethmoid cavity may be necessary to reduce polyp recurrence.[2,3] In these patients it may be necessary to partially resect the lower half of the middle turbinate and the horizontal portion of the ground lamella. This marsupializes the posterior ethmoids and sphenoid sinus (after a large sphenoidotomy) into the posterior nasal cavity with improved postoperative aeration of these sinuses (**Fig. 8.10**). This also facilitates the penetration of topical medications and nasal douches postoperatively.

Lateralized Atrophic Middle Turbinate

In some patients, especially those with long-standing severe septal deflections into the nasal cavity, the turbinate may be underdeveloped, very floppy, and lateralized. In these patients part of the turbinate may be resected at the time of surgery.

Fig. 8.9 The upward continuation of the middle turbinate is indicated with *solid white arrows*. Note the opacity medial to this upward continuation of the lateral lamella of the middle turbinate.

Fig. 8.10 The horizontal portion of the ground lamella is indicated by a series of *solid white arrows*. If this structure is maintained in patients with extensive nasal polyps it may result in under-aeration of the posterior ethmoids and sphenoid.

Fig. 8.11 CT scan illustrating a severe septal deflection (*broken white arrow*) and corresponding underdevelopment and lateralization of the middle turbinate on the left (*solid white arrow*).

When part of the middle turbinate is resected then the horizontal portion of the middle turbinate should also be removed flush with the lateral nasal wall. This almost invariably exposes the middle turbinate branch of the sphenopalatine artery with resultant bleeding and requires bipolar cautery (**Fig. 8.11**).

Lateral Displacement of the Middle Turbinate with Narrowing of the Frontal Recess

Particularly in patients who have had previous surgery or in patients with substantial olfactory fossa polyps, lateral displacement of the middle turbinates may occur (**Fig. 8.12**). This narrows the outflow region of the frontal sinus substantially and creates two problems. The first is the very narrow lateral dimension of the frontal recess, which makes surgery in this region very difficult and increases the risk of damage to the lateral wall of the olfactory fossa. The degree of difficulty

of the dissection increases if there is bleeding during the surgery. The lateralized portion of the middle turbinate is often thin and lacks rigidity and stability and this may result in this segment of the middle turbinate becoming unstable during surgery with resultant increased likelihood of postoperative lateralization and obstruction of the frontal ostium. The second problem is that as the sinuses heal after surgery, the narrow lateral dimension increases the likelihood of blood clot with subsequent fibrosis that leads to obstruction of the frontal ostium and consequently recurrent frontal sinusitis. If there are large polyps in the olfactory recess these may need to be resected to remove the lateral pressure that the polyps place on the middle turbinate. Care should be taken to limit the amount of raw tissue in the olfactory fossa to prevent scar formation in the olfactory fossa. This is best achieved by keeping the opening of the microdebrider blade facing only superiorly thereby preventing any lateral or medial mucosal damage.

Fig. 8.12 Coronal CT scan (**A**) shows significant lateralization of both middle turbinates (*white arrows*). Note opacified olfactory recesses (**A,B**). The extent of the lateralization of the middle turbinates is again seen on the axial scan (**B**, *white arrows*). The frontal recess is narrowed by at least 50% by this lateralization.

Posterior Attachment of Middle Turbinate (Videos 23 to 27)

The horizontal ground lamella attaches to the lateral nasal wall posterior to the maxillary sinus. Branches of the sphenopalatine artery traverse this region supplying blood to the middle turbinate. If this part of the ground lamella is removed, these vessels may bleed. This region is always meticulously inspected at the end of surgery and any bleeders cauterized with the suction bipolar forceps. Although the vessel may clot during surgery, coughing or straining in the postoperative period may dislodge the clot with consequent significant postoperative epistaxis.

◆ Anatomical Configurations that Place the Patient at Risk During the Surgery

Certain anatomical variations need to be sought on the CT scans prior to the dissection taking place. Identification of these may help avoid possible complications during the dissection of the posterior ethmoids.

Low Skull Base

A low skull base narrows the vertical height of the posterior ethmoids significantly. This is important for the surgeon to recognize before surgery in the posterior ethmoids is commenced. If the surgeon is unaware that the skull base is low, he or she may think that there may still be superior cells due to the low vertical height of the posterior ethmoids. Attempts to dissect further may injure the skull base associated dura and cause a

cerebrospinal fluid leak (CSF) leak. To illustrate the difference in vertical height, a CT scan with a normal skull base height and a patient with a low skull base is shown in **Fig. 8.13**.

It is critical in a patient with a low skull base that the approach into the posterior ethmoids is low and medial. A high entry through the vertical portion of the ground lamella in a patient with a low skull base would certainly put the skull base at risk[1] (**Fig. 8.14**).

A Curved Posterior Skull Base

Normally the posterior skull base is flat and the surgeon can dissect from the lamina papyracea medially along the skull base to the insertion of the superior turbinate with a minimum of risk. However, some patients may have a significant curve to the roof of the posterior ethmoids and the surgeon should assess the CT scans prior to surgery to establish the status of the posterior ethmoid fovea ethmoidalis before surgery is performed in this area (**Fig. 8.15**). Failure to recognize this curvature may result in the surgeon thinking that there is another cell situated medially on the skull base and if removal is attempted, injury to the skull base can occur.

Sphenoethmoidal Cell (Video 23)

Previous descriptions of the sphenoethmoidal (Onodi) cell state that it is a pneumatization of the posterior ethmoid cell laterally[1,4] and that the incidence can be as high as 42%.[5] However, in most cases this is not true as the sphenoethmoidal (Onodi) cell is rather a posterior pneumatization of the

Fig. 8.13 (**A,B**) The skull base originates from a point almost halfway down the vertical height of the lamina papyracea of the orbit (*broken lines*) whereas the more normal configuration (**C,D**) is seen with the fovea ethmoidalis taking origin from the upper aspect of the lamina papyracea (*broken lines*). (**C,D**) The vertical height of the ethmoid cavity is greater than in (**A,B**).

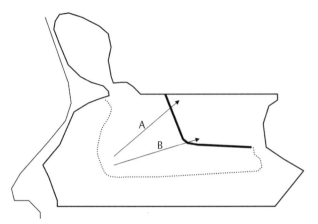

Fig. 8.14 This parasagittal diagram of the ground lamella of the middle turbinate illustrated the potential danger of entering the posterior ethmoids high on the vertical portion of the ground lamella (**A**, *arrow*) compared with the safety of entering the posterior ethmoids as low and medial as possible (**B**, *arrow*).

ethmoid cell over the sphenoid pushing the sphenoid inferiorly. To accurately identify a sphenoethmoidal (Onodi) cell, one must be able to recognize the transition from the posterior ethmoids to the sphenoid. This follows the theme of being able to recognize the transition from frontal sinus to anterior ethmoids (frontal recess), to recognize the transition from anterior to posterior ethmoids, and finally to be able to recognize the transition from posterior ethmoids to sphenoid sinus. If sequential coronal CT scans of the posterior ethmoids are evaluated, the transition from posterior ethmoids to sphenoid starts on the first CT scan that the posterior bony choanae can be seen (**Fig. 8.16**). Once the solid bony rim of the posterior choanae is identified, the cell sitting directly above this solid bone should be the sphenoid sinus. If there is any horizontal bony septation above this cell in this or subsequent more posterior coronal CT scans, this would be suspicious that there may be a sphenoethmoidal (Onodi) cell present (**Fig. 8.16**).

The posterior ethmoid cells should be followed in each sequential CT scan and one should establish whether a posterior ethmoid cell pneumatizes over the sphenoid. The parasagittal scan should always be checked as this can be very useful in recognizing a sphenoethmoidal (Onodi) cell. In **Fig. 8.16** one can clearly see how the posterior ethmoid cell pneumatizes over the top of the sphenoid (SPH) which in turn creates

the most useful characteristic of a sphenoethmoidal (Onodi) cell–the horizontal septum (HS) seen on a scan that is taken through the sphenoid. Thus, the transition from the posterior ethmoids to the sphenoid is critical to establish before the horizontal septation is sought. This septation is created by the anterior face of the sphenoid being pushed into a more horizontal plane by the sphenoethmoidal (Onodi) cell pneumatizing over the top of the sphenoid. **Figure 8.17** CT scans include a parasagittal scan and illustrate the horizontal plane taken by the anterior face of the sphenoid when a sphenoethmoidal cell is present. Axial scans are of little value in diagnosing a sphenoethmoidal (Onodi) cell.

It is important to identify an Onodi cell as this cell has the optic nerve in its posterosuperior region where it is vulnerable to injury during dissection. If the cell is not recognized the surgeon may not realize that the sphenoid sinus has been pushed inferiorly below the Onodi cell. If the access into the sphenoid is attempted through the Onodi cell, damage to the optic nerve, skull base, or carotid artery may result as these structures are adjacent to this cell while the sphenoid is below and more medial. The relationship between the Onodi cell and optic nerve can be clearly seen in **Fig. 8.17C**.

◆ **Sphenoidotomy (Videos 23 to 27)**

After dissection of the posterior ethmoids, the sphenoid can be entered. The sphenoid ostium is located medial to the superior turbinate in 83% of patients.[6] If the sphenoid is normal (without disease visible on the CT scan), the sphenoethmoidal recess can be inspected through the middle meatus by gently moving the superior turbinate laterally and visualizing the recess. If there is no disease in the sphenoethmoidal recess, the sphenoid ostium should be visible in most patients. If the sphenoethmoidal recess is diseased (inflamed hypertrophic mucosa or the presence of polyps), then consideration can be given to clearance of the recess usually with sphenoidotomy. If significant mucosal trauma is created in the recess by clearance of disease, then it is likely that the sphenoid ostium may be closed by scar tissue formation during healing and a sphenoidotomy should be performed to prevent this occurrence. If the sphenoid is diseased on the CT scan it should be opened. It is preferable to open the sphenoid through the posterior ethmoids rather than by

Fig. 8.15 The curved posterior ethmoid fovea ethmoidalis is indicated by the white arrow (**B**).

Fig. 8.16 The transition from the posterior ethmoids to the sphenoid occurs between (**B**) and (**C**). (**C**) The bony posterior choanae (*broken white arrow*) are seen. At the point where a complete bony posterior choana is identified, the sinus directly above this bony choanae should be the sphenoid sinus. The horizontal septation (*white arrow*) separates the sphenoid from the Onodi cell (*OC*) above it.

passing the instruments and endoscope medial to the middle turbinate as previously emphasized.[7] The medial to the middle turbinate route to the sphenoid ostium is only used when no middle meatal surgery is necessary such as a patient with isolated sphenoid disease or for pituitary surgery. In the transethmoidal route the already identified superior turbinate is used as the critical landmark for sphenoidotomy.[7,8] The lower one-third to half of the superior turbinate is removed either with a microdebrider or straight through-biting forceps. Once the turbinate is removed flush with the anterior face of the sphenoid, the microdebrider is used to palpate the face for the natural ostium of the sphenoid. It is usually found at the junction of the lower one-third and upper two-thirds but may be as high as the halfway point of the superior turbinate and is usually medial to the turbinate on the anterior face of the sphenoid[6] (**Fig. 8.18**).

In the majority of patients the natural ostium will be located using the landmarks described previously. However, in patients with a sphenoethmoidal (Onodi) cell, the natural ostium may be lower and more medial as the sphenoid is compressed by the sphenoethmoidal cell pneumatizing over the top of it. If the tip of the microdebrider does not fall into the natural ostium, a smaller straight suction is used to palpate this region. If the natural ostium can still not be located, then the CT scan is reviewed to confirm the position and size of the sphenoid sinus before proceeding further. If a sphenoid is present then the following measurement technique should be followed to open the sphenoid. The bony rim of

the posterior choana is located by passing the 4-mm microdebrider blade through the posterior ethmoids and into the nasopharynx. The tip of the microdebrider blade is pushed against the mucosa just above the bony choanae on the anterior face of the sphenoid. This creates a 4-mm indentation. Two further indentations are made above this one thereby measuring 12 mm from the bony rim of the posterior choana (**Fig. 8.19**).

A Freer elevator is then used to push through the anterior face of the sphenoid directly above the third indentation. The tip of the instrument is pushed through the bone and once it has penetrated the sphenoid cavity it is twisted to enlarge the opening. A microdebrider or Kerrison punch is then used to further open the sinus. The natural ostium is opened with the punch or microdebrider initially inferiorly toward the floor of the sinus and then toward the lamina papyracea and into the posterior ethmoids (**Fig. 8.20**).

There should be at least 8 to 10 mm of anterior face of the sphenoid still above this lateral opening and this newly created opening should therefore be well below the optic nerve. The opening can be further enlarged directly superiorly from the natural ostium, medially and inferiorly as well (**Fig. 8.20**). Opening of the natural ostium of the sphenoid invariably creates a circumferential raw surface around the natural ostium and therefore this opening needs to be enlarged into the posterior ethmoids to prevent postoperative stenosis. The anterior face of the sphenoid is removed up to the skull base and laterally to the lamina papyracea and then finally lowered

Fig. 8.17 (**A,B**) Indication of the value of the parasagittal scan in confirming the pneumatization of the sphenoethmoidal (Onodi) cell (*OC*) over the sphenoid with the formation of a horizontal septum (*HS*) in the coronal scan (**A**). (**A,C**) The optic nerve (*ON*) is identified and the relationship between this posterior sphenoethmoid cell (*OC*) and the ON can be seen.

Fig. 8.18 **(A)** On the left side the middle turbinate (*MT*), superior turbinate (*ST*), superior meatus (*SM*), and horizontal part of the ground lamella (*HGL*) are clearly identified before sphenoidotomy. In this figure the posterior ethmoids have not as yet been opened. Once the posterior ethmoids have been sequentially opened the superior turbinate is divided into the thirds. The lower one-third is removed with either a straight through-biting Blakesley or powered microdebrider up to the anterior face of sphenoid and the sphenoid ostium is identified before it is opened. **(B)** Cadaveric image taken with the endoscope within the superior meatus on the left side. The lower one-third of the superior turbinate has been removed revealing the natural sphenoid ostium. Note how the anterior face of the sphenoid sinus is contributed by the sphenoethmoidal recess (*SER*) and the posterior wall of a posterior ethmoid cell (*PE*).

to the floor of the sphenoid. The postnasal artery or vertical branch of the postnasal artery is often cut during widening of the sphenoid and requires bipolar cautery (**Fig. 8.20B**). In patients with significant new bone formation, an inferiorly based mucosal flap can be elevated and the underlying bone drilled away before the flap is replaced.[9] This interrupts the circumferential raw area and prevents stenosis.

If the superior turbinate has been completely or partially removed by previous surgery, the measurement technique described previously is used to locate the position of the natural ostium of the sphenoid sinus. Resection of part of the superior turbinate may possibly remove some olfactory neurons so as much of this turbinate as possible is preserved. Studies done on olfaction after this technique have not been shown to adversely affect the sense of smell of the patient after surgery.[10] Sphenoidotomy for pituitary surgery is discussed in Chapter 13.

Complications of Sphenoidotomy

Epistaxis

Bleeding is very common from the posterior nasal artery as it traverses the anterior face of the sphenoid on its way to the posterior septum. The posterior nasal artery is a branch of the sphenopalatine artery and travels horizontally just above the posterior choana (**Fig. 8.21**). It gives off a vertical branch that supplies the anterior face of the sphenoid. If this vertical branch is transected (and it often is as the sphenoid ostium is enlarged) a minor bleeder will be seen on the lower opening of the sphenoid. If the sphenoid ostium is further enlarged inferiorly toward the floor of the sphenoid sinus, the main trunk of the posterior nasal artery can be transected and result in a significant bleeder which usually spurts in a horizontal and medial direction. This is best managed with the suction-bipolar forceps* (Medtronic ENT) as the blood can be suctioned and cautery rapidly applied before the active bleeding results in blood

Fig. 8.19 Three sequential indentations are made with the blunt end of the 4-mm microdebrider blade starting at the medial upper limit of the posterior bony choana and moving directly superiorly medial to the cut edge of the superior turbinate.

A

B

Fig. 8.20 (A) The sphenoid ostium (*SO*) is first opened inferiorly (*black arrow*, **1**) then laterally (*black arrow*, **2**). This should afford a clear view into the sphenoid sinus and the remaining anterior face of the sphenoid can be removed up toward the optic tubercle (*OT*) but usually stopping short of the tubercle to lessen the potential risk to the optic nerve.

(B) A cadaveric image demonstrating technique for sphenoidotomy. Note how the sphenoid is opened down to the posterior nasal artery as it traverses the anterior face of the sphenoid on its way to the posterior septum. *SER*, sphenoethmoidal recess; *PE*, posterior ethmoid cell; *ST*, superior turbinate; *PNA*, posterior nasal artery.

vessel being covered in a blood and no longer visible for precise cautery. If a standard suction and standard bipolar forceps are used, the bleeder is usually so active that by the time that the suction is removed and the bipolar forceps positioned the vessel can no longer be seen. Because the

suction bipolar has integrated suction this problem can be rapidly overcome.

Damage to the Optic Nerve and CSF Leak

The most common cause of injury to the optic nerve during ESS is when a sphenoidotomy is attempted too high and too lateral and damage is caused to the orbital apex and optic nerve. In **Fig. 8.20** a diagrammatic view of the posterior ethmoids and superior turbinate is presented. Attempted entry into the sphenoid in the superior lateral region will take the surgeon onto the orbital apex and optic nerve and even into the anterior skull base. This can result in a devastating complication of a damaged optic nerve with visual loss and a CSF leak with potential intracranial damage. In general this situation begins when entry into the posterior ethmoids through the vertical portion of the ground lamella is made too high. The whole direction of surgery is then toward the skull base and if the surgeon is inexperienced and does not recognize this, he or she may assume that the structure in front of them is a sloping anterior wall of the sphenoid sinus rather than the sloping wall of the skull base. If the skull base is thinner than usual then entry into the anterior cranial fossa and/or damage to the optic nerve can occur. The key to preventing this devastating complication is to identify the superior meatus as the first step in the dissection of the posterior ethmoids immediately after the ground lamella is penetrated. This forces the surgeon to keep removing the ground lamella inferiorly until the superior meatus is clearly identified. If this dissection is continued and the anterior end of the superior turbinate is correctly identified, the surgeon is in the correct plane and place and so the risk

Fig. 8.21 Cadaveric image on the right side demonstrating the sphenopalatine artery (*SPA*) giving off the posterior nasal artery (*PNA*). This branch runs along the anterior face of the sphenoid, and can be inadvertently transected during sphenoidotomy. *PE*, posterior ethmoid cell; *ST*, superior turbinate; *SO*, sphenoid ostium.

of mistaking the skull base for the anterior face of the sphenoid should be minimized.

The other area that the optic nerve can be damaged is in the superolateral wall of the sphenoid sinus. The optic nerve is dehiscent in ~12%[5] of patients and inadvertent injury during surgery within the sphenoid sinus may lead to visual loss or blindness. It is tempting to use the microdebrider to remove polyps in the sphenoid but great care needs to be taken using the microdebrider in this sinus. In general the microdebrider should only be used along the floor and medial wall of the sphenoid and not in the superior or lateral region. Surgeons are also concerned when the sphenoidotomy is widened in a lateral direction. There are a few rules to follow during sphenoidotomy that can minimize the risk to the optic nerve. The natural ostium of the sphenoid is generally around the lower one-third of the superior turbinates' insertion into the anterior face of the sphenoid. The forward-biting Hajek Koffler punch is used to enlarge this natural ostium first inferiorly toward the floor and then laterally toward the orbit. As the orbit is approached the instrument should be well below the orbital apex and optic nerve (**Fig. 8.20**).

The second rule is that if the distal jaw of the biting mechanism of the Hajek Koffler punch can be placed behind a bony septation it is generally safe to remove. Even a septation arising from the optic nerve can be safely removed onto the nerve by allowing the punch to rest on the nerve while the septation is engaged between the jaws of the punch and cleanly removed from the surface of the nerve. However, the superolateral region of the anterior face of the sphenoid is very carefully removed to lessen any possible risk to the optic nerve (**Fig. 8.20**).

Damage to the Carotid Artery

The other major structure at risk during sphenoidotomy is the carotid artery. The bony wall covering the carotid is in most patients thin and dehiscent in 5 to 8%[5,11] of patients (**Fig. 8.22**).

Fig. 8.23 This axial CT scan shows the sphenoid sinus septum (*broken arrow*) inserting into the anterior face of the left carotid artery (*solid arrow*). Rotation of this septum during removal may result in a tear of the wall of the carotid artery.

This again emphasizes the risk of using a microdebrider with the cutting gate toward the lateral wall of the sphenoid. It only takes milliseconds for a dehiscent carotid artery wall to be damaged by the very effective cutting mechanisms in microdebriders with potentially catastrophic results. There are two other ways that the carotid artery may be damaged. In some patients the natural ostium of the sphenoid sinus is very small and the surgeon is unable to identify it and thus allow a safe entry into the sphenoid sinus. If a small or narrow instrument is pushed hard onto the face of the sphenoid in an attempt to penetrate into the sphenoid, the bone may suddenly give way with the instrument been driven into the sinus with considerable force. This instrument can then inadvertently penetrate the thin or dehiscent bone or dehiscent carotid with subsequent massive hemorrhage. In the operative technique previously described, a blunt Freer elevator is used to push through the anterior face of the sphenoid sinus. The entry into the sphenoid can be well controlled with this instrument and the surgeon can easily feel as the bone is penetrated without risk of the instrument slipping inadvertently into the sinus. Also the instrument has a large blunt surface and the penetration point is medial and inferior and is thus less likely to injure the carotid.

The second situation where a carotid injury may occur is if the intersinus septum of the sphenoid is attached to the anterior face of the carotid artery (**Fig. 8.23**).

If this septum needs to be taken down as is often the case during pituitary surgery and this attachment is grasped and rotated, it may fracture and bony spicules may damage the carotid wall. This can be avoided by using a through-biting instrument to sharply remove the septation. If the septation is too thick, then a diamond burr can be used.

Management of a carotid artery hemorrhage is discussed in Chapter 22.

Fig. 8.22 Left sphenoid with dehiscent carotid illustrated by *solid white arrows* and optic nerve illustrated with *solid black arrow*.

References

1. Edelstein DR, Liberatore L, Bushkin S, Han JC. Applied anatomy of the posterior sinuses in relation to the optic nerve, trigeminal nerve and carotid artery. Am J Rhinol 1995;9:321–333

2. Klossek JM, Peloquin L, Friedman WH, Ferrier JC, Fontanel JP. Diffuse nasal polyposis: postoperative long-term results after endoscopic sinus surgery and frontal irrigation. Otolaryngol Head Neck Surg 1997; 117(4):355–361

3. Dufour X, Bedier A, Ferrie JC, Gohler C, Klossek JM. Diffuse nasal polyposis and endonasal endoscopic surgery: long-term results, a 65-case study. Laryngoscope 2004;114(11):1982–1987

4. Elwany S, Elsaeid I, Thabet H. Endoscopic anatomy of the sphenoid sinus. J Laryngol Otol 1999;113(2):122–126

5. Kainz J, Stammberger H. Danger areas of the posterior rhinobasis. An endoscopic and anatomical-surgical study. Acta Otolaryngol 1992;112(5):852–861

6. Kim H-U, Kim S-S, Kang SS, Chung IH, Lee J-G, Yoon J-H. Surgical anatomy of the natural ostium of the sphenoid sinus. Laryngoscope 2001;111(9):1599–1602

7. Har-El G, Swanson RM. The superior turbinectomy approach to isolated sphenoid sinus disease and to the sella turcica. Am J Rhinol 2001;15(2):149–156

8. Bolger WE, Keyes AS, Lanza DC. Use of the superior meatus and superior turbinate in the endoscopic approach to the sphenoid sinus. Otolaryngol Head Neck Surg 1999;120(3):308–313

9. Donald PJ. Sphenoid marsupialization for chronic sphenoidal sinusitis. Laryngoscope 2000;110(8):1349–1352

10. Orlandi RR, Lanza DC, Bolger WE, Clerico DM, Kennedy DW. The forgotten turbinate: the role of the superior turbinate in endoscopic sinus surgery. Am J Rhinol 1999;13(4):251–259

11. Unal B, Bademci G, Bilgili YK, Batay F, Avci E. Risky anatomic variations of sphenoid sinus for surgery. Surg Radiol Anat 2006;28(2):195–201

9 Extended Approaches to the Frontal Sinus: The Modified Endoscopic Lothrop Procedure

Chronic frontal sinusitis has challenged surgeons for many years. In the past, frontal sinus obliteration through an osteoplastic flap (OPF) approach has been the gold standard for the management of recalcitrant frontal sinusitis.[1–3] Other external procedures such as frontoethmoidectomy have fallen into disfavor due to a failure rate of around 30%.[3,4] OPF and obliteration has a reported failure rate of around 10% but has a significant complication rate of around 65%.[3,5,6] The complications include cerebrospinal fluid (CSF) leak, frontal bossing, supraorbital neuralgia, chronic sepsis, mucocele formation, and chronic frontal bone osteitis with loss of the frontal sinus bone flap.[1–3,6] In recent years the modified endoscopic Lothrop (MEL) procedure—otherwise known as the Draf 3 or frontal drillout—has been proposed as an alternative to the OPF with obliteration.[7–20] The MEL procedure is based on the technique originally described by Lothrop in 1914.[21] This technique involves removal of the upper portion of the septum, the floor of the frontal sinus, and the intersinus septum. Removal of the floor is accomplished with the aid of a small external incision (similar to a Lynch incision) which creates a window through which the drill can be observed. Although this procedure was successful in 29 out of 30 patients, the technique was considered too technically difficult for most surgeons to master and it was not until Draf in 1991[7] and Gross in 1995[8,9] published series of patients using a modified version of the technique that interest was renewed. The major modification to the Lothrop technique is the absence of an external incision with the entire procedure performed endoscopically. The MEL can be used as an alternative to OPF with obliteration with recent publications[12] showing excellent short-term success rates with minimal complications. The indications for the MEL procedure should be the same as the indications for an OPF with obliteration and these are detailed in the following text.[12]

◆ Indications for Modified Endoscopic Lothrop Procedure

Failed Endoscopic Sinus Surgery

The MEL procedure is indicated in patients who have failed standard endoscopic sinus surgery (ESS) techniques.[12] These include clearance of the frontal recess and removal of cells obstructing the frontal ostium.[20] In those very rare cases where patients have a very large cell obstructing the frontal ostium (i.e., a type 4 cell that extends into the frontal sinus by more than 50% of the vertical height of the frontal sinus), management may include a primary MEL procedure if the surgeon is certain that the cell is causing significant obstruction and that it is not possible to remove the cell with standard ESS techniques discussed later.[20] All patients should have had a standard ESS approach with an attempt to remove obstructing cells from the frontal ostium and improve the drainage of the frontal sinus. It is only if such techniques fail that the MEL procedure should be considered for removal of a type 4 cell.[20] In **Fig. 9.1** the patient had undergone five previous standard ESS procedures and was still left with significant frontal sinus symptoms and a large type 4 cell obstructing the frontal sinus ostium. This patient underwent a successful MEL procedure.

Neo-Osteogenesis in the Frontal Recess and Frontal Ostium

Significant new bone formation in the regions of the frontal recess after ESS indicates probable osteitis. This can be difficult to manage with standard ESS techniques. The neo-osteogenesis results in a narrowed frontal sinus openings and increases vascularity in the region. Surgery to widen such

Fig. 9.1 (**A–D**) CT scans of a patient with a type 4 cell (*white arrow*) who had undergone multiple previous ESS procedures. (**D**) Note on the axial scan the significantly narrowed frontal sinus drainage pathway (*black arrow*) caused by the type 4 cell (**white arrow**).

narrowed ostia will often result in significant bleeding and loss of mucosa. The healing process may produce significant restenosis as ongoing low-grade osteitis and sinusitis continue to stimulate new bone formation and fibrosis. The MEL procedure overcomes this problem by drilling away a significant amount of the osteitic bone and creates the largest possible opening in the frontal sinuses. Even if some degree of restenosis occurs in the MEL procedure, this should not affect the function of the frontal sinuses.[22] Recent work done on the MEL procedure in our animal laboratory on the presence of neo-osteogenesis in a newly created frontal ostium suggests that most frontal ostia will restenose by an average of a third.[23,24] This figure was not affected by the presence of neo-osteogenesis which was found in 56% of animals. In addition, this restenosis did not affect the mucociliary drainage of the frontal sinuses as measured by the clearance of radioisotope from the frontal sinuses.[22] **Figure 9.2** shows a patient with significant neo-osteogenesis in the left frontal ostium. This patient had undergone six previous standard ESS procedures in an attempt to maintain a patent left frontal ostium. In all cases the restenosis was rapid and associated with a return of frontal sinus symptoms.

Frontal Recess Adhesions

In patients who have previously undergone multiple ESS procedures one will often find that the middle turbinates have been resected subtotally.[12] In this scenario the middle turbinate remnant may lateralize and become adhesive to the lateral nasal wall in the frontal recess. This results in significant narrowing of the frontal drainage pathway and, in some instances, complete obstruction of the frontal ostium (**Fig. 9.3**). Standard ESS techniques will usually fail to re-create a mucosalized opening of sufficient diameter into the frontal sinuses and a MEL procedure or OPF with obliteration should be considered.

Disease Processes with Resultant Loss of the Posterior Wall or Floor of the Frontal Sinus[18]

If the disease process results in bony erosion of either the posterior wall or floor of the frontal sinus, the mucosa of the sinus becomes adherent onto the dura or orbital

Fig. 9.2 (**A,B**) Coronal CT scans of a patient with multiple previous ESS procedures with neo-osteogenesis in the left frontal recess (*black arrow*) with associated chronic frontal sinusitis.

periosteum.[18] OPF with obliteration becomes extremely difficult in these patients as the mucosa cannot be safely or completely removed from the dura or orbital periosteum and a recurrence of a mucocele is likely if the sinus is obliterated. These patients often have long-term severe chronic sinusitis and may have disease with a high incidence of recurrence such as fungal sinus disease. It is important to keep the frontal ostia open as obstruction of the frontal ostium may lead to either orbital or intracranial complications (**Fig. 9.4**).[18]

Fig. 9.3 (**A–C**) This patient has undergone previous middle turbinate resection and the stump (*black arrow*) has lateralized blocking the frontal ostium. (**C**) In addition, new bone formation can be seen above the middle turbinate.

Fig. 9.4 (A–D) This patient with chronic frontal sinusitis with loss of the roof of the orbit and loss of the posterior table of the frontal sinus developed an abscess (*black arrow*) with associated cellulitis around the orbit and depression of the left globe. (**C,D**) In addition, this abscess had eroded the posterior table of the frontal sinus and compressed the anterior cerebral hemisphere. This was managed by a MEL procedure with the creation of a large communal frontal ostium.

Failed Previous OPF with Obliteration with Mucocele Formation[13]

Frontal sinus obliteration has been the gold standard for the management of recalcitrant frontal sinusitis for many years. However, severe mucosal disease such as that seen in patients with Samter's triad (aspirin sensitivity, asthma, and nasal polyposis), allergic fungal sinusitis, and aggressive recurrent nasal polyposis is best managed endoscopically rather than with an OPF and obliteration.[14–18] There is now widespread agreement in the literature that the MEL procedure should be the operation of first choice in this difficult group of patients.[14–18] One of the major problems with OPF and obliteration is the tendency for the adipose tissue placed in the frontal sinuses to resorb. Weber et al.,[14] in a large study of 82 patients who underwent OPF and obliteration, showed that the majority of patients had less than 20% of the sinus obliterated after a median of 15.4 months.[14] In this patient group who aggressively form polyps, such space can be rapidly filled by even the smallest amount of residual mucosa inadvertently left in the frontal sinuses. In the postoperative period this group tends to develop thick inspissated mucus among the regrowing polyps. Without a wide opening or marsupialization of the affected sinus, this mucus cannot be removed in the office. The inability to pass a large suction through the sinus ostium into the sinus cavity prevents this very tenacious mucus from being removed. A course of systemic prednisolone may loosen the mucus and lessen its tenacity facilitating its removal. Clearance of this toxic material allows shrinkage of the polyps and reestablishment of the nasal airway with control of polyp growth. In most patients it is a relatively simple procedure to create a wide maxillary antrostomy, completely remove all ethmoid cells, and open widely the anterior face of the sphenoid sinus. However, the frontal sinuses are extremely difficult to access without the wide opening that the MEL procedure creates. Naturally sized frontal ostia tend to be quickly obstructed by thickened mucosa and this results in a buildup of thick mucus in the frontal sinuses which may be resistant to aggressive prednisolone therapy and attempted suction clearance. One of the difficulties with OPF and obliteration in this group of patients is when there is loss of bone over the orbit or dura. Due to the aggressive nature of the polyposis and in some cases aggravated by repeated surgeries, there may be loss of the anterior or posterior bony frontal sinus wall. This brings the mucocele lining

in direct contact with the orbital periosteum and/or dura and makes it impossible to remove all the mucosa from these structures without resection.[15] Even microscopic mucosal remnants left on the periosteum or dura will lead to the development of a mucocele in the obliterated cavity (**Fig. 9.5**).

Fig. 9.5 (**A**) CT scan shows frontal sinus opacification with an orbital roof dehiscence (*white arrow*). (**B**) T2-weighted MRI shows a frontal sinus mucocele (*broken white arrow*). (**C**) CT scan shows both orbital and posterior table dehiscences where the mucocele is in contact with the orbital periosteum and the dura. (**D**) Axial CT scan shows previous osteotomies in the anterior table of the frontal sinus and MRI scan (**E**) shows the frontal sinus mucocele (*broken white arrow*) and the extensive nasal polyp formation in the nasal cavity (*solid white arrow*).

Another contraindication to OPF and obliteration is when the patient has very large pneumatized frontal sinuses.[15,18] In these patients it is extremely difficult to eradicate all the mucosa from the lateral and posterior recesses of the frontal sinus and this residual mucosa will form mucoceles which, if left untreated, will erode the bony walls of the sinus and may well give rise to either intracranial or orbital complications (**Fig. 9.6**). Mucoceles that form in a previously obliterated frontal sinus can be treated by an MEL procedure.[13,14,18] The mucocele should be sufficiently large that it can be accessed through the frontal recess and marsupialized into the frontal recess (**Fig. 9.6**).[13,18] Mucoceles confined to the far lateral aspect of previously well-pneumatized sinuses may be difficult to reach and, if the intervening space is filled with scar tissue, may be difficult to keep open postoperatively.

Patients who have previously undergone an OPF with obliteration often present with frontal pain and it can be quite difficult to ascertain whether their pain is from a frontal sinus mucocele or from other causes. All these patients undergo magnetic resonance imaging (MRI) to ensure that there is indeed a mucocele present. If there is no mucocele present surgery is usually not offered and the patient is given treatment for neuralgic pain or myofascial pain syndrome. To assess if the pain is neuralgic or myofascial in origin, a trial of low dose amitriptyline (10 mg per night) is prescribed for 6 weeks. If neuralgia or myofascial pain syndrome is contributing to the patient's pain, there should be an improvement in symptoms on this treatment.[19] Most patients will also undergo radioisotope screening to exclude osteomyelitis of the previous bone flap. If the radioisotope scan is positive, consideration may have to be given to removal of this bone flap.

Tumor Removal from the Frontal Sinus (Video 43)

The MEL procedure is useful for the removal of benign tumors from the frontal sinuses. These tumors include osteomas and inverting papillomas. Fairly large osteomas can be removed

Fig. 9.6 This patient has extensive pneumatization of the frontal sinuses. (**A–C**) OPF with obliteration failed with resultant superior and lateral mucocele formation (*black arrows*). This was addressed with a MEL. (**D**) The postoperative picture at 3 years is presented, with *black arrow* indicating one of the opened mucocoeles.

through the MEL opening.[12,15,18] **Figure 9.7** illustrates a patient with a large frontal osteoma which has blocked the pathway of the right frontal sinus and resulted in the formation of a large lateral mucocele. This mucocele had eroded the bone over the roof of the orbit with the lining of the mucocele in contact with a large proportion of the orbital periosteum (**Fig. 9.7**).

The patient underwent a MEL procedure with removal of 90% of the osteoma and drainage of the mucocele. A free mucosal graft was placed on the circumferential raw area created after removal of the osteoma. The patient is now 3 years postsurgery and has a nicely healed and patent right frontal sinus with free drainage of the lateral mucocele into the nose (**Fig. 9.8**).

The MEL procedure is also suitable for removing inverting papilloma from the frontal sinus.[12,15,20] **Figure 9.9** shows a recurrent inverting papilloma entering the frontal sinus on the left. This had previously been removed via a lateral rhinotomy procedure. The tumor is seen in the left frontal recess and sinus.

The entire tumor was removed after a MEL procedure until direct visualization. As a large area of frontal sinus mucosa was removed in association with the tumor, a free mucosal graft was placed. **Figure 9.10** shows the patient 1 year after the procedure. There still remains a little edema of the frontal ostium. Biopsies were negative for recurrence. Excellent visualization of the site of the tumor is provided by the large frontal ostium and recurrences can be detected early (**Fig. 9.10**).

Fig. 9.7 (A,B) CT scans and **(C,D)** MRI scans (T2-weighted) showing the osteoma (marked with a *black arrow*) and the right-sided lateral mucocele (marked with *white arrow*) with associated proptosis and inferolateral displacement of the eye. **(B)** Intraoperative images seen on the image-guidance system of the large frontal osteoma (*white arrow*) occupying the vast majority of the frontal sinuses. The laterally based mucocele is under the cross-hairs which are formed from the tip of the suction. (*continued*)

E

Fig. 9.7 (*continued*)

Fig. 9.8 Endoscopic view of the frontal ostium created after removal of the large frontal osteoma shown in **Fig. 9.7**. The *white arrow* indicates the lateral pathway created into the laterally based mucocele indicated in **Fig. 9.7A,B**.

◆ Relative Contraindications for the Modified Endoscopic Lothrop Procedure

Poorly Pneumatized Frontal Sinuses

In patients who have poorly developed (pneumatized) frontal sinuses the bone of the frontal beak and the intersinus septum is very thick (**Fig. 9.11**).[12,18,20] This can make creation of a large frontal sinus ostium difficult as more bone needs to be taken away. In most cases this results in a larger raw bony surface as there is less residual mucosa in the region of the frontal sinus. In the postoperative period there is a tendency for the frontal ostium to cicatrize. We routinely now harvest a free mucosal graft from the region where the septal window is created and place this in the neo-ostium. No glue is used to hold it there as it sticks well within a few hours. This free graft prevents the circumferential laying down of fibroblasts and results in less postoperative stenosis than leaving the bone bare. In **Fig. 9.11** the patient has very underdeveloped frontal sinuses with a thick frontal beak and intersinus septum.

If the postoperative frontal ostium is viewed after 24 months (**Fig. 9.12**), the smaller-than-usual frontal ostium can be seen. This case illustrates the importance of creating

Fig. 9.9 (**A–C**) CT scans show recurrent inverting papilloma on the lamina papyracea entering the frontal sinus (*white arrows*). (**D**) This is confirmed with an MRI scan which shows that the opacity within the frontal sinus is not just retained secretions.

Fig. 9.10 This endoscopic view shows the patient from Fig. 9.9 4 years postoperatively with a nicely healed common opening into both frontal sinuses. The entire area of previous tumor involvement can be easily surveyed endoscopically for any recurrences.

the largest possible bony ostium at the time of surgery and that although underdeveloped frontal sinuses may be a relative contraindication, the patient can still have a successful MEL procedure if these principles are adhered to.

Narrow Anteroposterior Depth of the Frontal Sinus[12,18,20]

In some patients the skull base comes farther forward than normal and narrows the anteroposterior width of the frontal sinus. This in turn limits the anteroposterior width that can be created during surgery and increases the likelihood of postoperative scarring and closure of the frontal ostium. In **Fig. 9.13A–D** the patient has a very narrow anteroposterior diameter of the frontal sinus. This limits the opening that can be surgically created.

◆ Surgical Technique[12,13,17,18,25–28] (Videos 28 to 30 and 43)

It is currently our routine to use image-guidance equipment for all our MEL procedures.[12,13,18,20,26] Image guidance helps to identify the olfactory fossa projections and aids

Fig. 9.11 (A–C) Series of three CT scans (**A,** right parasagittal; **C,** left parasagittal) illustrating the thick frontal beak (*white arrows*) resulting from underpneumatized frontal sinus (*white arrow*).

in the creation of the largest possible frontal sinus ostium. This ability to create the largest possible opening is critical for the success of this procedure. Image guidance is set up before surgery. Once the accuracy of the system is verified surgery begins. The first step is to surgically revise, as necessary, the maxillary, ethmoid, and sphenoid sinuses. It is important that this is done before the frontal sinus surgery as the frontal sinus component can be relatively time-consuming and the surgical field tends to worsen progressively as the operation proceeds. Visualization of the anatomy of the maxillary, ethmoid, and sphenoids can be difficult due

Fig. 9.12 This is the postoperative picture taken of the patient shown in **Fig. 9.11** 3 years after surgery. The *black arrow* reveals a small granulation on the anterior skull base which was subsequently removed. The *white solid arrow* indicates the frontal intersinus septum and the *broken white arrow* indicates a small amount of mucus present in the right frontal sinus. The patient is currently asymptomatic.

to excessive bleeding if this is left to the end of the surgical procedure.

Infiltration with lidocaine and adrenaline is performed in the region above the axilla of the middle turbinate and the vault of the nose. The adjacent septum anterior to the middle turbinate is also infiltrated. A zero-degree scope is used for the majority of the dissection and a 30-degree scope is used when the floor of the frontal sinus is removed. The first step is to remove the mucosa above the middle turbinate up to the roof of the nose with a powered microdebrider exposing the underlying bone.[12] The mucosa of the septum anterior to the middle turbinate adjacent to the roof of the nose is removed over a 3 × 2 cm area (**Fig. 9.14**). This step is performed bilaterally. Alternatively this mucosa is harvested as a free mucosal graft on both sides and this mucosa is placed on the anterior surface of the neo-ostium as a free graft at the end of the procedure. We have found that this speeds up the healing process postoperatively and decreases the amount of granulation tissue during the healing period. The cartilage and bone in the septal window is removed. An instrument should be able to be passed from the one side of the nose through the septal window and under the axilla of the middle turbinate on the other side (**Fig. 9.14**).[12]

If this is not possible, the septal window should be lowered until this can be easily done. If there is a pathway between the frontal sinus and the frontal recess (i.e., there is no mucocele present with complete separation of the frontal sinus and frontal recess), a frontal sinus mini-trephine is placed in each frontal sinus. Flushing the frontal sinus mini-trephine will result in fluorescein-stained saline being seen under the axilla of the middle turbinate. This step is done early as it increases the safety of the dissection. Regular flushing of the frontal sinus will result in fluorescein flowing through the frontal ostium allowing the surgeon to have a constant posterior reference point and thus keep the dissection away from the skull base. The fluorescein-stained saline delineates the frontal ostium and we can therefore dissect the bone anterior to the ostium (but not medial) knowing that the dissection is anterior to the skull base (**Fig. 9.15**).

Fig. 9.13 (**A**) This image taken from the computer-assisted surgery (CAS) navigation system shows the very narrow anteroposterior dimension of the frontal sinuses. The *black arrow* on the operative view indicates the relatively large area of bone removed from the forward extending anterior skull base. The only residual mucosa in this newly created frontal ostium is in the posterolateral regions. (**B**) The anterior and posterior free mucosal grafts (*black arrows*) that were put in place at the end of the surgery. (**C**) The frontal ostium after 3 months. The adhesion between the upper and lower grafts is indicated by the *black broken arrow.(continued)*

D

Fig. 9.14 Drawing after creation of the septal window with the middle turbinates (*MT*) and septum (*S*) on view. The *arrow* indicates that the septal perforation needs to be lowered until an instrument can be passed from one side of the nose (in this case the right side) across the septal perforation under the axilla of the opposite middle turbinate (in this case the left).

Fig. 9.13 *(continued)* (**D**) The frontal ostium at 5 years postsurgery with the adhesion indicated by the *black arrow*. This adhesion can be seen in the early postoperative period (**C**), marked by the *broken black arrow*. The patient is currently asymptomatic.

Fig. 9.15 Diagram illustrating the positioning of the frontal cannula (*C*) through the skin of the forehead just medial to the eyebrow into the lumen of the frontal sinus (*FS*). A fronto-ethmoidal cell (*FEC*) and an agger nasi cell (*ANC*) are indicated in the diagram. *MT*, middle turbinate; *UP*, uncinate process.

The computed tomography (CT) scans of both frontal recesses are viewed in three planes and the anatomy of the frontal recess is reconstructed using the building block technique previously described.[27,28] The 3.2-mm cutting burr is used to remove the frontal process of the maxilla directly above the axilla (**Fig. 9.16**). In the initial stages of this dissection the burr is swept from the frontal ostium anterior across the frontal process of the maxilla removing both anterior and lateral bone. This opens the access to the frontal ostium in a funnel shape. This process is analogous to performing a front-to-back mastoidectomy by removing the outer cortical bone and creating a funnel-shaped access to the antrum. As this lateral and superior bone removal continues anterior and superior to the axilla of the middle turbinate a small amount of skin is exposed to define the lateral extent of the dissection.

Dissection is continued superiorly using regular flushes of the fluorescein to identify the anterior lip of the frontal ostium and to allow the bone anterior to the frontal ostium (the bone which forms the frontal "beak") to be removed. Care is taken to ensure that drilling is done in only a superior and lateral direction without drilling medially as this may endanger the skull base. It is important to accurately define the lateral extent of the dissection by exposing a small area of skin. As long as the exposure of the skin is done directly above the axilla of the middle turbinate, the drill will be anterior to the orbit. This dissection is in the same coronal plane as the lacrimal sac and the lacrimal sac may be exposed if bone is removed laterally within 8 mm of the axilla of the middle turbinate. The skin exposure is done bilaterally to define the lateral limits of dissection and to ensure achievement of maximal ostial width. Drilling continues superiorly until the floor of the frontal sinus is entered and the frontal sinus can be seen. Further removal of this floor and

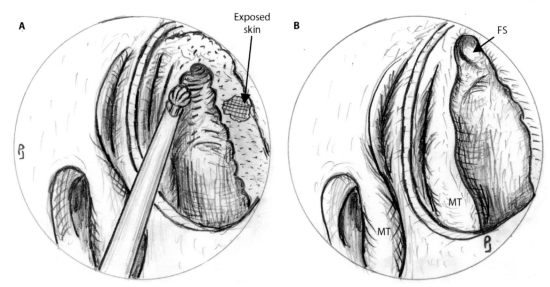

Fig. 9.16 The 3.2-mm cutting burr is used to remove the bone above the axilla of the middle turbinate. (**A**) The anterior wall of the agger nasi cell and the beak of the frontal process of the maxilla are removed until the frontal sinus is entered. Note the small lateral area of exposed skin which marks the lateral extent of the dissection. (**B**) The frontal sinus (*FS*) has been entered. *MT*, middle turbinate.

of the beak of the frontal process of the maxilla (the anterior wall of the dissection) is facilitated by using an angled burr (**Fig. 9.17**). Once the floor of the frontal sinus is opened on one side, the endoscope and drill are transferred into the opposite nostril and the process repeated until the floor of the second frontal sinus is exposed. Note that up until this point no medial dissection has taken place. If the dissection is brought medially before the frontal sinus is entered, the surgeon is likely to damage the forward projections of the olfactory fossae and cause a CSF leak. Once the floor of the frontal sinus is entered the straight burr is usually

changed to an angled burr and the telescope to a 30-degree scope (**Fig. 9.17**).

The dissection is now brought medially from both sides until the frontal intersinus septum is seen (**Fig. 9.18**). Note that this medial dissection takes place at the upper limit of the opening of the frontal sinuses and that drilling in a medial direction lower down can still potentially endanger the skull base. This dissection is alternated from side to side thereby connecting the two frontal sinuses. The last structure to be removed is the intersinus septum. Once this is done the frontal sinus opening is in the shape of a crescent (**Fig. 9.18**).

Fig. 9.17 The frontal sinus (*FS*) has been opened bilaterally. The angled burr is used to remove the "beak" or anterior wall of the frontal sinus further enlarging the frontal ostium.

Fig. 9.18 The medial dissection is done at the upper limits of the opened frontal sinuses as indicated by the *block arrows*. Once the intersinus septum is reached the opening is in the shape of a crescent.

Fig. 9.19 The maximum lateral opening has been created and the bony beak removed until there is a smooth transition from the frontal sinus anterior wall into the nose without bony ridges. The frontal "T" (*FT*) is formed by the junction of the middle turbinates and the septum. An olive-tipped suction pushes the mucosa posteriorly exposing the first olfactory neuron (*black arrow*).

The aim of the surgery is now to transform this crescent opening into an oval opening thereby creating the largest possible anteroposterior (AP) and lateral diameters for the frontal ostium. The first step is to remove the intersinus septum as high as possible, right up to the roof of the frontal sinus. Once this is done the anterior frontal bone is removed until there is no longer an anterior ridge or lip of bone separating the frontal sinus from the nasal cavity. When the anterior table of the frontal sinus is viewed with a 30-degree scope, the transition from the frontal sinus to nasal cavity should be smooth. Any bony ridges should be removed (**Fig. 9.19**).

The final and most dangerous step of the operation is to remove the bone over the forward projection of the skull base. This forward projection forms the frontal "T." The "T" is made up by the two middle turbinates attaching to the septum (**Fig. 9.18**). The frontal sinus intersinus septum, nasal septum, and associated middle turbinates are drilled posteriorly toward the skull base. At the "T" the olfactory fossae project forward from the skull base and great care needs to be taken so that the "T" is lowered as far as possible without exposing the dura of these olfactory projections. These projections can most clearly be seen on the axial scan (**Fig. 9.20**).

Fig. 9.20 (**A–C**) Sequential axial CT scans illustrating the frontal beak (*black arrow*) and the forward projection of the olfactory fossa into the transition area between the frontal recess (**A**) and the frontal sinus (**C**). The skull base is indicated by the *broken white arrows*. For the maximum anteroposterior diameter to be created the bone of the frontal beak should be drilled down to a thin layer and the bone overlying the forward projections of the olfactory fossae (*white arrow*) drilled back as close as possible to the skull base.

Fig. 9.21 This intraoperative photo demonstrates the first olfactory neuron (*ON*) as the mucosa is peeled away from the skull base during widening of the frontal sinus ostium. The intersinus septum (*ISS*) and left middle turbinate (*LMT*) can be seen.

Fig. 9.22 This intraoperative photo illustrates the wide frontal sinus ostium achieved at the end of the endoscopic modified Lothrop procedure. The *black arrow* indicates the frontal sinus septum and the *white arrows* indicate the anterior extensions of the olfactory fossa. Note how the bone over the fossae has been lowered onto the skull base giving an oval-shaped opening rather than a crescent-shaped opening into the frontal sinuses. The *white broken line* indicates the large anteroposterior extent of the frontal ostium. The 4-mm olive-tipped suction is placed in the picture as a size reference.

The position of these forward projections or horns can be identified in two ways. First the image-guidance suction can be used to determine the exact position of these forward projections of the skull base. However, these should always be clinically correlated by sliding a suction Freer elevator between the bone and mucosa in the roof of the nose and gently pushing the mucosa downward. The anterior ethmoidal nerve and first olfactory fibers are easily visible and indicate the most anterior position of the olfactory bulb (**Fig. 9.21**). It is important to clinically correlate findings of the image guidance as the head frame can shift with resultant inaccuracies.

Once the position of the forward projections of the anterior skull base are located, the bone over the anterior skull base is lowered to within 1 mm of the olfactory fibers. This is done either with a diamond burr or with the 3.2-mm straight cutting burr. If a cutting burr is used, the bone should be lightly brushed with the burr spinning at maximum revolutions (12000 rpm). The technique is similar to that used when removing the final bone from the facial nerve during facial nerve decompression. Lowering this forward projection of the olfactory fossa is crucial for the largest possible opening to be created into the frontal sinuses. Failure to remove this projection gives a narrow AP dimension and a crescent-shaped opening which has a greater tendency to stenose. Lowering the bone over the olfactory fossa gives the widest possible AP dimension to the new common frontal sinus ostium (**Fig. 9.22**).

In most patients an oval-shaped frontal sinus ostium is created. The average dimensions should be ~18 mm in the AP plane and 20 to 24 mm from side to side. The size of the opening is determined by the patient's anatomy but should be made as large as possible.

At the end of the procedure, the suction bipolar forceps are used to achieve hemostasis. Particular attention is paid to the posterior edge of the septal window and anterior ends of the middle turbinates. If the middle turbinates are unstable, they are sutured with a dissolving suture through the septum. This allows their lateral surfaces to heal before the suture dissolves and they lateralize. This prevents adhesions from forming.

◆ **Postoperative Care**[12,13,18]

The frontal sinus cannulae are left in place for 3 days. Frontal sinus saline douches are started through the frontal cannulae within 2 hours of completion of the operation. This will wash any blood clot out of the frontal ostium. Saline nasal washes are also performed with the 240-mL squeeze bottle wash four to six times a day. Patients are instructed to place half the bottle through each nostril with the top half of the body parallel to the floor with the head tilted down—this position maximizes frontal sinus penetration. In the last saline wash of the day, one 2-mL ampule of budesonide 1 μg/mL (Pulmicort Respules; AstraZeneca, Wilmington, DE) is added to the saline in the bottle before douching. The Pulmicort wash is continued once daily for a few months postoperatively until the sinuses have healed. Immediately prior to removal of the frontal sinus cannulae, 5 mL of steroid and antibiotic cream (NOT ointment) is injected through each cannula. This coats the newly created frontal sinus ostium and tends to decrease the amount of adherent crusts that form in this region in the postoperative period. The patients are reviewed again at 2 weeks when all crusts, residual cream, and blood clots are meticulously removed from the frontal sinus ostium. This process is crucial because if these adherent clots are left they form the framework into which collagen is laid encouraging fibrosis of the frontal sinus ostium. In our animal model, postoperative douching of the frontal sinus after a MEL procedure tended to improve the mucociliary drainage of the frontal sinuses at 2 and 4 months after surgery.[22] This trend was not statistically significant.

◆ Stenosis of the Frontal Neo-Ostium[23,24]

In both studies done on the sheep animal model and on long-term review of 80 MEL patients, the frontal ostium narrowed to about a third of its original size.[23,24] It was also apparent that this narrowing occurred within the first 12 months after surgery and that thereafter the frontal ostium was stable.[24] The time course of how the frontal ostium narrows is presented in **Fig. 9.23**.

The only significant factor in the patients who eventually developed frontal ostial stenosis was the size of the original ostium at the time of the initial surgery.[24] Other factors such as aspirin sensitivity, fungal sinusitis, and nasal polyposis were found not to influence the development of stenosis. This emphasizes the importance of creating the largest possible opening at the time of the original surgery and underlies the significant effort that is made to create the largest possible opening during surgery (exposure of skin on each side and complete removal of the frontal beak). These results also emphasize the success that the MEL has in the management of patients with these very difficult conditions. One would expect that aspirin triad and fungal sinusitis that aggressively form polyps would develop postoperative stenosis as the high likelihood of polyp regrowth in these conditions would narrow the frontal ostium significantly, necessitating reoperation. In our most recent long-term study with significant follow-up, this was shown not to be the case with these conditions having no statistical influence on the development of postoperative stenosis.[24] It appears that MEL is one operation that can break the ongoing cycle of repeated polyp regrowth and revision surgery. This may be due to the surgeon's ability to remove the fungal mucin from the frontal sinuses and clear the frontal sinus in the office. If the patient is then given a course of prednisolone, the mucosa of the frontal sinus and ethmoids may return to normal. Repeated

suction clearance and prednisolone may be required and as long as the patient is having four or fewer courses of prednisolone every 12 months, this regimen is continued and gives good control of the patient's symptoms. Once the patient requires more than four courses of prednisolone a year, revision surgery is offered.

◆ Results[12,13,18,24]

Our department has published the largest series of MEL procedures to date.[12,13,18,24] The first study[12] involved 83 consecutive patients who underwent the MEL procedure for several indications.[12] Their presenting symptoms and etiology are shown in **Table 9.1**.[12]

Of this group of 83 patients, 6 patients developed stenosis of the frontal ostium and required revision of the MEL procedure. In a subsequent study[24] with significantly longer follow-up, 10 patients out of 80 (12.5%) required revision surgery indicating that the long-term stenosis rate remained low.[24] **Figure 9.24** shows a patient with frontal ostial stenosis.

The patency rate of the frontal ostium after MEL procedure was 93% at 21 months follow-up[12] and in the second study was 87.5% with a mean follow-up of 29.4 months. This second study measured the frontal ostium at surgery and at time intervals after surgery and showed that the size of the frontal ostium remained stable after 12 months. Three patients (4%) continued to deteriorate after 12 months. Thus, the overall incidence of frontal ostium stenosis (12.5%) is low if attention is paid to creating the largest possible frontal sinus opening at the time of surgery. **Figure 9.25** shows three examples of healthy frontal sinus ostia at more than 12 months after the MEL procedure.

As far as symptoms are concerned, the success rate was not as high as the patency rate. There were 21 out of the 83 patients who continued to have symptoms from their sinuses. This is summarized in **Table 9.2**.[12] It should be kept in mind that this group of patients is part of a highly recalcitrant group of patients who have undergone multiple previous operations and often have diseases such as aspirin

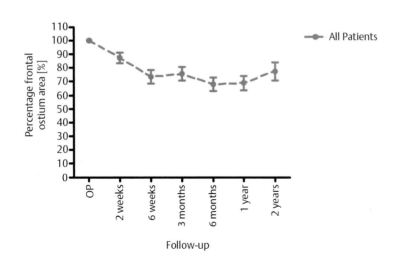

Fig. 9.23 Time course for 80 patients in whom the frontal ostium was measured at the time of surgery and at regular time points in the postoperative period. All patients start with the biggest possible frontal ostium (100%) and each subsequent reading is a percentage of this original measurement. (From Tran K, Beule A, Singhal D, Wormald PJ. Frontal ostium restenosis after the endoscopic modified Lothrop procedure. Laryngoscope 2007; 117(8):1457–1462.)

Table 9.1 Summary of Pathology, Presenting Symptoms, Disease Severity, and Complications of Patients Having Endoscopic Modified Lothrop Procedure

Pathology	n	Preop Frontal Pain	Preop Complications	Mean Lund & Mackay score	No Communication Between Frontal & Nose	Neo-osteogenesis in Frontal Ostium Region
Chronic sinusitis	10	10	1 orbital	1.5	0	7
Chronic fungal sinusitis	16	13	2 intracranial	2	0	3
Allergic fungal sinusitis	8	7	3 intracranial 1 orbital	2	0	0
Nasal polyps	3	3	0	1.5	0	0
ASA and polyps	15	13	0	2	0	0
Mucoceles	8	8	2 orbital	2	8	8
Previous osteoplastic flap with mucocele	17	17	2 intracranial 2 orbital	2	17	17
Frontal osteoma	2	2	0	1.5	0	2
Previous frontal sinus trauma	4	4	1 orbital 1 intracranial 1 CSF leak	1	2	2
Total	83	77	17*	1.72	27	39

*One patient had two and another had three complications.

Abbreviations: ASA, acetylsalicylic acid; CSF, cerebrospinal fluid.

Source: Used with permission from Wormald PJ. Salvage frontal sinus surgery: the Modified Lothrop Procedure. Laryngoscope 2003, 113:276–283.

sensitivity, polyps, and asthma and fungal sinusitis that have high recurrence rates.

Note that there was one CSF leak. This occurred in a patient who underwent drainage of an orbital abscess associated with the superior rectus muscle in an already blind eye. Also

associated with this abscess was a traumatic meningocele extending into the orbit from a fracture in the roof of the orbit. Once the abscess was drained, a flush of CSF was seen. This was repaired using a fat-plug and the "bath-plug" technique. To date there have been no CSF leaks caused during the drillout procedure or during lowering the bone over the projections of the olfactory fossae.

Fig. 9.24 Patient has undergone significant frontal ostium stenosis until the residual ostium (marked with a *black arrow*) is only 2 × 4 mm. This will cause retention of secretions within the frontal sinuses and symptoms and needs to be revised.

◆ Revision Surgery

Revision MEL procedure is conducted along similar lines to the primary surgery. Frontal trephine cannulae are placed early into the frontal sinuses and fluorescein in saline used to delineate the skull base. The frontal ostium is widened by removal of all scar tissue. If the repeat CT scan shows any areas of bone which are still significantly thick, then these are lowered until the maximum sized frontal sinus ostium is created. Postoperative care is similar to what has been described previously except that all patients receive prednisolone drops after every second saline douche. If a circumferential raw area is created, free mucosal grafts are placed in the ostium. We have also found the use of CHITODEX gel* (Medtronic ENT, Jacksonville, FL) to be very helpful in maintaining patency in this group of patients.[29,30] This gel is made up of chitosan and dextran, and it is important to remove all crusts and blood clots at the 2-week postoperative visit. CHITODEX gel has been shown both in vitro and in vivo in human trials to be very successful in preventing scar tissue formation. Failure to properly debride and clean the frontal ostium at this point can lead to the formation of adhesions which may in turn contribute to long-term closure of the frontal ostium.

A, B   C

Fig. 9.25 Three patients post-MEL procedure with oval-shaped frontal ostia and healthy frontal sinuses.

Table 9.2 Summary of the Outcomes of Patients Having Modified Endoscopic Lothrop Procedure

Pathology	n	Intraoperative Complications	Postop Symptoms	Frontal Ostium Closed	Revision Lothrop Surgery	Average Follow-up (months)
Chronic sinusitis	10	0	2 recurrent infections	2	1 at 4 months	22.9
			1 continued frontal pain		1 at 8 months	
Fungal sinusitis	16	0	3 recurrent fungus	1	1 at 7 months	21
			1 continued frontal pain			
Allergic fungal sinusitis	8	0	5 recurrent fungus	3	1 at 6 months	13.1
					2 at 12 months	
Nasal polyps	3	0	0	0	0	33
ASA and polyps	15	0	3 recurrent polyps	0	0	24
			2 recurrent infections			
Mucoceles	8	0	0	0	0	19.3
Previous osteoplastic flap with mucocele	17	0	1 recurrent infections	0	0	23
			3 continued frontal pain			
Frontal osteoma	2	0	0	0	0	23.5
Previous frontal sinus trauma	4	1 CSF leak from meningoenceph-alocele	0	0	0	17.5
Total	**83**	**1**	**21**	**6**	**6**	**21.9**

Abbreviations: ASA, acetylsalicylic acid; CSF, cerebrospinal fluid.

Source: Used with permission from Wormald PJ. Salvage frontal sinus surgery: the Modified Lothrop Procedure. Laryngoscope 2003;113:276–283.

References

1. Casiano RR, Livingston JA. Endoscopic Lothrop procedure: the University of Miami experience. Am J Rhinol 1998;12(5):335–339
2. Becker DG, Moore D, Lindsey WH, Gross WE, Gross CW. Modified transnasal endoscopic Lothrop procedure: further considerations. Laryngoscope 1995;105(11):1161–1166
3. Wormald PJ. The axillary flap approach to the frontal recess. Laryngoscope 2002;112(3):494–499
4. Close LG, Lee NK, Leach JL, Manning SC. Endoscopic resection of the intranasal frontal sinus floor. Ann Otol Rhinol Laryngol 1994;103(12):952–958
5. Alsarraf R, Kriet J, Weymuller EA Jr. Quality-of-life outcomes after osteoplastic frontal sinus obliteration. Otolaryngol Head Neck Surg 1999;121(4):435–440
6. Catalano PJ, Lawson W, Som P, Biller HF. Radiographic evaluation and diagnosis of the failed frontal osteoplastic flap with fat obliteration. Otolaryngol Head Neck Surg 1991;104(2):225–234
7. Draf W. Endonasal micro-endoscopic frontal sinus surgery, the Fulda concept. Oper Tech Otolaryngol Head Neck Surg 1991;2:234–240
8. Gross WE, Gross CW, Becker D, Moore D, Phillips D. Modified transnasal endoscopic Lothrop procedure as an alternative to frontal sinus obliteration. Otolaryngol Head Neck Surg 1995;113(4):427–434
9. Gross CW, Gross WE, Becker D. Modified transnasal endoscopic Lothrop procedure: frontal drillout. Oper Tech Otolaryngol Head Neck Surg 1995;6:193–200
10. Schlosser RJ, Zachmann G, Harrison S, Gross CW. The endoscopic modified Lothrop: long-term follow-up on 44 patients. Am J Rhinol 2002;16(2):103–108
11. Ulualp SO, Carlson TK, Toohill RJ. Osteoplastic flap versus modified endoscopic Lothrop procedure in patients with frontal sinus disease. Am J Rhinol 2000;14(1):21–26
12. Wormald PJ. Salvage frontal sinus surgery: the endoscopic modified Lothrop procedure. Laryngoscope 2003;113(2):276–283
13. Wormald PJ, Ananda A, Nair S. Modified endoscopic Lothrop as a salvage for the failed osteoplastic flap with obliteration. Laryngoscope 2003;113(11):1988–1992
14. Weber R, Draf W, Keerl R, et al. Osteoplastic frontal sinus surgery with fat obliteration: technique and long-term results using magnetic resonance imaging in 82 operations. Laryngoscope 2000;110(6):1037–1044
15. Javer AR, Sillers MJ, Kuhn FA. The frontal sinus unobliteration procedure. Otolaryngol Clin North Am 2001;34(1):193–210
16. Hosemann W, Kühnel T, Held P, Wagner W, Felderhoff A. Endonasal frontal sinusotomy in surgical management of chronic sinusitis: a critical evaluation. Am J Rhinol 1997;11(1):1–9
17. Weber R, Draf W, Kratzsch B, Hosemann W, Schaefer SD. Modern concepts of frontal sinus surgery. Laryngoscope 2001;111(1):137–146
18. Wormald PJ, Ananda A, Nair S. The modified endoscopic Lothrop procedure in the treatment of complicated chronic frontal sinusitis. Clin Otolaryngol Allied Sci 2003;28(3):215–220
19. West B, Jones NS. Endoscopy-negative, computed tomography-negative facial pain in a nasal clinic. Laryngoscope 2001;111(4 Pt 1):581–586
20. Wormald PJ, Chan SZX. Surgical techniques for the removal of frontal recess cells obstructing the frontal ostium. Am J Rhinol 2003;17(4):221–226
21. Lothrop HA. XIV. Frontal sinus suppuration: the establishment of permanent nasal drainage; the closure of external fistulae; epidermization of sinus. Ann Surg 1914;59(6):937–957
22. Rajapaksa SP, Ananda A, Cain T, Oates L, Wormald PJ. The effect of the modified endoscopic Lothrop procedure on the mucociliary clearance of the frontal sinus in an animal model. Am J Rhinol 2004;18(3):183–187
23. Rajapaksa SP, Ananda A, Cain TM, Oates L, Wormald PJ. Frontal ostium neo-osteogenesis and restenosis after modified endoscopic Lothrop procedure in an animal model. Clin Otolaryngol Allied Sci 2004;29(4):386–388
24. Tran K, Beule A, Singhal D, Wormald PJ. Frontal ostium restenosis after the endoscopic modified Lothrop procedure. Laryngoscope 2007;117(8):1457–1462
25. Gross CW. Surgical treatments for symptomatic chronic frontal sinusitis. Arch Otolaryngol Head Neck Surg 2000;126(1):101–102
26. Loehrl TA, Toohill RJ, Smith TL. Use of computer-aided surgery for frontal sinus ventilation. Laryngoscope 2000;110(11):1962–1967
27. Wormald PJ. The agger nasi cell: the key to understanding the anatomy of the frontal recess. Otolaryngol Head Neck Surg 2003;129(5):497–507
28. Wormald PJ. Surgery of the frontal recess and frontal sinus. Rhinology 2005;43(2):82–85
29. Athanasiadis T, Beule AG, Robinson BH, Robinson SR, Shi Z, Wormald PJ. Effects of a novel chitosan gel on mucosal wound healing following endoscopic sinus surgery in a sheep model of chronic rhinosinusitis. Laryngoscope 2008;118(6):1088–1094
30. Valentine R, Athanasiadis T, Moratti S, Robinson S, Wormald PJ. The efficacy of a novel chitosan gel on hemostasis following endoscopic sinus surgery in a sheep model of chronic rhinosinusitis. Am J Rhinol Allergy 2009;23(1):71–75

10 Sphenopalatine Artery Ligation and Vidian Neurectomy

Epistaxis may be classified clinically into anterior and posterior bleeds.[1] If the vascular supply of the nose is reviewed, it is apparent that anterior epistaxis would originate from the vascular anastomosis of vessels around Little's (or Kiesselbach's) area or from the anterior ethmoidal artery. Little's plexus is formed by branches from the sphenopalatine artery (SPA; via the posterior nasal artery branch) anastomosing with branches from the greater palatine, nasolabial (a branch of the facial artery), and anterior ethmoidal arteries. Bleeding from Little's area is usually easily visible and managed by either local cautery or an anterior nasal pack. Bleeding from the anterior ethmoidal artery is rarely spontaneous and usually seen after trauma with associated skull base fractures or intraoperative injury. Posterior bleeding is often seen from under the inferior turbinate where branches of the SPA anastomose with branches from the pharyngeal artery. This area is termed Woodruff's area. Bleeders in this region can be difficult to visualize due to their location under the posterior end of the inferior turbinate. Other posterior bleeders may arise from the lateral nasal wall, posterior choana, or posterior septum.

◆ Postoperative Epistaxis

Significant postoperative epistaxis (as opposed to the blood-stained ooze usually seen in the first 24 hours after nasal surgery) typically occurs when a vessel of significant diameter bleeds. Logically this would be either in the region of the SPA or anterior ethmoidal artery. Intraoperative damage to the anterior ethmoidal artery is almost always visible during surgery and would in most patients need to be dealt with immediately as the resultant bleeding usually obscures the surgical field making further surgery difficult if not impossible. However, vessels divided in the region of the SPA may bleed for a short period of time and then undergo spasm and thrombose. As these vessels are located posteriorly, the blood will drain into the nasopharynx and not come to the notice of

the surgeon who may then not seek out the bleeding vessel and cauterize it. By the time the surgery is completed, the vessel may either be in spasm or thrombosed. If the patient strains or becomes hypertensive in the immediate postoperative period, significant epistaxis can result which may necessitate the placement of a nasal pack or return to theater to cauterize the bleeding vessel. On occasions epistaxis may occur days or even weeks postoperatively. In this situation the patient has likely developed a postoperative infection with increased vascularity and, if the blood clot detaches from the vessel or is dislodged by coughing or straining, epistaxis may result.

To prevent postoperative epistaxis, close inspection of the region of the SPA is performed at the end of surgery. Particular attention is paid to the region of the horizontal insertion of the ground lamella into the lateral nasal wall especially if the ground lamella has been resected and to the lateral nasal wall in the superior meatus (**Fig. 10.1**). In addition, close inspection is made of the anteroinferior region of the sphenoid at the lower edge of the sphenoidotomy. If the sphenoid has been widely opened then the posterior nasal artery or its vertical branch may have been divided (**Fig. 10.1**). Bipolar cautery is applied with the suction bipolar forceps* (Medtronic ENT, Jacksonville, FL) until the field is dry. If the patient is still hypotensive at this stage the anesthesiologist is asked to raise the blood pressure into the normal range before the patient is awakened. During this time this region is inspected regularly on both sides and any vessels that bleed as the pressure is raised are cauterized.

Comorbidities for Spontaneous Epistaxis

The majority of patients (69%) presenting with severe epistaxis have associated comorbidities.[1] These usually include hypertension, cardiovascular disease, and clotting abnormalities. Over 60% of patients managed in our series were either on aspirin or on warfarin as part of their ongoing medical treatment.[1] As the effects of aspirin and aspirin-like

Fig. 10.1 (**A**) The vessels branching from the sphenopalatine artery (*SPA*) commonly bleed after endoscopic sinus surgery. Branches supplying the horizontal portion of the ground lamella (*HGL*) and the anterior wall of the sphenoid (posterior nasal artery [*PNA*]) need to be cauterized using a suction bipolar at the end of surgery to ensure that no bleeding occurs in the postoperative period. (**B**) Cadaveric image on the right side demonstrating the SPA, within the pterygopalatine fossa, giving off the PNA. This branch runs along the anterior face of the sphenoid and can be inadvertently transected during sphenoidotomy. *PE,* posterior ethmoid cell; *ST,* superior turbinate; *SO,* sphenoid ostium; *MT,* middle turbinate.

drugs are not immediately reversible, no specific treatment is given for these clotting abnormalities. However, in patients who are on warfarin, this is stopped and, if necessary, a transfusion of fresh frozen plasma is given to rapidly lower the international normalized ratio (INR; below 2) before proceeding to surgery.

◆ Indications for Sphenopalatine Artery Ligation

Before SPA ligation is considered, it needs to be established that the bleeding is coming from the posterior region of the nose. Patients who are assessed for possible SPA ligation are asked to forcefully blow their nose to expel all blood clots from the nose. The nose is then sprayed with a combination of lidocaine and epinephrine. The patient keeps their head forward after the nose blowing thereby allowing blood to drip into a kidney dish held below the nose. A rigid nasal endoscope and suction are then passed into the nose to assess where the bleeding is coming from. If the vessel is clearly visible, cautery is attempted.[2] If the vessel in not visible but bleeding is confirmed to be posterior, then an inflatable or expanding posterior nasal pack is placed and the patient is prepared for surgery.

Surgical Technique (Videos 31 and 32)

This procedure can be performed under either local anesthetic or general anesthetic. The first step is to put the bleeding vessel into spasm. A pterygopalatine block is placed transorally. The greater palatine canal is located by palpation

of the hard palate. A finger is passed along the hard palate until the junction of the hard and soft palate is felt. The finger is slowly slid anteriorly along the midpoint between the midline and teeth. The depression created by the greater palatine foramen is felt. This is usually opposite the second molar tooth (**Fig. 10.2**).[1,3]

With the finger still on the mucosal depression an endoscope is slid into the mouth and the location of the depression endoscopically confirmed. The finger is then removed while the endoscope position is maintained. A 2-mL syringe with 1:80 000 lidocaine and adrenaline is attached to a 25-gauge needle that has been bent at 25 mm from the tip at a 45-degree angle. The detailed anatomy of the greater palatine canal is presented in Chapter 2. The greater palatine canal is, on average, 18 mm long and the overlying soft tissue has an average depth of 7 mm. Therefore, bending the needle at 25 mm ensures that the needle does not enter the pterygopalatine fossa for any significant distance.[3] This lessens the risk of damage to the maxillary nerve or artery by the needle. The foramen and canal are located with the tip of the needle and the needle slid up into the canal to the bend. After aspiration has been performed, 2 mL of lidocaine and adrenaline are injected. Spasm of the SPA with cessation of active bleeding was achieved in all the patients in our published series who were actively bleeding at the time of surgery.

The nasal cavity is decongested using the combination of cocaine and adrenaline-soaked neuropatties. The lateral wall of the nose anterior to the posterior end of the middle turbinate is infiltrated with lidocaine and adrenaline. A right-angled suction is used to palpate the membranous posterior fontanelle of the maxillary sinus and the junction of the vertical portion to the palatine bone. Once the palatine bone is identified a U-shaped incision is made onto bone (**Figs. 10.3** and **10.4**). The incision is started under the

Fig. 10.2 (A) The location of the left greater palatine canal is indicated with a solid black arrow. A blood stain from the pterygopalatine injection is visible in this region. The second molar tooth is indicated with a *broken black arrow*. **(B)** The posterior edge of the hard palate is indicated with a *solid white arrow*. This is the first landmark. The finger is slid anteriorly until the depression of the greater palatine canal is felt (*broken white arrow*).

Fig. 10.3 (A) The right angled curved suction palpating the posterior fontanelle of the maxillary sinus. **(B)** The U-shaped incision extending from the inferior surface of the horizontal part of the middle turbinate to just above the insertion of the inferior turbinate. **(C)** Cadaveric dissection with right-angled ball probe palpating the posterior fontanelle (*PF*). *MT*, middle turbinate.

Fig. 10.4 (**A**) A suction Freer elevator is used to elevate the mucosal flap in the subperiosteal plane keeping the initial dissection low, just above the insertion of the inferior turbinate, until the anterior face of the sphenoid is reached. As the dissection is taken superiorly the ethmoidal crest (*EC*) and sphenopalatine artery (*SPA*) are seen. (**B**) A cadaveric image of a U-shaped incision from the middle turbinate to just above the inferior turbinate. This image clearly identifies the suture between the maxilla and the palatine bone (*S*). (**C**) Further dissection with the posterior maxillary sinus wall removed revealing the sphenopalatine artery (*SPA*) within the pterygopalatine fossa (*PPF*). The ethmoid crest (*EC*) is seen directly anterior to the sphenopalatine foramen (*SPF*). *MT*, middle turbinate; *IT*, inferior turbinate; *PT*, posterior fontanelle.

horizontal portion of the ground lamella, down the palatine bone, and continued along the insertion of the inferior turbinate posteriorly.[1]

The suction Freer elevator is used to elevate the mucosal flap. It is important to establish the subperiosteal plane at the point of incision as this allows a relatively bloodless dissection and also allows the periosteum to be stripped off the underlying bone in a manner similar to that used in raising a subperichondrial flap during a septoplasty. The initial elevation is done in the inferior region of the flap just above the insertion of the inferior turbinate on the lateral nasal wall (**Fig. 10.4A,C**).[1]

Keeping the dissection low initially keeps the surgeon under the SPA. This dissection should be carried posteriorly until the anterior face of the sphenoid is reached. This is an important landmark as it allows the surgeon to be sure that the dissection has been carried far enough posterior before the dissection is taken superiorly. As the flap is lifted superiorly, the SPA is visualized exiting the sphenopalatine foramen. It is tented by the flap (**Fig. 10.5**).[1]

An additional landmark that can be sought is the ethmoidal bony process/crest of the palatine bone.[4,5] This bony projection is seen directly anterior to the sphenopalatine foramen (**Figs. 10.4** and **10.5**). It can be curetted away to improve visualization of the foramen. The artery is contained within the tissues exiting the foramen. Dissection with the suction Freer elevator is performed above the pedicle and the artery identified within the pedicle (**Fig. 10.5**). Once it is clearly delineated, two Ligar clips are placed on the artery. Care should be taken to ensure that the clip is placed all the way across the pedicle. The artery may divide before exiting the foramen and it is not uncommon for there to be a posterior branch exiting the foramen behind the anterior branch.[5] This posterior branch may exit through its own foramen in up 16% of patients.[5] This branch (called the posterior nasal artery) travels across the posterior choana to the posterior aspect of

A

B

Fig. 10.5 **(A)** The flap is elevated superiorly and the sphenopalatine artery (*SPA*) is tented as it exits the sphenopalatine foramen. The ethmoidal crest (*EC*) of the palatine bone has been curetted to further expose the sphenopalatine foramen (*SPF*) and SPA. **(B)** The U-shaped mucosal flap has been elevated in a mucoperiosteal plane, and the contents of the sphenopalatine foramen (*SPF*) have been dissected demonstrating the nasopalatine nerves (*NPN*) and the SPA.

the septum to supply the majority of the blood to the septum (**Fig. 10.1**). Endoscopic Ligar clip applicators should be used as they are easier to manipulate in the posterior region of the nasal cavity. The Ligar clip should be placed across the pedicle and the front of the clip applicator pushed until it touches the anterior face of the sphenoid. As the clip is closed the tips are moved slightly anterior to the sphenoid face so that they do not rub against the bone during closure. If, despite this maneuver, the clip does not sit properly across the pedicle then further dissection may be needed before more clips are applied. When the pedicle is first exposed, there is too great a volume of tissue to be clipped and the vessels should be dissected out and clipped individually. A malleable suction Freer elevator or standard suction Freer elevator can be of value for this as the pedicle tends to ooze during this dissection before the clip is applied. Continuous suction through the instrument allows dissection to continue despite any oozing of blood. Clipping is recommended in spontaneous epistaxis as the caliber of the SPA is large in these patients and bipolar cautery alone may not be as effective. However, the vessel is usually cauterized after clipping to make sure no bleeding results if the clip is dislodged during the dissection for the posterior nasal artery (PNA). The PNA is sought in all patients as it may significantly contribute to a spontaneous posterior bleed and, if not sought, may contribute to failure of the procedure. Such dissection may dislodge the clip from the SPA and, if the artery had not been cauterized in addition to being clipped, may result in a significant bleed that can be difficult to manage. Once the PNA is identified it is cauterized with the suction bipolar. It is difficult to clip as it sits on the anterior face on the sphenoid and so the clip will often not sit over the vessel properly. The mucosal flap is replaced and held in place by a 2 × 2 cm piece of fibrillar Surgicel (Ethicon, Somerville, NJ). This is used because a considerable proportion of patients are either on aspirin or warfarin and it helps control oozing from the incision. No other packing is placed in the nose. The patient is discharged soon after recovery if no further bleeding is noted.

Results

In a recently published series of 13 consecutive patients,[1] four patients underwent SPA ligation under local anesthetic and nine under general anesthetic. The four who had local anesthetic were considered to be at risk if given general anesthetic. The average age was 55.9 years (range 23–79) with an approximate equal sex distribution (males, seven; females, six). All patients presented with intractable posterior epistaxis and underwent SPA ligation. One patient developed further epistaxis during the 12-month follow-up period resulting in a 92% primary success rate in the treatment of the epistaxis.[1] The patient who rebled was on aspirin and had a platelet abnormality with widespread ecchymosis on his arms and legs.

To date a further 26 patients have undergone SPA ligation in our department. Similar incidences of comorbidities and anticoagulation were seen. The success at 12-month follow-up remains in the region of 90%.

Bleeding From a Large Vessel in the Nose or Sinuses

A spurting artery in the region of the frontal recess will usually indicate damage to the anterior ethmoidal artery. The region should be packed with neuropatties soaked in adrenaline and cocaine. After waiting several minutes, the area can be checked. If the bleeding is from the skull base or from the region of the orbital periosteum associated with the skull base, suction bipolar cautery can be used to control the bleeding. Unipolar diathermy should not be used as it can arc to exposed dura and cause a cerebrospinal fluid (CSF) leak. If the bleeding is from the medial region of the frontal recess, Surgicel and Gelfoam (Pharmacia and Upjohn Company, Kalamazoo, MI) soaked in thrombin should be placed over the artery and the area firmly packed. Our preference is to use ribbon gauze soaked with bismuth, iodoform, and paraffin paste (BIPP). This allows pressure to be placed over the Gelfoam and Surgicel. The BIPP gauze can be removed after a day or two. Cautery (bipolar or unipolar) should be avoided as there is a significant risk that any cautery (higher risk with unipolar) may burn a hole through the dura and cause a CSF leak.

Arterial spurting from the region of the SPA should be controlled with suction bipolar forceps* (Medtronic ENT). If this is not available, a pterygopalatine fossa block will usually put the vessel in spasm and allow bipolar diathermy (without suction) to be used to control the bleeder (Chapter 2). Arterial bleeding is usually from the posterior nasal artery or the SPA (**Fig. 10.1**).

Key Points

The management of intractable epistaxis can either be with a nasal pack and postnasal balloon or ligation of the artery. If packing is used the balloon will usually occlude the nasopharyngeal airway.[6] In elderly patients this may produce hypoxic episodes which may in turn precipitate fatal arrhythmias.[7-10] The alternative to endoscopic SPA ligation is ligation of the maxillary artery through a Caldwell Luc approach.[11-13] Although this has a good success rate (87–90%), there are significant coassociated morbidities, with cheek and teeth pain and paresthesia being the most common (28%).[11-13] The nonsurgical option of management is to embolize the bleeding vessel.[13] Again, this is usually a successful procedure but has significant associated comorbidities including hemiplegia, facial pain, facial paraesthesia, ophthalmoplegia, and blindness.[11,13] The overall complication rate of this procedure is 29%. The advantages of endoscopic SPA ligation is that it can be done under either local or general anesthetic, it is relatively quick and straightforward with minimal associated comorbidity, and has a good success rate. Our policy is that the nose should not be packed after the procedure and, if possible, the patient should be discharged from the hospital within 12 hours of the procedure. This dispenses with the need to keep patients in the ward with a packed nose, resulting in a better utilization of hospital resources.

◆ Vidian Neurectomy

Vidian neurectomy was established by Golding-Wood in the 1960s for the management of intractable vasomotor rhinitis, allergic rhinitis, and for nasal polyposis.[14] The vidian nerve supplies the nasal cavity with parasympathetic secretomotor fibers and sectioning of this nerve was found to improve symptoms of rhinorrhea, sneezing, postnasal space discharge, and nasal obstruction.[14-16] The initial enthusiasm for this technique was tempered by recurrence of symptoms after a 2-year follow-up and by complications. The surgical technique for severing the nerve has varied[14-16] and, in some cases, the nerve was never accurately identified before it was either cut or cauterized.[16] It is interesting that even though there have been several reports regarding the success of this technique over many years[13-18] in the management of chronic rhinorrhea and in some cases of nasal polyposis, that this technique has not been widely adopted. One of the reasons for this may be the lack of a reliable and safe surgical technique for identifying and sectioning the nerve.

The Anatomy of the Vidian Canal

The vidian canal connects the foramen lacerum with the pterygopalatine fossa, and is formed just anterior to the foramen lacerum where the carotid artery turns vertically up toward its vertical segment in the sphenoid sinus. The greater superficial petrosal nerve and fibers from the sympathetic plexus around the carotid artery join to form the vidian nerve which then enters the vidian canal just anterior to the foramen lacerum. To aid understanding of the course of the vidian canal a series of coronal computed tomography (CT) scans are presented starting in the foramen lacerum and progressing forward allowing the vidian canal to be identified and followed anteriorly and slightly medially to where the canal opens in a funnel fashion into the pterygopalatine fossa (**Fig. 10.6**). If the parasagittal CT scan of this region is viewed the vidian canal can be clearly seen traversing the floor of the sphenoid sinus into the pterygopalatine fossa (**Fig. 10.6**).

Understanding the anatomy of the vidian canal is very important in the endoscopic management of tumors infiltrating the pterygopalatine fossa and particularly in the management of juvenile nasopharyngeal angiofibromas (JNA). JNA tend to track down the vidian canal and widen the canal toward the carotid artery. If this is not looked for both on the imaging and during surgical removal of JNA, residual tumor can be left in the canal and may form the nidus for tumor regrowth. **Figure 10.7** demonstrates the anatomical relationship between the vidian canal, the pterygopalatine fossa, and the carotid artery. This dry bone dissection illustrates the relationship between the vidian canal, floor of the sphenoid sinus, and carotid artery (**Fig. 10.7**). In this specimen the carotid artery has been exposed. The vidian canal can be seen as it travels along the floor of the sphenoid from the vidian canal foramen to the paraclival carotid artery.

Figure 10.8 illustrates the palatovaginal canal and how this can be confused with the vidian canal if their close relationship is not recognized.

Surgical Technique (Video 32)

The nasal preparation and injection of the pterygopalatine fossa through the mouth is performed as previously described (Chapter 2). The mucosal incisions for vidian neurectomy

Fig. 10.6 (**A–I**) The series of coronal CT scans begin with scan (**A**) through the foramen lacerum (*white arrow*) and, as the scans move anteriorly (**B–H**), the Vidian canal can be followed along the floor of the sphenoid (*white arrows*) into the pterygopalatine fossa (**G,H**). *(continued)*

are the same as for SPA ligation. The artery is localized and cauterized with the suction bipolar diathermy forceps. Cautery is preferred as the clips tend to slip off or are knocked off as the surgery progresses to the area behind the sphenopalatine foramen. The SPA is significantly larger in patients with active epistaxis than in patients undergoing elective surgery

(vidian neurectomy) and therefore bipolar cautery is effective for obtaining hemostasis in the latter cases.

Once the SPA foramen is identified, the mucosal flap is raised behind the foramen until the face of the sphenoid sinus is identified (**Fig. 10.9**). One of the first structures seen as this flap is elevated is the posterior pharyngeal nerve

Fig. 10.6 *(continued)* Note the foramen rotundum (**G**, *black arrow*) and the infraorbital fissure (**H**, *black arrow*). (**I**) A parasagittal scan of the Vidian canal from the foramen lacerum to the pterygopalatine fossa (*white arrow*). Note how the canal funnels outward as it enters the fossa.

emanating from the pterygopalatine ganglion and running superficial to the vidian canal laterally into the palatovaginal canal (PVC). This nerve can easily be mistaken for the vidian nerve (**Fig. 10.9**). The posterior pharyngeal nerve travels through the PVC (**Fig. 10.9**) and then onto the pharynx to provide sympathetic and parasympathetic fibers to this region (**Fig. 10.9**).

If a successful vidian neurectomy is to be performed it is vitally important to understand the relationship between the PVC and the vidian canal. These two canals both transmit sizable nerves and both travel along the floor of the sphenoid sinus, emanating from the anterior aspect of a widening vidian canal as it approaches the pterygopalatine fossa and are separated by only a few millimeters. Important differences allowing accurate identification of each of these structures are the more medial position of the PVC, the relatively smaller nerve passing through the PVC, and the significantly smaller diameter of the PVC compared with the vidian canal (**Figs. 10.9** and **10.10**).

The posterior pharyngeal nerve is divided and the anterior face of the sphenoid is identified and perforated with a Freer elevator (**Fig. 10.11A**). This opening is enlarged until a clear view into the sphenoid sinus is obtained and the floor of the

sphenoid sinus is identified. This gives certainty regarding the horizontal location of the vidian canal as it always runs along the floor of the anterior aspect of the sphenoid sinus (**Fig. 10.8**). The key landmark is the palatine bone. If a line is drawn vertically up the posterior aspect of the palatine bone and another drawn through the floor of the sphenoid sinus, the intersection of these two lines marks the vidian canal (**Fig. 10.10**). Check the coronal CT scans in **Fig. 10.6** and the cadaver dissection in **Fig. 10.9** to confirm this.

To expose the vidian canal the posteroinferior margin (sphenoidale process of the palatine bone) of the spheno-palatine foramen needs to be removed (**Fig. 10.12M**). This is best done with either a straight through-biting Blakesley forceps or a forward biting 2-mm Kerrison punch. This will remove the medial wall of the pterygopalatine fossa and allow the vidian canal to be clearly identified. In some patients this bone can be thick and difficult to remove and can be removed with a dacryocystorhinostomy diamond burr. Note that the periosteum overlying the pterygopalatine fossa is still intact and if this is torn the yellow fat within the fossa should be visible. This should be expected and should not be confused with orbital fat. Removal of the posteroinferior wall of the sphenopalatine foramen will allow identifica-

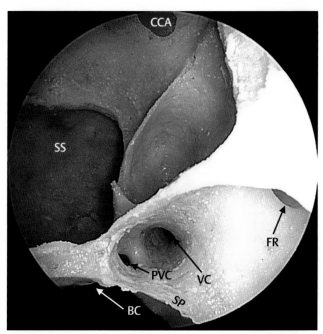

Fig. 10.7 (**A**) This dry bone image of the sphenoid sinus within the body of the sphenoid. It clearly demonstrates how the vidian canal (*VC*) communicates with the pterygopalatine fossa (*PPF*) anteriorly and the foramen lacerum posteriorly. The vidian canal runs in the floor of the sphenoid sinus, and frequently has a sphenoid sinus septation (*S*) attaching to the roof of the canal. The foramen lacerum is the location of the supralacerum genu of the carotid artery, where the horizontal petrous carotid artery turns upward to become the paraclival carotid artery (*PCA*). The vidian canal and nerve is a vital landmark in surgical dissection in this area. *PF*, pituitary fossa; *FR*, foramen rotundum; *CCA*, anterior genu of the cavernous carotid artery.

Fig. 10.8 This dry bone specimen has had the sphenoidale process (*SP*) of the palatine bone drilled (the posterior bony contribution to the sphenopalatine foramen). This allows visualization of the palatovaginal canal (*PVC*) and vidian canal (*VC*), both running along the floor of the sphenoid sinus (*SS*) and emanating at the anterior face of the sphenoid sinus. Note the more medial position of the PVC, and the smaller diameter when compared with the VC. Also note the gutter formed from the SP and indicated underlying the letter VC as this forms the floor as the vidian canal widens as it enters the pterygopalatine fossa. *FR*, foramen rotundum; *BC*, bony choana; *CCA*, anterior genu of the carotid artery.

Fig. 10.9 (**A**) The anterior face of the sphenoid sinus (*SPH*) is exposed and the outline of the sinus marked (*SSO*) with *dotted lines*. The palatovaginal canal (*PVC*) is seen with the posterior pharyngeal branch of the pterygopalatine ganglion entering the canal. (**B**) Cadaveric picture of the sphenoid sinus (*SS*) opening that has been maximized down to the floor of the sphenoid. The sphenopalatine foramen is made up of the sphenoidale process (*SP*) and the orbital process (*OP*) of the palatine bone, and drilling these allows wide exposure of the medial contents of the pterygopalatine fossa. The pharyngeal nerve (*PN*) is the first nerve visualized and is the most medial nerve, running to the pterygopalatine ganglion (*PPG*). Just lateral to this the vidian nerve (*VN*) can also be seen joining the PPG. *GPN*, greater palatine nerve; *VA*, vidian artery.

Fig. 10.10 (**A**) Freer elevator is used to perforate the anterior face of the sphenoid sinus just above the floor of the sinus. This opening is enlarged and a clear view into the sphenoid sinus obtained so that the floor of the sphenoid sinus (*FSS*) can be clearly seen. (**B**) A line is drawn in continuation with the posterior margin of the palatine bone (*PBL*).

tion of the floor of the funnel-shaped opening of the vidian canal. This floor forms a "gutter" in which the vidian nerve runs (see **Fig. 10.9**). A sickle knife is used in the subperiosteal plane to slide from the removed edge of the foramen along the "gutter" to the lateral wall of the funnel-shaped opening of the vidian canal. Once this maneuver has been performed the vidian nerve lies directly above the sickle knife.

A sickle knife is again used to stay on the bone of the anterior face of the sphenoid above the vidian canal and to continue this subperiosteal dissection over the vidian nerve until the lateral aspect of the canal is identified. The fat of

Fig. 10.11 The posteroinferior region of the SPA foramen (sphenoidal process) needs to be removed to identify the vidian canal (*block arrow*).

the pterygopalatine fossa is exposed and the sickle knife is used to probe the fat and expose the vidian nerve. Note that the nerve is large (3–4 mm in diameter). Also note that the vidian canal travels directly posteriorly toward the vertical part of the carotid artery. If there are additional septations within the sphenoid sinus these septations will in most cases attach to the roof of the vidian canal in the floor of the sphenoid sinus (providing an additional landmark; **Fig. 10.7**). The nerve is usually immediately visible after it exits the vidian canal at the level of the floor of the sphenoid sinus. It is dissected free until it is seen to move laterally toward the pterygopalatine ganglion in the pterygopalatine fossa (**Figs. 10.9** and **10.12**).

Extensive lateral dissection can allow the maxillary nerve to be visualized but this not recommended for the standard vidian nerve section (**Fig. 10.12**). Once the nerve is identified, confirmation that it is the vidian nerve is made by following the nerve into the vidian canal. This canal runs in an anteroposterior direction and the nerve can be visualized exiting the canal. The normal procedure to cut the nerve is to either use the sickle knife with the tip tracking subperiosteally along the gutter until the nerve sits in the natural curve of the sickle knife and then to cut upward or to use a curved skull base scissors* (Medtronic ENT) angled from medial to lateral to cut the nerve. A 2- to 3-mm section of the nerve is removed and the remaining nerve exiting the vidian canal is cauterized with bipolar diathermy. Unipolar diathermy is not recommended as the infraorbital canal and maxillary nerve are in relative close proximity and damage can occur with injudicious usage of unipolar diathermy in this region. Optic nerve injury has also been described after blind attempts were made to cauterize the vidian nerve. Therefore we advocate clear visualization and positive identification followed by section of the nerve and bipolar diathermy of the nerve root (**Fig. 10.13**). To ensure that the nerve has been

A

B

Fig. 10.12 **(A)** The vidian nerve is seen exiting the vidian canal running toward the sphenopalatine foramen before moving laterally toward the maxillary nerve in the pterygopalatine fossa. Cadaver dissection **(B)** shows more extensive dissection. The superior third of the clivus and the planum sphenoidale have been drilled and dura removed, along with exposure of the junction between the lateral sphenoid wall and the pterygopalatine fossa. The floor of the sphenoid sinus has been drilled up to the vidian nerve (VN). The VN can be visualized running slightly laterally, after it exits the vidian canal, to join the pterygopalatine ganglion (PPG), as opposed to the pharyngeal nerve (PN) which runs in a lateral direction to join the PPG. The PPG can be seen to hang medially off the maxillary nerve just after it exits the skeletonized foramen rotundum (FR). IT, inferior turbinate; LCM, longus capitis muscle; PCC, paraclival carotid artery; CCA, anterior genu of the cavernous carotid artery; SPF, sphenopalatine foramen; GPN, greater petrosal nerve.

cut, 360 degrees of bone must be visible around the vidian canal with the cut nerve end clearly visible in the canal. Once this is achieved the mucosal flap is replaced. If it tends to fall away from the lateral nasal wall a small piece of Gelfoam is placed under the middle turbinate over the flap to hold it in place. No other packing is placed in the nose.

Fig. 10.13 The vidian nerve (VN) has been cut and the entire bone of the vidian canal (VC) around the nerve can be seen. The stump of the nerve should then be cauterized with a bipolar forceps. The pharyngeal nerve (PN) and fat of the pterygopalatine fossa can be seen.

Results[19]

Over the past 5 years, nine patients have undergone 14 operations. The mean follow-up was 25 months. Most of the patients suffered intractable rhinorrhea (80%) with nasal obstruction (72%), postnasal drip (64%), and sneezing (57%) also prominent. Postoperatively there was a significant improvement in rhinorrhea and nasal obstruction at the last follow-up (mean > 2 years). In three patients there was a worsening of sneezing postoperatively. In addition, 35% of patients suffered a variable amount of dry eye and 28% had nasal crusting. Half of the vidian neurectomies were deemed to be highly successful by the patients at a mean follow-up time of 2 years.[19]

Key Points

Vidian neurectomy has been shown to result in significant histologic changes in the nasal mucosa including mast cell depletion.[20] The exact mechanism by which vidian neurectomy results in improvement in symptoms postoperatively is unknown. As most previous studies have not histologically confirmed the sectioning of the nerve, there may be patients who have not actually had their vidian nerve sectioned but have been included among patients who have undergone vidian neurectomy. A significant amount of research on the outcomes after vidian nerve neurectomy needs to be performed before the role of vidian nerve neurectomy in endoscopic sinus surgery is properly defined.

References

1. Wormald PJ, Wee DTH, van Hasselt CA. Endoscopic ligation of the sphenopalatine artery for refractory posterior epistaxis. Am J Rhinol 2000; 14(4):261–264

2. Sharp HR, Rowe-Jones JM, Biring GS, Mackay IS. Endoscopic ligation or diathermy of the sphenopalatine artery in persistent epistaxis. J Laryngol Otol 1997;111(11):1047–1050

3. Mercuri LG. Intraoral second division nerve block. Oral Surg Oral Med Oral Pathol 1979;47(2):109–113

4. Snyderman CH, Goldman SA, Carrau RL, Ferguson BJ, Grandis JR. Endoscopic sphenopalatine artery ligation is an effective method of treatment for posterior epistaxis. Am J Rhinol 1999;13(2):137–140

5. Wareing MJ, Padgham ND. Osteologic classification of the sphenopalatine foramen. Laryngoscope 1998;108(1 Pt 1):125–127

6. McGarry GW, Aitken D. Intranasal balloon catheters: how do they work? Clin Otolaryngol Allied Sci 1991;16(4):388–392

7. Jacobs JR, Dickson CB. Effects of nasal and laryngeal stimulation upon peripheral lung function. Otolaryngol Head Neck Surg 1986;95(3 Pt 1): 298–302

8. Shaheen OH. Epistaxis in the Middle Aged and Elderly. Thesis, London: University of London

9. El-Guindy A. Endoscopic transseptal sphenopalatine artery ligation for intractable posterior epistaxis. Ann Otol Rhinol Laryngol 1998;107(12): 1033–1037

10. Papsidero MJ. The role of nasal obstruction in obstructive sleep apnea syndrome. Ear Nose Throat J 1993;72(1):82–84

11. Metson R, Lane R. Internal maxillary artery ligation for epistaxis: an analysis of failures. Laryngoscope 1988;98(7):760–764

12. Premachandra DJ, Sergeant RJ. Dominant maxillary artery as a cause of failure in maxillary artery ligation for posterior epistaxis. Clin Otolaryngol Allied Sci 1993;18(1):42–47

13. Strong EB, Bell DA, Johnson LP, Jacobs JM. Intractable epistaxis: transantral ligation vs. embolization: efficacy review and cost analysis. Otolaryngol Head Neck Surg 1995;113(6):674–678

14. Golding-Wood PH. Observations on petrosal and vidian neurectomy in chronic vasomotor rhinitis. J Laryngol Otol 1961;75:232–247

15. Kamel R, Zaher S. Endoscopic transnasal vidian neurectomy. Laryngoscope 1991;101(3):316–319

16. Fernandes CM. Bilateral transnasal Vidian neurectomy in the management of chronic rhinitis. J Laryngol Otol 1988;102:894–895

17. Greenstone MA, Stanley PJ, Mackay IS, Cole PJ. The effect of vidian neurectomy on nasal mucociliary clearance. J Laryngol Otol 1988;102(10): 894–895

18. Krajina Z. Critical review of Vidian neurectomy. Rhinology 1989;27(4): 271–276

19. Robinson SR, Wormald PJ. Endoscopic vidian neurectomy. Am J Rhinol 2004; In press

20. Konno A, Togawa K. Vidian nerve neurectomy for allergic rhinitis. Arch Otorhinolaryngol 1979;225:67–77

11 Powered Endoscopic Dacryocystorhinostomy

Endoscopic dacryocystorhinostomy (DCR) was initially described by Caldwell in the 19th century.[1] However, it fell into disrepute as surgeons experienced problems with visualization of the surgical site. In the early 20th century, Toti described the external DCR procedure and, with a few modifications, this procedure remains largely unchanged from those early descriptions.[2] As the technique has developed, so the success rate for the external procedure has improved until today, in the hands of properly trained oculoplastic surgeons, success rates of between 90 and 95% can be expected.[3] As endoscopic sinus surgery (ESS) became popular in the late 1980s, there was renewed interest in endoscopic DCR with the initial descriptions having appeared in the late 1980s and early 1990s.[4–6] As could be expected of a new and developing technique, the initial success rates were lower than that of external DCR and varied between 65 and 90%.[4–6] Laser endoscopic DCR was promoted in the mid 1990s but success rates were disappointing and tended to be at the lower end of the spectrum (around 75%).[7–9] This was probably due to the technique creating only a small opening into the posterior inferior lacrimal sac through the thin lacrimal bone. It is well recognized within the literature on external DCR that a small ostium does not achieve the same success rates as a large opening of the lacrimal sac.[10]

The original endoscopic DCR technique was described as follows: a mucosal flap anterior to the middle turbinate was raised and the junction between the lacrimal bone and frontal process of maxilla established. A Hajek Koffler punch was used to remove what bone one could over the lacrimal sac.[4] In the early 1990s, I reviewed my own results with this technique and found a disappointing long-term patency rate of only 83%.[11] On review of the literature on external DCR, the critical factor necessary for achieving the 90 to 95% success rate was a wide bone removal so that the entire lacrimal sac was exposed.[10,12–14] Following this the mucosa of the lacrimal sac and nasal mucosa were anastomosed with sutures allowing primary intention healing without significant granulation. This raised the question—could the external DCR technique be duplicated by a similar intranasal technique? If this were to be done the first step was to define the intranasal anatomy of the lacrimal sac.[13] The early descriptions of the intranasal anatomy of the sac placed the sac anterior to the middle turbinate with minimal extension of the sac above the insertion of the middle turbinate on the lateral nasal wall (the so-called axilla of the middle turbinate as it resembles an armpit).[13,15,16] To investigate the precise location of the sac, a series of computed tomography (CT) dacryocystograms (DCGs) in patients undergoing DCR were performed and the relationship of the lacrimal sac and the axilla of the middle turbinate evaluated.[13] This study showed that the anatomy of the sac on the lateral nasal wall was significantly different to what had been previously described in the literature (**Fig. 11.1**). The sac was not only anterior to the middle turbinate but a significant proportion was located above the axilla of the middle turbinate. On average the sac extended 8 mm above the axilla of the middle turbinate.[13] Therefore, if the external DCR principles were to be applied to endoscopic DCR, a different technique was required. This led to the design of a new technique (powered endoscopic DCR) which is presented in the following text.[14,17,18]

◆ Preoperative Assessment of the Patient Presenting with Epiphora

Examine the Eye and Look for Other Causes of Watery Eye

Excess Tear Production

- *Conjunctival disease.* Patients with conjunctivitis present with sticky secretions or pus in the eye that is often worse when they awake in the morning. Antibiotic eye drops are used to treat bacterial infections and prevent colonization in patients with viral conjunctivitis.

Fig. 11.1 The *broken line* indicates the location of the sac prior to our studies on the intranasal anatomy of the lacrimal sac. The *shaded area* is the actual intranasal position of the lacrimal sac on the lateral nasal wall. Note it extends between 8 and 10 mm above the axilla of the middle turbinate.

- *Dry eye.* Patients may have significant dryness that will irritate the eye and produce tearing. Application of artificial tears is usually all that is necessary.
- *Lid malposition.* Ectropion or entropion cause the puncta to not be properly positioned in the tear lake. A floppy lower eyelid (increased lid laxity) may also place the puncta in a position where tear collection is impaired. Surgical repositioning or tightening of the lid is required.
- *Blepharitis.* Blepharitis causes a mucoid discharge from the eye. In this condition there is an alteration in the bacteriology of the mucous glands in the hair follicles of the eyelashes that results in a mucoid discharge from the eye. The vision will be blurred and the eye often burns. Treatment is to rub the eyelid margin with gauze soaked in warm soapy water twice a day. This will need to be done for ~3 months before the condition resolves.

Epiphora

- *Punctal stenosis.* Obliteration or narrowing of the superior or inferior punctum.
- *Canalicular stenosis or obstruction.* Superior or inferior canalicular stenosis or obstruction may follow trauma or viral infection.
- *Nasolacrimal duct blockage.* Usually from unknown cause.

Nasolacrimal Duct Obstruction

In epiphora caused by nasolacrimal duct obstruction (NLDO), tears will frequently run down the cheek. This is more noticeable in conditions that stimulate tear formation such as walking in a cold wind. During examination, the position and size of the puncta should be assessed. The lid laxity and

Fig. 11.2 **(A)** A soft stop is felt as the probe rests against a common canaliculus stricture or obstruction whereas in **(B)** a hard stop is felt as the probe comes to rest against the bone encasing the lacrimal sac.

positioning of the puncta in the tear lake should be determined. To assess the patency of the inferior, superior, and common canaliculi, the upper lacrimal system should be probed (**Fig. 11.2**). The punctum is dilated with a punctum dilator. A Bowman's lacrimal probe is then used to probe the inferior canaliculus and common canaliculus.

Differentiating between a soft and a hard stop on probing helps assess the patency of the canalicular system. If a common canaliculus stricture is present, it should be diagnosed preoperatively so appropriate steps can be taken to correct it during surgery. Additionally, the patient can be informed that the likelihood of a successful procedure is significantly less than is the case with a DCR performed for nasolacrimal duct obstruction.

Syringing of the lacrimal system will also help assess the patency of the nasolacrimal system. In NLDO there will be significant reflux through the upper punctum with no saline penetration into the nose. In partial NLDO there will be reflux through the upper punctum with saline penetration into the nose but only with increased syringing pressure. Penetration into the nasal cavity without reflux through the upper punctum indicates a patent (but not necessarily functional) lacrimal system. It is sometimes confusing to determine exactly where the saline is refluxing as some may reflux from the punctum that has been injected, or from the other punctum or a combination.

Examine the Nasal Cavity

Rigid nasal endoscopy is performed on all patients presenting with epiphora. A significant proportion (15%) of patients require surgery for nasal pathology at the same time as the DCR. Mostly this is for associated chronic sinusitis. All patients need to be questioned regarding nasal symptoms and endoscopy performed to assess the nasal cavity. If there is evidence of nasal and sinus disease, appropriate investigations are performed and treatment instituted. If medical therapy fails to resolve the problem, surgery is performed at the same time as the DCR.

Dacryocystogram and Lacrimal Scintillography

We routinely perform a DCG to assess the patency of the canalicular system and penetration of dye into the nasolacrimal sac.[17] If the patient has a hard stop on probing with a blocked

Fig. 11.3 Right nasolacrimal duct (NLD) obstruction with reflux through the superior punctum into the conjunctiva with patent left NLD system.

Fig. 11.4 Obstruction of the left common canaliculus–sac junction with reflux of dye into the conjunctival region.

system on syringing, this investigation can be omitted. Filling of the sac but failure of the dye to penetrate the nasal cavity confirms the diagnosis of NLDO (**Fig. 11.3**).

Patency of the NLD system without reflux through the canalicular system normally indicates an anatomically patent system (left side, **Fig. 11.3**). Failure of the dye to penetrate the lacrimal sac may indicate a common canalicular obstruction (**Fig. 11.4**).

To assess the function of the NLD system, lacrimal scintillography is performed. DCG assesses anatomy but not function. A radioisotope is placed in the conjunctival fornix and regular scanning performed for 30 minutes. If the isotope penetrates the lacrimal sac and not the nasal cavity, NLDO exists (**Fig. 11.5**).

In some patients the DCG may show no filling of the lacrimal sac, whereas scintillography shows filling of the sac (**Fig. 11.6**). This may occur when the sac is full of mucus and the distended sac kinks the common canaliculus just before it enters the sac.

Scintillography also helps identify a functional obstruction when the DCG is normal (patent) in a symptomatic patient. If the scintillography confirms lack of nasal cavity

penetration of the isotope, then a functional NLDO exists (**Fig. 11.7**). These patients can be managed by performing an endoscopic DCR but the outcome is not as successful as with anatomical obstruction of the NLD system (see results of functional NLDO).

◆ Surgical Technique[14,17–19] (Videos 33 and 34)

After nasal decongestion with neuropatties and infiltration with lidocaine and adrenaline, a no. 15 scalpel blade is used to make the initial mucosal incisions. It is important that these incisions are correctly placed as they form the borders for the subsequent bone removal and lacrimal sac exposure. The first incision is made horizontally 8 to 10 mm above the axilla of the middle turbinate, starting ~3 mm posterior to the axilla and coming forward ~10 mm onto the frontal process of the maxilla (bony prominence in the lateral nasal wall just anterior to the middle turbinate). The blade is then turned vertically and a vertical incision made to about two-thirds of the vertical height of the middle turbinate, stopping just above the insertion of the inferior turbinate into the lateral nasal wall (**Fig. 11.8**). The blade is turned horizontally

A

B

Fig. 11.5 DCG shows nasolacrimal duct obstruction (NLDO) on the right side. The scintillography shows penetration of the radioisotope on the left into the nasal cavity but shows holdup on the right with no nasal cavity penetration. This confirms the diagnosis of NLDO.

Fig. 11.6 Obstruction of left common canaliculus on DCG with radioisotope penetrating the lacrimal sac on scintillography indicating likely distention of sac kinking common canaliculus–sac junction.

Fig. 11.7 If the left side is examined on the DCG the system appears normal. However, on the scintillography although the sac fills nicely with radioisotope, no penetration of the nasal cavity occurs. Later time points need to be checked to ensure that this continues to be the case. This is an anatomical obstruction of the nasolacrimal system on the right side and a functional obstruction on the left side.

Fig. 11.8 (**A**) Mucosal incisions 8 to 10 mm above and anterior to the axilla of the middle turbinate. (**B**) Cadaveric dissection demonstrating the horizontal and vertical incisions. The horizontal superior incision is made 8 to 10 mm above the axilla of the middle turbinate (MT), and started 3 mm behind the axilla of the MT, and continued 10 mm in front. The vertical incision is continued for two-thirds of the MT height. (**A** adapted with permission from Wormald PJ. Powered endoscopic DCR. Otolaryngol Clin North Am 2006;39:539–549.)

and the inferior incision is started at the insertion of the uncinate process and brought forward to meet the vertical incision (**Fig. 11.9**).

Using a 30-degree endoscope a suction Freer elevator is used to elevate the mucosal flap while ensuring that the tip of the instrument always maintains contact with the bone (**Fig. 11.10**). Be particularly careful to keep the tip of the suction Freer on bone as it rides over the prominence of the frontal process of the maxilla as the bone contour can fall away abruptly and contact with the bone and surgical plane can be lost. At this point the bone should be palpated so that the junction of the soft lacrimal bone and hard bone of the frontal process can be identified (**Fig. 11.10C**). This is a key landmark and must be sought in all primary surgeries. Note that the lacrimal bone is sought at the bottom of the region from which the mucosal flap has been raised, just above the insertion of the inferior turbinate. The thin lacrimal bone is 2 to 5 mm wide before the insertion of the uncinate process is reached (**Fig. 11.11**). Dissection stops at the uncinate and the uncinate insertion should not be disturbed. A round knife (from the standard ear tray of

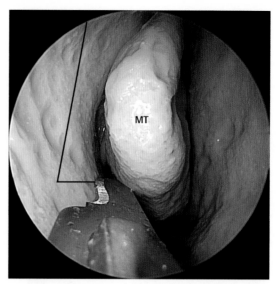

Fig. 11.9 Cadaveric image of left nasal cavity demonstrating the inferior horizontal incision. This incision begins from the insertion of the uncinate process (*UP*) forward to meet the vertical incision.

Fig. 11.10 (A) Illustrates elevation of the flap with a suction Freer elevator. Note the round knife removing the thin lacrimal bone in the inferior region of the dissection. The cadaveric photo (**B**) shows the suction Freer hard against the frontal process (*FP*), elevating the mucoperiosteal flap. (**C**) At the junction where the hard frontal process can fall away to become the soft lacrimal bone (*LB*), care must be taken when elevating in this region. *MT*, middle turbinate. (**A** adapted with permission from Wormald PJ. Powered endoscopic DCR. Otolaryngol Clin North Am 2006;39: 539–549.)

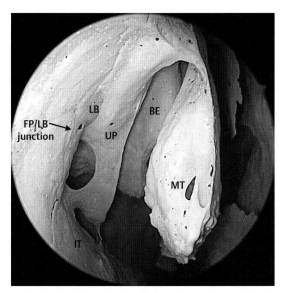

Fig. 11.11 Dry bone image demonstrating the junction between the hard frontal process (*FP*) and soft lacrimal bone (*LB*). The common boundary shared between the lacrimal bone and the uncinate process (*UP*) can be clearly visualized. *IT*, inferior turbinate; *MT*, middle turbinate; *BE*, bulla ethmoidalis.

instruments) is used to flake the soft lacrimal bone away from the posteroinferior region of the sac. If this is difficult, the frontal process can be removed first before the lacrimal bone is flaked away.

Once the lacrimal bone has been removed, a forward biting Hajek Koffler punch is used to remove the lower portion of the frontal process of the maxilla (**Fig. 11.12**). The tip of the punch is used to push the lacrimal sac away before the punch is engaged and the bone is removed. The lacrimal sac may be inadvertently grasped as the punch is closed. The punch should be opened after the initial bite to allow any sac wall that may have been pinched in the jaws of the punch to be released.

After this maneuver the punch is closed over the loose bone and this bone removed. This avoids tearing the sac with the punch. Bone removal continues both anteriorly and superiorly until the punch can no longer be seated on the bone. Removal of the frontal process of the maxilla uncovers the anteroinferior portion of the lacrimal sac (**Fig. 11.12**), and only stops when the bone becomes too thick for the punch to engage. At this point a 25-degree curved 2.5-mm rough diamond burr (Medtronic ENT, Jacksonville, FL) is attached to the microdebrider and used to remove the rest of the bone up to the superior mucosal incision (**Fig. 11.13**). In the vast majority of cases an agger nasi cell is present and the mucosa of this cell will be exposed as the sac is followed superiorly above the axilla of the middle turbinate (**Fig. 11.12B**). The diamond burr can be brought into light contact with the lacrimal sac lining without damaging the sac. Significant pressure by the diamond burr on the sac will cause damage. A cutting burr will remove the bone faster; however, it does cause significant damage to the sac wall and will often result in a hole in the sac wall. The bone is removed until the entire sac is exposed. The sac should stand proud of the lateral nasal wall so that when the sac is incised and the mucosal flaps are rolled out, they will lie flat on the lateral nasal wall (**Fig. 11.13**). Thus the sac will be marsupialized into the wall rather than an ostium being created in the sac.

Next the inferior punctum is dilated with a punctum dilator and a Bowman's lacrimal probe is passed into the sac (**Fig. 11.14**). When the probe is moved up and down in the sac its tip should be able to be seen moving behind the sac wall. This confirms that the probe is indeed within the sac (**Fig. 11.15**). Movement of the sac without visualization of the tip of the probe usually indicates that the probe is still at the common canaliculus-sac junction and the lateral wall is being pushed onto the medial wall with some movement of the medial wall. Cutting down on the probe, if it is not in the sac lumen, can result in damage to the common canaliculus opening. With the tip of the probe visible through the sac wall, a DCR spear knife* (Medtronic ENT) is used to make a vertical incision as far

Fig. 11.12 (**A**) A cadaveric image of the right side showing removal of the bone of the frontal process (*FP*) of the maxilla by Hajek Koffler punch (lower end) and DCR diamond burr (upper end). (**B**) The exposure of the lacrimal sac (*LS*) with exposure of the agger nasi cell (*AN*) mucosa. *MP flap*, mucoperiosteal flap.

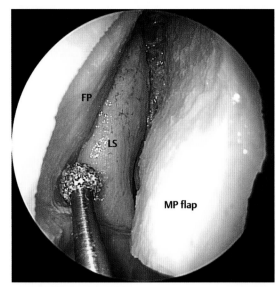

Fig. 11.13 Cadaveric photo of the right side demonstrating further exposure of the lacrimal sac (*LS*) by drilling the frontal process (*FP*) of the maxilla superiorly. *MP flap*, mucoperiosteal flap.

posteriorly as possible through the sac wall (**Fig. 11.15**). This results in the largest possible anterior flap. The tip of the spear knife is pushed into the tented sac wall just underneath the region of the probe and the sac wall is opened using a rotating motion (**Fig. 11.15**). Do not place the entire blade of the spear knife into the sac but rather cut with the anterior two-thirds of the blade. The sac is slit from top to bottom. The DCR minisickle knife* (Medtronic Xomed) is used to make upper and lower releasing incisions in the anterior flap so that the flap can be rolled out on the lateral nasal wall (**Fig. 11.16**).

Three millimeter soft tissue scissors from the skull base set (Medtronic ENT) are used to make upper and lower releasing incisions in the posterior flap and this flap is also rolled out (**Fig. 11.16**). The sac should now be completely marsupialized and lie flat on the lateral nasal wall.

To determine the width of the mucosal flaps, the amount of raw bone above and below the sac is estimated. The

original mucosal flap is repositioned over the opened sac so that the areas of raw bone can be measured up against the original flap. Once the width of flap is determined, the flap is trimmed with a pediatric through-biting Blakesley forceps leaving the upper and lower limb of this flap the same thickness as the exposed bone above and below the marsupialized sac (**Fig. 11.17**). Most of the middle section of the original flap is removed to allow the posterior wall of the flap and mucosal edge of the mucosal flap to be approximated. The posterosuperior region of lacrimal and nasal mucosa is difficult to approximate because the middle turbinate holds the nasal mucosal flap away from the sidewall. In this region the agger nasi cell is opened and the mucosa from this cell approximated to this region of the lacrimal mucosa. This results in a U-shaped flap and the surgeon should aim to achieve approximation of lacrimal and nasal mucosa superiorly, posteriorly, and inferiorly. This mucosal flap can be difficult to fashion with standard through-biting Blakesley forceps so the pediatric Blakesley forceps are kept for DCR surgery alone and only used on this flap. This keeps them sharp and allows the mucosa to be cut without tearing of the mucosa and losing the flap. Approximating the lacrimal and nasal mucosa should result in a first intention healing rather than a secondary intention healing and should reduce the formation of granulation tissue and scarring and therefore lessen the potential risk of closure of the sac and failure of the surgery (**Fig. 11.18**).

Next the tightness of the common canaliculus is evaluated by placing a Bowman's canalicular probe through the common canaliculus and the probe is visualized entering the sac through the common canaliculus. If the common canaliculus holds the probe tightly then lacrimal tubes should be placed to dilate the common cannaliculus.[20] If the probe passes easily through the common canaliculus and is not firmly gripped then no tubes are placed. If the gripping of the probe is equivocal then tubes are placed in patients with functional NLDO and not placed in patients with anatomical NLDO. For placement of tubes the puncta are dilated and silastic lacrimal intubation tubes (O'Donoghue tubes) are placed through the upper and lower puncta and retrieved

A, B   C

Fig. 11.14 Cadaveric images of the right lower eyelid. (**A**) The punctum dilator has been passed into the inferior punctum. (**B**) When passing the dilator, and then the lacrimal probe, it is important to first pass the probe 90 degrees to the lower eyelid. (**C**) Then the probe is rotated parallel with the lower lid and inserted until the probe tip is seen within the lacrimal sac.

A, B

C

Fig. 11.15 (**A**) Bowman's lacrimal probe tenting the flap to facilitate incision with the DCR spear knife. Cadaveric dissection demonstrating the lacrimal probe (*LP*) tenting (**B**) the lacrimal sac (*LS*), and DCR spear knife incision (**C**) posteriorly to allow for the largest anterior lacrimal flap. This incision should be made along the posterior third of the tented sac wall to ensure the largest possible anterior flap. (Adapted with permission from Wormald PJ. Powered endoscopic DCR. Otolaryngol Clin N Am 2006;39: 539–549.)

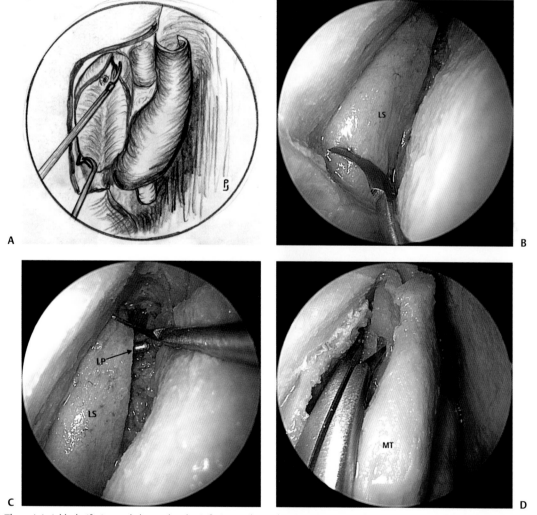

A

B

C

D

Fig. 11.16 (**A**) The mini-sickle knife is used the make the inferior and superior releasing incision on the anterior mucosal flap to allow the flap to be rolled out onto the frontal process of the maxilla. The superior and inferior releasing incisions are cut in the posterior flap with the scissors from the skull base set. Cadaveric dissection images showing the mini-sickle knife being used to perform the inferior (**B**) and superior (**C**) releasing incision on the anterior lacrimal flap, with superior and inferior incision on the posterior flap performed with skull base scissors (**D**). *LS*, lacrimal sac; *MT*, middle turbinate; *LP*, lacrimal probe. (**A** adapted with permission from Wormald PJ. Powered endoscopic DCR. Otolaryngol Clin North Am 2006;39:539–549.)

A

B

Fig. 11.17 (A) The mucosal flap is trimmed with the pediatric through-biting forceps. The superior and inferior mucosal flaps are matched to the raw bone above and below the opened lacrimal sac (*block arrows*). The agger nasi cell (*ANC*) mucosa is exposed and opened to allow apposition in this area. **(B)** Cadaveric dissection image demonstrating the trimming of the mucosal flap (*MF*) centrally to allow for raw bone coverage superiorly and inferiorly. This allows mucosal apposition between the posterior (*PLF*) and anterior lacrimal sac mucosa to the nasal mucosal and primary intention wound healing. (**A** adapted with permission from Wormald PJ. Powered endoscopic DCR. Otolaryngol Clin N Am 2006;39:539–549.)

endosnasally (**Fig. 11.19A**). A square of Gelfoam (Pharmacia and Upjohn Company, Kalamazoo, MI) is slid over the tubes into the nasal vestibule (**Fig. 11.19B**). A spacer of silastic tubing is slid over the tubes and used to push the Gelfoam onto the mucosal flaps (**Fig. 11.19C,D**). This spacer is ~10 mm long and 4 mm in diameter. This tubing acts as a spacer below which Ligar clips are placed to secure the tubes (**Figs. 11.19D and 11.20**). Before placing the clips ensure a loop of tubing is pulled in the medial canthus of the eye so that the tubes are not tight (**Fig. 11.21**). If the loop is tight the tubes can cheese-wire through the puncta.

Before cutting the silastic tubes a square of MeroGel (Medtronic ENT) is slid up the tubing and placed over the flaps to hold them in position. The silastic tubing is cut and the Gelfoam/MeroGel gently lifted off the flaps and the position of the flaps checked before it is replaced (**Fig. 11.22**). The postnasal space is cleared of blood.

◆ Postoperative Care

Saline nasal spray is started within 3 to 4 hours of surgery. This aids in clearing any residual blood clots and keeping the nasal cavity moist and clear of secretions. Gentle blowing of the nose is allowed without closing the nasal vestibule. The patient is placed on broad-spectrum antibiotics for 5 days and antibiotic eye drops are used for 3 weeks. If O'Donoghue tubes were placed, they are removed in the clinic after 4 weeks and the patency of the nasolacrimal system checked by placing a drop of fluorescein in the conjunctiva and endoscopically monitoring the flow of fluorescein from the conjunctiva to the nose. It is rare to see any granulations but if they are present they should be removed. The patient is reviewed for a further 18 months before discharge.

◆ Results

The results of this technique have been published in peer-reviewed journals.[14,17–22] When discussing the success rate of DCR it is important to clearly define "success." In many

Fig. 11.18 Cadaveric dissection image on the right side showing both the anterior (*ALF*) and posterior (*PLF*) lacrimal flaps opened and lying along the lateral nasal wall. Apposition of the mucosal flap (*MF*) with the lacrimal sac mucosa, both anterior and posterior lacrimal flaps, can be seen. *MT*, middle turbinate.

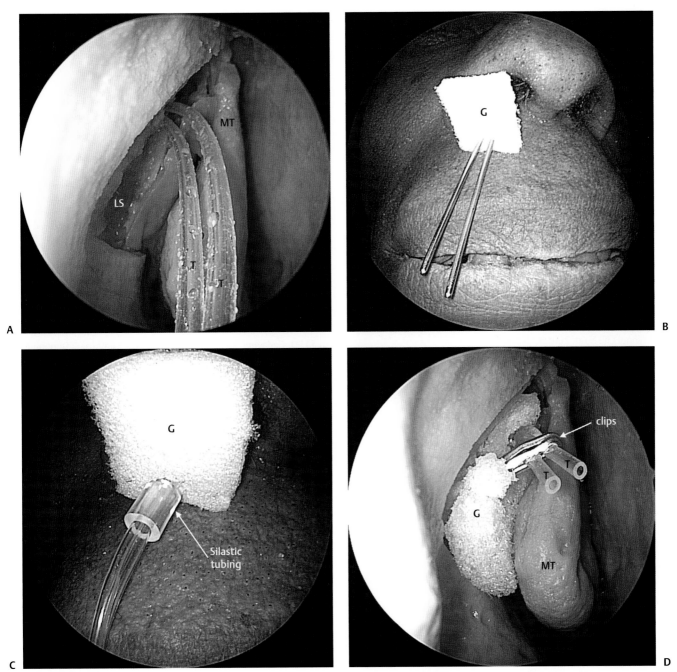

Fig. 11.19 Cadaveric dissection images taken on the right side. O'Donoghue lacrimal intubation tubes (*T*) have been passed through the superior and inferior canaliculus, then through the common canaliculus, the nasal cavity (**A**), and then the right nostril (**B**). (**C**) The lacrimal tubes (*T*) are passed through a small square of Gelfoam (*G*) followed by a 10-mm piece of 4-mm silastic tubing. (**D**) The silastic tubing and Gelfoam are then passed up into the middle meatus so that the Gelfoam square secures the lacrimal flaps and mucosal flap into position. Ligar clips are then placed below the silastic tubing to hold the Gelfoam in position.

previous studies "success" has been defined as either a symptomatic improvement, a complete absence of symptoms, or as an anatomically patent nasolacrimal system after surgery. For a DCR to be called successful both criteria (symptoms and anatomical patency) need to be fulfilled: the patient should be completely asymptomatic and there should be an endoscopically confirmed patent nasolacrimal system. The lacrimal sac should be marsupialized and well healed forming

part of the lateral nasal wall (**Fig. 11.23A**). Once fluorescein has been placed in the conjunctiva it should be visualized immediately in the marsupialized sac (**Fig. 11.23B**).

One of the recent published series included 162 consecutive DCRs with a minimum follow-up of 12 or more months.[18] Patients who had a nonfilling lacrimal sac on DCG which may suggest a common canaliculus problem but had otherwise normal canaliculi were included. Only patients who had a

Fig. 11.20 Placement of the silastic O'Donoghue lacrimal intubation tubes with a silastic sleeve space and Ligar clips to hold the tubes in place. The superior and inferior mucosal flaps are indicated with black arrows. (Adapted with permission from Wormald PJ. Powered endoscopic DCR. Otolaryngol Clin N Am 2006;39:539–549.)

Fig. 11.21 Cadaveric image of the right medial canthus. O'Donoghue lacrimal intubation tubes (*T*) have been placed through the superior (*SP*) and inferior puncta (*IP*). Care is taken to ensure that tubes are not positioned too tight, making eye opening difficult.

3 to 4 mm long obliteration of the common canaliculus on both DCG and probing were excluded. There were four patients who were excluded for significant common canaliculus stenosis/obstruction. Patients who have a nonfilling lacrimal sac on DCG may have a large or distended lacrimal sac which may cause the common canaliculus to kink at its insertion to the sac. These patients can be successfully managed with an

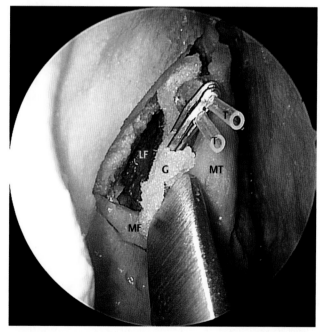

Fig. 11.22 Cadaveric dissection image of the right side demonstrating that the Gelfoam square (*G*) is lifted and the position of the lacrimal (*LF*) and mucosal flaps (*MF*) are checked after the O'Donoghue tubes (*T*) have been cut. *MT*, middle turbinate.

endoscopic DCR. To examine the results of this technique the patients were divided into those who underwent a primary DCR (no previous surgery), revision DCR, and those who filled the criteria for a pediatric DCR (less than 10 years old).

Results in Primary DCR[14,17,18,20,21]

In one of the larger series[18] with 162 patients, 126 were primary DCRs, 19 revision DCRs, and 18 pediatric DCRs. In the primary DCR group, there were 115 patients who had a successful outcome (90%). Of the 11 patients considered failures, six had an anatomically patent nasolacrimal system with a free flow of fluorescein from the conjunctiva to the nose (such as demonstrated in **Fig. 11.23B**). This gives an anatomical patency rate of 96% (121/126). However, symptomatic patients are still classified as failures even if the surgery was technically successful. The primary DCR patient group can be further divided into anatomical or functional obstruction according to their preoperative investigations (DCG and scintillography). In the anatomically obstructed group the success rate was 95% whereas in the functional group it was 81%. This functional group still had a 95% anatomical patency but a few patients with a patent system still had symptoms and were therefore classified as failures. If success is defined as complete absence of symptoms with anatomical patency, functional obstruction of the lacrimal system does not have as good a prognosis as anatomical obstruction and this should be kept in mind when consenting patients with functional obstruction. An important caveat to this is that all patients who had residual postoperative symptoms in the functional group stated that the symptoms were significantly improved after the DCR.

A B

Fig. 11.23 (**A**) Lacrimal sac marsupialized into the lateral nasal wall in a patient that had ESS. (**B**) Fluorescein seen draining freely into the opened lacrimal sac.

Results and Technique Modifications in Revision DCR[14,17,18] (Video 35)

There were 19 revision DCRs performed in this series. The success rate was 83% but increased to 89% with a second revision operation. The surgical technique for revision DCR is the same as for primary DCR with a few minor modifications. A variably sized bony ostium was created at the time of the primary DCR. The sac remnant may be significantly smaller and scarred than is the case with a primary DCR and this may make the creation of nasal mucosa and lacrimal sac mucosa apposition more difficult. The initial mucosal incisions are still placed as previously described with the reservation that the anterior vertical incision must be placed anterior to the previously created bony ostium. In other words the anterior vertical incision must be placed onto bone. If you are unsure of the anterior limit of the previous bony ostium, palpate the frontal process of the maxilla. Start anteriorly on the frontal process and move posteriorly until the junction of the hard bone and soft ostium can be palpated. Once the initial mucosal incisions have been made, use the suction Freer elevator to elevate the mucosal flap from the bone anteriorly, above and below the previous bony ostium. The plane of the already elevated mucosa should be continued posteriorly using a scalpel. Sharp dissection is necessary as the mucosa is attached to the underlying sac by fibrous tissue. Once the mucosal flap is raised, bony removal and the rest of the DCR technique is as previously described.

Results and Technique Modifications in Pediatric DCR[14,17-23]

In the most recent series there were 21 consecutive pediatric DCRs. The success rate was 92%. Patients included in this group were under the age of 14 years. In the pediatric age group, especially the patients in the 18 months to 6 year age group, there are important anatomical differences that the surgeon needs to be aware of. The nasal vestibule is much smaller and there can be some initial difficulty getting a 4-mm endoscope and an instrument in the nasal cavity simultaneously. The same sized scopes and instruments are used for the pediatric and adult endoscopic DCRs with the exception of the Hajek Koffler punch which is replaced by a 2-mm Kerrison forward biting punch. However, as surgery continues, the nasal vestibule stretches and its narrowness was never more than an initial concern. The other anatomical variation is the underdevelopment of the turbinates with a relatively small vertical height of the nasal cavity. This puts the axilla of the middle turbinate in relative close proximity to the skull base and increases the risk to the skull base. The initial mucosal incisions remain similar to those described in adults and the superior incision is still placed ~8 mm above the axilla. This will be just below the skull base in a 2-year-old so the surgeon must be aware of this proximity while removing bone from over the sac. The remainder of the procedure is the same as was previously described. Pediatric DCR is a very successful operation with 100% anatomical success rate in our series[20] (patency of the lacrimal ostium on endoscopy). However, only 92% of these patients were completely symptom free.[20] The postoperative management for patients younger than 10 years of age is different to that previously outlined. We electively do a postoperative evaluation under general anesthesia after 4 weeks. The intranasal lacrimal ostium is evaluated and the O'Donoghue tubes are removed. There may be granulations around the ostium especially on the anterior wall as this is the region where lacrimal and nasal mucosa are most difficult to approximate and there is often a little exposed bone after draping of all

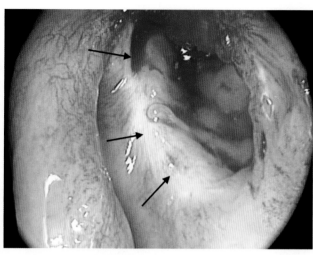

A

B

Fig. 11.24 **(A)** The lacrimal ostium after 4 weeks in an 18-month-old patient with granulations on the anterior lip of the ostium (*black arrows*). **(B)** The lacrimal ostium after removal of these granulations. The posterior region of primary intention healing without granulation tissue is marked with *black arrows*. The patient continued to heal well and was asymptomatic at follow-up.

the mucosal flaps (**Fig. 11.24**). These granulations should be removed and this region should subsequently heal well. In some patients there may be minor adhesions between the lateral nasal wall and septum and these are also divided. This occurs because the nasal cavity is small and we do not perform a septoplasty unless there is significant septal deviation. In those patients with significant septal deviation, a Killian's incision is performed and the septum mobilized from the maxillary crest and from the bony septum. No cartilage or bone is excised. This mobilization is usually sufficient and allows surgery to proceed in the previously obstructed nasal cavity. Mobilization without tissue resection also lessens the risk of disturbing the septum's further growth and consequently altering facial features.

◆ Rationale for the Insertion of O'Donoghue Tubes[20]

O'Donoghue tubes are placed after endoscopic DCR if the common canaliculus is tight and this is done in an attempt to dilate the common canaliculus opening into the lacrimal sac. The tubes are not placed in an attempt to keep the sac open as the sac is so widely marsupialized with lacrimal and nasal mucosa apposition it would be unnecessary. The aim of the O'Donoghue tube insertion is to dilate the common canaliculus opening by placing silastic tubes for 4 weeks. Over many years of observing the Bowman's lacrimal probe entering the lacrimal sac it was apparent that the mucosal fold that forms the valve of Rosenmüller can be tight and that this may contribute to symptoms in some patients. It did not make sense to create a large lacrimal ostium but fail to address a potential more proximal obstruction. We have recently done research into placement of tubes only in those patients in whom the common canaliculus was tightly gripping the Bowman probe and found that the success rate in patients with a loose common canaliculus did not change whether tubes were placed

or not.[20] We do think it more likely in patients who, on DCG, do not have penetration of the dye into the sac but on scintigraphy have penetration of the radioisotope into the sac. We also found that in functional nasolacrimal obstruction we have a lower threshold for placing tubes as these patients have a lower success rate and the common canaliculus may be contributing to this. The radioisotope has more time to slowly penetrate the valve then the dye does and may indicate a tight common canaliculus opening. In **Fig. 11.25** we present two examples of tight valves of Rosenmüller and it can clearly be seen how the mucosal fold grips the end of the probe.

◆ Ancillary Procedures

Septoplasty was necessary in 47% of patients. This was done endoscopically through a Killian's incision. The area of obstructing septal deflection directly adjacent to the anterior end of the middle turbinate was removed whereas the anterior cartilage was kept intact. In 15% of patients ESS was necessary for ongoing nonresponsive chronic sinusitis or nasal polyposis.

◆ Complications

Complications in powered endoscopic DCR are very rare. There were three cases of postoperative hemorrhage giving a complication rate of 1.9%. No other complications occurred. Serious complications can occur if the surgeon loses anatomical landmarks. These include damage to the orbit and orbital contents and damage to the anterior cranial fossa with a cerebrospinal fluid (CSF) leak. If the landmarks described previuosly are kept in mind and the surgeon stays anterior to the insertion of the uncinate, penetration of the orbit is unlikely. Dissection posterior to the uncinate, however, will usually result in orbital fat exposure. Should this

Fig. 11.25 **(A)** In the first patient, the common canaliculus grips the single O'Donoghue tube tightly. **(B)** The tip of the probe is tightly held by the valve. **(C)** In the second patient, the silastic tube and probe are tightly held by the valve and **(D)** the two tubes are seen to dilate the valve.

occur it should be left alone and not manipulated in any way. As the bone is removed above the middle turbinate the mucosa of the agger nasi cell will be exposed. The diamond burr should be kept in contact with the bone directly above the sac and bone removal should continue to the mucosal incision. If there is any doubt as to exactly which part of mucosa is sac wall and which is skin or agger nasi cell mucosa, a DCR light pipe* (Medtronic ENT) is introduced into the sac and the sac transilluminated. If the surgeon stays in close proximity to the sac while removing the bone the likelihood of damage to the skull base with a subsequent CSF leak is very small.

◆ Key Points

It is beneficial when starting to do endoscopic DCRs that the sinus surgeon develops a close liaison with an ophthalmologist.[11] Both have expertise in different areas and the

combination of this expertise helps in both the workup for surgery and during the surgical procedure. Our team consists of an ENT surgeon and an oculoplastic surgeon. We assess patients together in the lacrimal clinic. The oculoplastic surgeon helps with the assessment of other causes of epiphora such as blepharitis, entropion, ectropion, lid laxity, etc. and will be able to teach the sinus surgeon how to syringe and probe the lacrimal system. The sinus surgeon is able to endoscopically assess the nasal cavity, septum, and any ancillary sinus disease that may be present. At surgery the sinus surgeon has the endoscopic skills to deal with the septum and expose the lacrimal sac. The oculoplastic surgeon has the expertise in probing the lacrimal system and passing O'Donoghue tubes and dealing with lid laxity, entropion, or ectropion. Both surgeons should learn to be comfortable with all aspects of assessment and surgery and we routinely alternate our roles during surgery.

The key to success in powered endoscopic DCR is being able to picture the anatomy of the lacrimal sac as it will be encountered when the sac is approached from the nasal cavity. Understanding the anatomical relationships allows complete exposure of the sac and marsupialization of the sac into the lateral nasal wall. In addition preservation of mucosa with fashioning of mucosal flaps allows the nasal and lacrimal mucosa to be opposed with first intention rather than second intention healing. This decreases the risk of granulation tissue and scar formation and gives a reliable and reproducible result.

References

1. Caldwell G. Two new operations for obstruction of the nasal duct, with preservation of the canaliculi, and with an incidental description of a new lacrymal probe. Am J Ophthalmol 1893;10:189–193

2. Toti A. Nuovo Metodo conservatore dicura radicale delle suppurazione croniche del sacco lacrimale (dacricistorhinostomia). Clin. Moderna (Firenza) 1904;10:385

3. Hartikainen J, Antila J, Varpula M, Puukka P, Seppä H, Grénman R. Prospective randomized comparison of endonasal endoscopic dacryocystorhinostomy and external dacryocystorhinostomy. Laryngoscope 1998;108(12):1861–1866

4. McDonogh M, Meiring JH. Endoscopic transnasal dacryocystorhinostomy. J Laryngol Otol 1989;103(6):585–587

5. Metson R. Endoscopic surgery for lacrimal obstruction. Otolaryngol Head Neck Surg 1991;104(4):473–479

6. Steadman MG. Transnasal dacryocystorhinostomy. Otolaryngol Clin North Am 1985;18(1):107–111

7. Gonnering RS, Lyon DB, Fisher JC. Endoscopic laser-assisted lacrimal surgery. Am J Ophthalmol 1991;111(2):152–157

8. Massaro BM, Gonnering RS, Harris GJ. Endonasal laser dacryocystorhinostomy. A new approach to nasolacrimal duct obstruction. Arch Ophthalmol 1990;108(8):1172–1176

9. Woog JJ, Metson R, Puliafito CA. Holmium:YAG endonasal laser dacryocystorhinostomy. Am J Ophthalmol 1993;116(1):1–10

10. Linberg JV, Anderson RL, Bumsted RM, Barreras R. Study of intranasal ostium external dacryocystorhinostomy. Arch Ophthalmol 1982;100(11):1758–1762

11. Wormald PJ, Nilssen E. Endoscopic DCR: the team approach. Hong Kong J of Ophthalmol 1998;1:71–74

12. Welham R, Wulc A. Management of unsuccessful lacrimal surgery. Br J Ophthalmol 1987;71(3):152–157

13. Wormald PJ, Kew J, Van Hasselt A. Intranasal anatomy of the nasolacrimal sac in endoscopic dacryocystorhinostomy. Otolaryngol Head Neck Surg 2000;123(3):307–310

14. Wormald PJ. Powered endoscopic dacryocystorhinostomy. Laryngoscope 2002;112(1):69–72

15. Unlü HH, Gövsa F, Mutlu C, Yücetürk AV, Senyilmaz Y. Anatomical guidelines for intranasal surgery of the lacrimal drainage system. Rhinology 1997;35(1):11–15

16. Rebeiz EE, Shapshay SM, Bowlds JH, Pankratov MM. Anatomic guidelines for dacryocystorhinostomy. Laryngoscope 1992;102(10):1181–1184

17. Wormald PJ, Tsirbas A. Investigation and endoscopic treatment for functional and anatomical obstruction of the nasolacrimal duct system. Clin Otolaryngol Allied Sci 2004;29(4):352–356

18. Tsirbas A, Wormald PJ. Endonasal dacryocystorhinostomy with mucosal flaps. Am J Ophthalmol 2003;135(1):76–83

19. Wormald PJ. Powered endoscopic DCR. Otolaryngol Clin North Am 2006;39:539–549

20. Callejas CA, Tewfik MA, Wormald PJ. Powered endoscopic dacryocystorhinostomy with selective stenting. Laryngoscope 2010;120(7):1449–1452

21. Leibovitch I, Selva D, Tsirbas A, Greenrod E, Pater J, Wormald PJ. Paediatric endoscopic endonasal dacryocystorhinostomy in congenital nasolacrimal duct obstruction. Graefes Arch Clin Exp Ophthalmol 2006;244(10):1250–1254

22. Mann BS, Wormald PJ. Endoscopic assessment of the dacryocystorhinostomy ostium after endoscopic surgery. Laryngoscope 2006;116(7):1172–1174

23. Tsirbas A, Davis G, Wormald PJ. Revision dacryocystorhinostomy: a comparison of endoscopic and external techniques. Am J Rhinol 2005;19(3):322–325

12 Cerebrospinal Fluid Leak Closure

The traditional management of anterior skull base cerebro-spinal fluid (CSF) leaks was via an anterior craniotomy and intracranial repair of the leak. This was usually done by elevating the frontal lobes in the region of the suspected site of the leak and laying a sheet of fascia lata over this area. The success rate of this technique was around 70% but usually left the patient with some loss of smell. In addition, frontal lobe retraction is associated with the risk of postoperative epilepsy. In the late 1980s and early 1990s endoscopic closure of CSF leaks was first reported. Since then many published series have reported success rates of above 90%.[1–3] This high success rate and the very low associated morbidity are the major advantages of the endoscopic technique.[1] A variety of materials have been used to close these leaks.[3,4] Free mucosal grafts, pedicled mucosal grafts, fat, fascia, muscle, and synthetic materials such as hydroxyapatite have all been described with similar success rates.[3,4] In a recent review Hegazy et al.[3] felt that the type of material did not appear to make a significant difference to the success rate of the closure. Although this may indeed be the case in small CSF leaks, the purely on-lay technique may not be as suitable for larger leaks.[3,4] The techniques proposed in this chapter (the bath-plug closure and fascia lata repair) have been used in a large series of patients and have been found to be reliable for both large and small leaks.[5,6] In our experience if the on-lay technique alone is used for medium or large defects with a free flow of CSF, the graft tends to be pushed away from the skull base and hence from the dural defect and the flow of CSF resumes. Although the leak may be sealed at the end of the operation, coughing or straining in the postoperative period may raise the CSF pressure sufficiently to cause the leak to start again. An analogy of patching these high flow CSF leaks with on-lay technique alone is trying to patch a plastic bag of water by applying a patch to the outside of the bag.[5,6] The bath-plug technique allows the plug to be placed on the inside of the bag and uses the pressure from the water to increase the seal on the plug. The other techniques presented (underlay alone or underlay and on-lay fascia grafting) and the indications for these techniques also overcome this problem of the CSF pressure

pushing the graft away from the skull base because the fascia is placed intracranially and the CSF pressure again helps create the seal. This chapter does not attempt to describe all the alternative techniques but will concentrate on the bath-plug and underlay fascia techniques as we have considerable experience in a wide variety of situations with these techniques and have found them to be both versatile and reliable.[5,6]

◆ Etiology of Cerebrospinal Fluid Leaks

Anterior skull base CSF leaks can be divided into four broad categories according to their etiology. In a recent large series from our department, there was a fairly even spread between leak types: skull base trauma, spontaneous, meningoencephaloceles, and iatrogenic leaks.

Traumatic Cerebrospinal Fluid Leaks

Traumatic CSF leaks usually follow an anterior skull base fracture. The initial management is conservative as most of these leaks will cease within 10 days of the injury. However, leaks that persist longer than 10 days should be closed. One of the major causes of continued CSF leakage is rotation of a bony spicule which continues to hold the edges of the torn dura apart as demonstrated in this traumatic CSF leak of the sphenoid in **Fig. 12.1**. If the bone fragment is freely mobile, then this should be removed at the time of closure of the leak. More common than traumatic CSF leaks of the sphenoid are those seen in the fovea ethmoidalis or at the fovea ethmoidalis-olfactory fossa junction (**Fig. 12.2**).

Less frequent are fractures in the posterior table of the frontal sinus. Fortunately these leaks from the base of skull fractures rarely need closure but if they persist, access is usually only possible with an endoscopic modified Lothrop procedure or an osteoplastic flap. The endoscopic modified Lothrop procedure allows most of the posterior table of the frontal sinus

Fig. 12.1 (A,B) CT scans of patient with a fracture through the clinoid (**A**, *white arrow*) with a displaced bony fragment (**B**, *white arrow*) and a CSF leak. Note the fluid level in the sphenoid.

to be accessed and the CSF leak can be closed under direct visualization (**Fig. 12.3**). The reason that skull base fractures tend to heal spontaneously as opposed to injuries created during endoscopic sinus surgery (ESS) is that, although the dura is torn, there is usually no bony displacement so there is no prolapse of the torn dura preventing sealing. Where there is bony fragment displacement, surgical closure of the CSF leak should be done expeditiously and not watched expectantly. CSF leaks during ESS almost always have associated bony loss and dural prolapse so all are closed expeditiously without any conservative management prior to surgery.

Spontaneous Cerebrospinal Fluid Leaks

Spontaneous CSF leaks are usually seen either in the cribriform plate or lateral wall of the sphenoid sinus. Cribriform

fossa leaks often result from a dilation of the dural sheath around the olfactory fibers. A small prolapse of dura may result which may leak CSF (**Fig. 12.4**).

Spontaneous CSF leaks in the sphenoid sinus are usually seen in well-pneumatized sphenoid sinuses where the sinus pneumatizes into the sphenoid wing under the maxillary nerve. This brings this region of the sphenoid sinus in contact with the temporal lobe region of the middle cranial fossa with only thin bone separating the two. One theory as to why the skull base becomes eroded in this region is that arachnoid granulations in the floor of the middle cranial fossa often do not have a venous connection. When these arachnoid sacks fill with CSF and pulsate they may gradually erode the bone eventually leading to a prolapse of dura and arachnoid into the sphenoid with an associated leak.[7-10] In addition it is thought that several of these patients may have undiagnosed benign raised intracranial pressure as part of the etiology. In

Fig. 12.2 CT scan of patient following head trauma with a fracture through the fovea ethmoidalis (*white arrow*) and with an associated CSF leak. Note the fluid level in the adjacent ethmoid sinus.

Fig. 12.3 CT scan of a patient with a fracture through the posterior table (*white arrow*) of the frontal sinus with an associated CSF leak.

Fig. 12.4 A coronal CT illustrating a triangular dilation of the cribriform plate around an olfactory neuron (confirmed at surgery).

Fig. 12.5 Defect in left lateral wing of sphenoid with prolapse of dura through the defect.

Fig. 12.5 a defect is seen in this lateral aspect of this well-pneumatized sphenoid with associated opacity (prolapsing meninges and CSF).

Meningoencephaloceles with Associated Cerebrospinal Fluid Leaks

Meningoencephaloceles may either be spontaneous (congenital or acquired) or associated with a previous traumatic event. Congenital meningoencephaloceles usually present within the first few years of life. The meningoencephalocele consists of meninges and dura containing CSF with a variable amount of brain tissue prolapsing through the skull base defect into the nasal cavity or sinuses. The brain tissue within the encephalocele is usually nonfunctional and is usually resected as the first step

of the procedure. Posttraumatic meningoencephaloceles often have a funnel-shaped defect in the skull base and this needs to be recognized during the repair process as this affects the ability of the surgeon to properly visualize the edges of the bony skull base defect as well as the intracranial cavity. The funnel-shaped bony defect is caused by the intracranial contents protruding through the defect and pushing the edges of the bony defect downward into the nasal cavity/sinuses (**Fig. 12.6**).

Iatrogenic Cerebrospinal Fluid Leaks

Iatrogenic leaks will frequently be seen on the lateral wall of the olfactory fossa and fovea ethmoidalis. The lateral wall of the olfactory fossa forms the medial limit of the dissection of the frontal recess. It can be very thin varying from 0.1 to

Fig. 12.6 (**A**) CT shows the bevelling of the edges of the meningoencephalocele (*white arrow*). (**B**) Three-dimensional reconstruction also illustrates the funnel shape of the skull base defect through which the meningoencephalocele protrudes (*black arrow*).

Fig. 12.7 Intraoperative iatrogenic injury to the anterior fovea ethmoidalis (*white arrow*) on the right side.

1 mm in thickness and is perforated by the anterior ethmoidal artery. Damage to this lateral wall of the olfactory fossa may occur if the dissecting instruments are turned medially during surgery in this region. Laceration of the anterior ethmoidal artery with bleeding may prompt the use of diathermy in an attempt to obtain hemostasis. Unipolar diathermy, if used to cauterize a bleeding vessel, may burn through the bone and dura causing a CSF leak. The remaining skull base (fovea ethmoidalis) may be damaged if the surgeon loses orientation and fails to recognize that the dissection has reached the skull base. If cells are assumed to be present on the skull base, an attempt to remove these "cells" may damage the skull base with an associated CSF leak (**Fig. 12.7**). Generally these leaks are readily apparent at the time of surgery and can be fixed with the bath-plug technique described.

◆ Preoperative Assessment

This is performed if the patient presents with a suspected CSF leak. Intraoperative CSF leaks should be dealt with at the time of the surgery. The most reliable method of confirming a CSF leak is to test the clear watery secretions from the nose for β2 transferrin (β2 transferrin is only present in CSF).[4,5,7,11] Once the CSF leak has been confirmed, the site of the leak is sought by performing a high resolution fine cut computed tomography (CT) scan of the sinuses.[5,11] On this scan dehiscences of the anterior skull base are sought. Depending on the suspected cause, different areas in the anterior skull base are thoroughly scrutinized for bony defects. An additional clue may be the presence of fluid in the sinuses indicating that the leak is in the region of the opacified sinuses. Patients with spontaneous CSF leaks without evidence of any bony dehiscences on CT scan and without any opacification of any sinuses should have the cribriform plate region carefully examined intraoperatively for the CSF leak as it has been our experience that this is the most likely source of the leak (**Fig. 12.4**).

If the site of the leak is not apparent on the CT scan a high resolution T2-weighted magnetic resonance imaging (MRI) scan may allow visualization of fluid within the sinuses and, if the patient is leaking at the time of the MRI, it may allow identification of the site of the leak.[5,11] All patients with suspected meningoceles or meningoencephaloceles should have a preoperative MRI. This allows brain tissue within the meningoencephalocele to be identified and the opinion of the neurosurgeon should be sought whether the resection of this tissue transnasally is considered reasonable and safe (**Fig. 12.8**).

Although in the past there have been other investigations used to identify CSF leaks, the discussed investigations are the only ones recommended. Intrathecal contrast does not

Fig. 12.8 (A) A CT scan showing the skull base defect of a congenital meningoencephalocele (*white arrow*) whereas (**B**) is a T2-weighted MRI showing a large CSF-filled sac filling the nasal cavity with an associated stalk of brain tissue prolapsing through the skull base defect (*white arrow*). This meningoencephalocele was managed endoscopically.

improve the sensitivity of the detection of the site of a CSF leak. Intrathecal radioisotope may confirm the presence of CSF in the nasal cavity, but does not add additional information to that obtained by a positive β2 transferrin test.[3] If the site of the leak is not able to be determined with the previously listed investigations, the patient is taken to theater and intrathecal fluorescein is injected into the CSF space and the site of the leak sought while the patient in under general anesthetic.[5,11,12]

◆ Surgical Technique (Videos 36 to 38)

Broad-spectrum intravenous antibiotics are given with induction of anesthesia.

Intrathecal Fluorescein

Most patients undergoing elective CSF leak repair will have intrathecal fluorescein injected before surgery.[4,5,11,12] Patients who have a CSF leak during surgery will have the leak repaired at the time of the surgery without the placement of fluorescein intrathecally. All our patients with suspected CSF leak preoperatively sign a separate consent form designed specifically to explain the risks of the administration of intrathecal fluorescein. The most common side effects are paresthesias and tingling in the hands and feet and convulsions. These side effects were reported when significantly higher concentrations of fluorescein were used and have not been seen in our series or other very large patient series.[4–6,11–15] In elective CSF leak closure the lumbar drain is placed while the patient is awake. Ten milliliters of CSF is removed from the intrathecal space. A 40 to 60-kg person will have 0.2 mL of 5% fluorescein mixed with the 10 mL of CSF administered whereas patients 60 kg and above have 0.25 mL of 5% fluorescein mixed with the 10 mL of CSF administered.[4,5,11,12] The fluorescein-stained CSF is reinjected through a filter into the intrathecal space at a rate of 1 mL/min. This is done while the patient is awake so that any possible side effects can be identified. Once the fluorescein-stained CSF has been reinjected, the patient is kept in the theater recovery area for 1 to 2 hours in the head-down position to allow for the fluorescein to enter the cranial cavity and mix with the CSF around the brain. If there is a significant flow of CSF at this time, the appearance of fluorescein within the CSF is fairly rapid (within 20 minutes) but may take significantly longer in low flow CSF leaks or where there is a relative paucity of CSF within the system. Once the patient is anesthetized they are placed in the head-down position during preparation of the patient's nose with local anesthetic solution. This draping and setup of the theater equipment usually takes about 10 to 20 minutes, allowing additional time for the fluorescein to penetrate the intracranial cavity.

Intrathecal fluorescein can be invaluable for locating those difficult to find CSF leaks. Fluorescein can help identify the site of a small CSF leak or a leak that is intermittent or that has recently stopped leaking (usually just prior to the surgery). If a blue light filter is used on the light source even the smallest quantities of fluorescein can be visualized intraoperatively and the leak can then be closed.[5,6] If at this stage the leak is still not visible, the patient should be placed in the head-down position and a forced inspiration maneuver (Valsalva-like) performed by the anesthesiologist. This should be repeated several times while the surgeon examines the most likely sites for the CSF leak. If no leak is seen the patient should be placed head down and ventilated for a further 30 minutes before the nasal cavity and sinuses are reexamined for fluorescein-stained CSF.[6] Again the blue light filter can be very useful. If the site of the leak is still not apparent, manipulation of the CSF space is attempted. The lumbar drain is attached to an arterial pressure monitor with a three-way tap. The CSF pressure is measured (normal 0 to 15 mm water). Twenty milliliters of Ringer's lactate is injected into the intrathecal space through the lumbar drain and the pressure remeasured. After 40 mL have been injected, the head-down forced inspiration maneuver is repeated with the blue light filter to see if the leak is visible. The Ringer's lactate aliquots can be repeated but the intrathecal pressure must be measured after each aliquot to ensure that it does not go over 30 mm of water. In our series one patient required 120 mL of Ringer's before the leak became apparent.[6]

A cornerstone of this procedure is the identification of the site of the CSF leak. The leak cannot be closed if the site cannot be identified.

Another major advantage of the fluorescein-stained CSF is the ability of the surgeon to test if the CSF leak closure is watertight once the leak has been repaired.[5] After the repair has been performed as described next, the patient is placed head down and the forced inspiration maneuver repeated. The smallest leak of CSF can be easily seen as the CSF is a bright yellow/green color.

Bath-Plug Technique for Cerebrospinal Fluid Leak Repair (Video 36)

This technique forms the mainstay for the closure of CSF leaks with over 90% of our patients undergoing this technique. Once the site of the CSF leak has been identified, the dural defect is enlarged until the bony rim of the skull base can be clearly seen. As the dural defect is enlarged, a strong flow of fluorescein-stained CSF is usually apparent. It is important to remove the prolapsed dura and meninges and not to attempt repair of a dural or meningeal defect without identifying the surrounding bone as the dura and meninges provide no support for the tissue used to repair the defect. The bone of the skull base is solid and if the repair is based around this solid support a good result is more likely. On occasion the bone of the skull base may be fractured and unstable. If small pieces of bone are visible, these should be removed before repair. Large pieces of bone should be left in place and the dura opened to the edge of these large pieces. If large bony fragments are present, the bath-plug technique is still suitable but the graft needs support as the suture is pulled after intracranial placement of the graft. Once the bony rim of the defect has been identified, the nasal mucosa around the defect is stripped away for at least 5 mm. This allows the free mucosal graft to stick to the bone and ultimately a better seal is achieved (**Fig. 12.9**).

Fig. 12.9 The bony margins of the defect in skull base are identified, prolapsing dura removed, and the mucosa circumferentially stripped away from edge of defect for ~5 mm (*black arrow*).

Fig. 12.10 Demonstration of the fat plug (*black arrow*) relative to the size of the defect. Note that the fat plug is the same diameter as the defect.

The skull base defect is measured using a curette. For example the defect may be two curettes wide and three long. If a 3-mm curette is used, the defect would be 6 × 9 mm. A 6 × 9 mm fat graft is then harvested from the earlobe. If the defect is larger than 12 mm, fat is obtained either from the region of the greater trochanter of the thigh or from the abdomen. If possible, the earlobe is the preferred region for obtaining the fat graft as the fat globules are tightly knitted and easy to work with. However, if there have been multiple piercings of the earlobe, or the defect is large, then the greater trochanter region is preferred as the fat globules in this region are again more fibrous and tightly knitted than the fat from the abdomen. The fat plug should be the same diameter as the defect (otherwise there will be difficulty introducing it through the defect) and ~1.5 to 2 cm long (**Fig. 12.10**).

A 40 Vicryl suture (Ethicon, Somerville, NJ) is knotted through one end of the fat plug and the suture passed down the length of the fat plug (**Fig. 12.11**).

A free mucosal graft is harvested from the lateral nasal wall (usually on the opposite side to that which has the CSF leak). The mucosa is taken from the lateral nasal wall anterior to the middle turbinate and is usually ~3 × 3 cm (larger if the defect is large). The fat plug is placed below the defect and the malleable frontal sinus probe (Medtronic, Jacksonville, FL) is used to gently introduce the fat plug through the defect. The malleable frontal sinus probe does not have a ball-tip on the end which aids the introduction of the fat plug. If a probe with a ball-tip is used, the fat tends to stick to the ball and as the probe is pulled back after introducing fat intracranially, fat is pulled with the probe and this results in difficulty introducing the fat plug intracranially.[5] The important part of this technique is to introduce only a very small amount of fat through the defect with each maneuver. If a large amount of fat is introduced

through the defect with one maneuver, significant pressure may be required and the probe can slip a significant distance into the intracranial cavity with the potential to injure intracranial structures.[5] If small amounts of fat are introduced with each maneuver then greater safety is achieved as the probe does not need to enter the intracranial cavity by more than a few millimeters with each maneuver (**Fig. 12.12**).[4,5]

Consideration needs to be given to the possibility that there may be a vessel present in the region where the fat plug is introduced. This likelihood is increased with repair of meningoencephaloceles as vessels are present that supply blood to the prolapsed brain and dura. In addition the brain tissue that prolapses into the defect is often adherent to the edges of the defect, decreasing the amount of intracranial space available for introduction of the fat plug. In these situations the technique of placing one layer of facia lata intracranially and the second layer as an on-lay or closed with a pedicled septal flap is preferred. However, if the fat plug is manipulated gently into the intracranial cavity the likelihood of damage of intracranial structures is very small. In our large series, no such injuries occurred.

Once the fat plug has been safely introduced through the defect, the plug is stabilized with the probe and the Vicryl suture is gently pulled. This expands the fat plug on the intracranial side of the defect and allows the CSF pressure to increase the seal of the fat in the defect (much like the water pressure of the bath sealing the bath plug in the drain) (**Fig. 12.13**).

The seal is tested by placing the patient head down and asking the anesthesiologist to perform a forced inspiration (Valsalva) maneuver. No fluorescein-stained CSF should be seen. This maneuver further pushes the fat plug into the defect and a little prolapse of fat through the defect is normal. The patient is placed head up (15 degrees) and the free

Fig. 12.11 The 40 Vicryl suture is knotted at one end of the fat plug before being passed along the length of the fat plug.

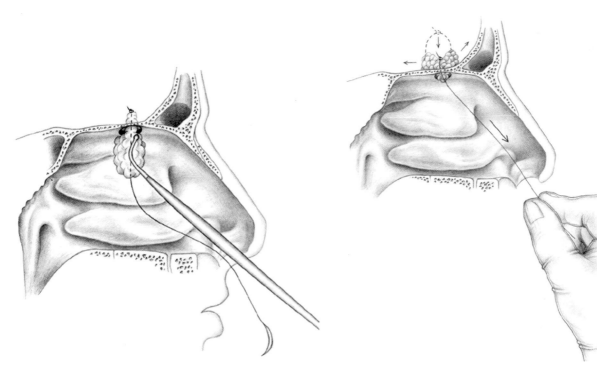

Fig. 12.12 The fat plug is gently manipulated through the skull base defect into the intracranial cavity. Only a small piece of fat is introduced with each maneuver.

Fig. 12.13 The Vicryl suture is gently pulled while the fat graft is supported. This expands the fat graft on the intracranial surface and pulls the fat into the defect giving a solid seal of the defect.

Fig. 12.14 The free mucosal graft is slid up the Vicryl suture to cover the slightly protruding fat plug and skull base defect.

Fig. 12.15 This patient presented with a right sided spontaneous CSF leak and, at surgery, a 1.5 cm × 8 mm defect was found in the olfactory fossa. The brain was adherent to the dura around the defect and needed to be carefully mobilized before the fascia lata graft was placed. This photo shows the fascial graft in place as an underlay (*white arrows* mark the limits of the defect). No fluorescein can be seen and a solid seal has been achieved. This graft was covered with a free mucosal graft and fibrin glue and Gelfoam. No nasal pack was placed.

mucosal graft is slid up the Vicryl suture until it covers the defect. Ensure that the graft is correctly orientated with the mucosal surface facing the nasal cavity (**Fig. 12.14**).

Fibrin glue is applied and the Vicryl suture is cut. Gelfoam (Pharmacia and Upjohn Company, Kalamazoo, MI) is placed over the free mucosal graft and fibrin glue reapplied. Several layers can be placed in this manner. No other nasal packing is used.

Special Situations

Meningoencephaloceles with a Cerebrospinal Fluid Leak (Video 38)

The meninges and protruding brain tissue are resected up to the skull base. This is normally done with a powered microdebrider. If significant brain tissue is seen on the MRI prolapsing into the nasal cavity or sinuses, a neurosurgical consultation should be sought regarding the safety of resection of the brain tissue. After resection the dural edges are cauterized with a suction bipolar forceps to ensure hemostasis. Exposure of the bony limits of the skull base defect is important as proper closure of the defect cannot be achieved by placing grafts against prolapsed dura and such a repair is doomed to failure. Once the bone of the skull base defect is clearly exposed and surrounding mucosa on the nasal surface gently removed from the edges of the bony defect the prolapsing brain tissue can be addressed. The brain tissue is shrunk using the suction bipolar until the stump of remaining brain tissue lies within the intracranial cavity. At this point an assessment needs to be made as to whether the edges of the prolapsed brain tissue are in contact with the edges of the skull base defect and whether it is adhesive to the dura around the defect. This is often the case and in these patients a fat plug graft is not suitable because there is insufficient space on the intracranial surface of the defect to

place the fat plug. This is especially true in defects larger than 5 mm as greater amounts of brain tissue tends to prolapse into the larger defects with a greater chance of this prolapsed brain becoming adherent to the dura around the defect. The first step is to use the suction bipolar forceps to shrink the brain tissue adherent to the edges of the defect. Any small blood vessels visualized are cauterized with the suction bipolar. The malleable suction Freer elevator from the frontal sinus malleable set* or from the skull base set* (Medtronic ENT) is bent to the appropriate angle and the brain tissue gently mobilized from the dural edges around the defect to create sufficient space circumferentially around the bony defect. The fascia lata graft is measured to be ~20 mm larger than the defect's diameter so that there is at least 5 mm of graft to be slid into this space between brain and dura around the whole circumference of the defect. In some instances the two-surgeon approach can be useful. The second surgeon can gently push the prolapsing brain tissue intracranially to allow the graft to be placed. The CSF and brain tissue then seals this graft into place and, in most cases, no further fluorescein-stained CSF should be visible (**Fig. 12.15**).

For large skull base defects (> 2 cm) either a second layer of fascia lata is placed on the nasal surface or a pedicled septal flap is rotated to close the defect followed by fibrin glue. In smaller defects a free mucosal graft with the mucosa harvested from the middle turbinate or floor of the nose is placed over this intracranial graft followed by fibrin glue. Defects from the posterior wall of the frontal sinus up to the anterior face of the pituitary and from lamina papyracea to lamina papyracea have been successfully closed using this two-layer facia lata or septal flap approach. When large defects are closed, the fibrin glue is covered by Gelfoam and then a nasal pack is placed in the nose for 5 days. No lumbar drain is used in large defects as this is likely to result in air being sucked into the intracranial cavity rather than improving the chances of a seal. **Figure 12.16** illustrates the postoperative

Fig. 12.16 The skull base defect is outlined by the black arrows and the frontal sinus ostia by the white arrows. Note the re-mucosalization of the region of the defect.

view of the skull base after a large defect was closed with the two-layered fascia lata technique.

Some authors have recommended the use of bone or cartilage in the repair of large skull base defects but we have found this to be unnecessary. If cartilage or bone is introduced intracranially, it pushes the fat plug or fascia away from the dura and bony rim of the defect and does not allow for a solid seal. In patients in whom we placed bone or cartilage in an attempt to provide a solid reconstruction of the skull base, these were removed intraoperatively because the defect could not be adequately sealed and CSF continued to leak. In none of the patients who have undergone large defect reconstructions of their skull base have we seen any recurrence of encephaloceles over many years of follow-up. The argument that bone or cartilage is needed to provide stability to the skull base to prevent encephalocele development is false.

Defects in the Lateral Wall of a Very Pneumatized Sphenoid Sinus: The Transpterygopalatine Fossa Approach

In this series there were four patients who had a defect in the lateral wall of a very pneumatized sphenoid sinus.[6] All presented with meningoceles or meningoencephaloceles with associated CSF leaks (**Fig. 12.17**).

In three of the four patients multiple previous attempts at closure had been made at other institutions usually by attempting to obliterate the sphenoid with fat. These had failed and the patients were referred to our department for closure. To close these leaks adequate exposure of the lateral wall of the sphenoid is required. This is achieved by removal of the posterior wall of the maxillary sinus and removal of the contents of the medial region of pterygopalatine fossa with preservation

Fig. 12.17 Defect in the right lateral wing of the sphenoid (*white arrow*) with CSF-filled sphenoid sinus.

of the maxillary nerve. The vidian nerve and pterygopalatine ganglion may need to be sacrificed during this exposure. The posterior wall of the pterygopalatine fossa (which is also the anterior wall of the sphenoid) is removed and direct access through the pterygopalatine fossa is achieved. This will usually involve division of the sphenopalatine artery and other branches of the maxillary artery. Division of such a large artery is preceded by cauterization with the suction bipolar forceps* (Medtronic ENT) otherwise significant bleeding may result. The posterior wall of the pterygopalatine fossa is thick and is resected with the high speed skull base diamond burr. Care is taken not to injure the maxillary nerve as it traverses the pterygopalatine fossa. Once direct access is achieved in this manner, the meningocele or meningoencephalocele is dealt with in the same manner as described previously.

◆ Postoperative Care

The patient is given broad-spectrum antibiotics for 5 days postoperatively. Saline nasal spray is started immediately after the operation. The patient is instructed not to blow their nose for at least 2 to 3 weeks postoperatively. The lumbar drain is kept on free drainage at the level of the shoulder. With this arrangement, CSF should only drain if the intracranial pressure rises and so the lumbar drain serves as a safety valve for the first 24 hours. If the lumbar drain drains more than 5 to 10 mL per hour it is raised above the shoulder to slow the drainage. After 24 hours the lumbar drain is removed and the patient is slowly mobilized over the following 24 hours and then discharged.

◆ Results

To date 39 patients have been managed with this technique.[4,5] If these patients are divided into the four broad categories, there were 7 traumatic CSF leaks, 8 spontaneous CSF leaks, 12 meningoencephaloceles, and 12 iatrogenic CSF leaks. The average age was 40 years and the male-to-female ratio was 1.2:1.

Table 12.1   Summary of Patients Treated with the Bath-Plug Closure for Cerebrospinal Fluid Leak Repair[6]

No.	Site	Size (mm)	Follow-up (months)	Second Closure Required	Successful
Traumatic CSF Leaks					
1	Lateral wall of sphenoid	4 × 3	28	No	Yes
2	Around carotid in sphenoid with bony fragment	4 × 3	5	No	Yes
3	Posterior table of frontal sinus	3 × 3	6	No	Yes
4	Cribriform plate	6 × 4	5	No	Yes
5	Ethmoid	3 × 3	26	No	Yes
6	Sphenoid	7 × 5	26	No	Yes
7	Sphenoid	6 × 6	18	No	Yes
Iatrogenic CSF Leaks					
1	Posterior ethmoid in association with skull base dehiscence from previous trauma	3 × 2	15	No	Yes
2	Posterior wall of frontal sinus; sinus previously cranialized with mucocele formation	6 × 4	28	Yes	Yes
3	Posterior ethmoids	4 × 3	32	No	Yes
4	Posterior ethmoids after resection of adenocarcinoma; previous CSF leak at same spot with previous resection of adenocarcinoma	4 × 5	12	No	Yes
5	Posterior ethmoids	6 × 4	4	No	Yes
6	Posterior ethmoids	5 × 5	12	No	Yes
7	Adjacent to anterior ethmoidal artery	3 × 3	74	No	Yes
8	Sphenoid after intracranial meningioma removal	3 × 3	15	No	Yes
9	Post craniofacial surgery in anterior ethmoids	3 × 3	20	No	Yes
10	Post adenocarcinoma resection anterior ethmoid	2 × 3	12	No	Yes
11	Post adenocarcinoma resection anterior ethmoid	3 × 3	10	No	Yes
12	Ethmoid roof (appeared to have an abnormally thin fovea ethmoidalis on both sides and had primary surgery at another institution)	16 × 12	16	No	Yes
Spontaneous CSF Leaks					
1	Cribriform plate	6 × 3	11	No	Yes
2	Cribriform plate	2 × 1	12	No	Yes
3	Cribriform plate	3 × 2	38	No	Yes
4	Lateral wall of sphenoid	6 × 4	7	No	Yes
5	Cribriform plate	5 × 5	64	No	Yes
6	Roof of sphenoid	12 × 8	70	No	Yes
7	Posterior ethmoid	8 × 6	68	No	Yes
8	Sphenoid	1 × 2	8	No	Yes
Meningoencephaloceles associated with a CSF leak					
1	Sphenoid meningocele on lateral wall of very pneumatized sphenoid; two previous attempted closures failed; mild intracranial hypertension	8 × 6	5	Yes	Yes
2	Cribriform plate meningoencephalocele	10 × 8	58	No	Yes
3	Meningoencephalocele found 2 years after cribriform plate trauma as a neonate	12 × 10	8	No	Yes
4	Sphenoid meningocele in lateral wall of very pneumatized sphenoid	8 × 6	7	No	Yes
5	Frontal sinus meningoencephalocele	6 × 4	28	No	Yes
6	Cribriform plate meningocele	3 × 3	11	No	Yes
7	Cribriform plate meningoencephalocele	4 × 4	30	No	Yes
8	Sphenoid meningoencephalocele on the lateral wall of a very pneumatized sphenoid	4 × 4	26	No	Yes
9	Anterior ethmoid meningoencephalocele	13 × 8	62	No	Yes
10	Cribriform plate meningoencephalocele	14 × 8	75	No	Yes
11	Posterior cribriform plate meningoencephalocele after craniofacial surgery 2 years previously	12 × 9	30	No	Yes
12	Sphenoid meningocele on the lateral wall of a very pneumatized sphenoid sinus	8 × 8	6	Yes	Yes
Totals					
39		5.9 × 4.5	23.5	3	39

Table 12.1 summarizes the site, size, and success of the closure of the bath-plug technique.

Eight of the iatrogenic CSF leaks were referred to our department from outside institutions for closure. Thirty-six of the 39 leaks were closed at the first operation giving a primary success rate of closure of 93%. The mean follow-up time for all patients was 28 months (standard deviation = 23), ranging from 14 months to 95 months. The three patients that failed surgery were revised and all are currently successfully closed. Two of these patients had CSF leaks in the lateral wall of the sphenoid sinus and both had undergone multiple previous attempts at closure before referral to our department.[4,5] These patients were examined for evidence of raised intracranial pressure and, in one patient, there was mild left papilledema. This patient probably has mild idiopathic interventricular hypertension and is currently being monitored to ensure no other problems develop. The third patient had a previous cranialization of the frontal sinus and developed a CSF leak in the posterior wall of the cranialized frontal sinus. Access was achieved by a modified endoscopic Lothrop procedure but the leak was high and lateral in the frontal sinus and difficulty was had with the placement of the fat plug. The patient started leaking within 48 hours of the repair and was taken back to theater where the fat plug was found to be partially extruded. A new fat plug was placed and closure was successful.

The technique and results of the closure of large skull base defects after the endoscopic removal of large sections of the skull base to provide access to the intracranial cavity for tumor removal are not included in these results but discussed in the later chapters on skull base surgery. For non–skull base surgery related defects we have found that two layers of fascia lata with one placed intracranially and the other on the nasal surface of the skull base or in association with a pedicled septal flap in combination with fibrin glue, Gelfoam, and nasal packing gives a reliable closure. The one leak we have had in this patient group was the first patient operated on in whom we closed a large 3 × 3 cm defect with fat and fibrin glue alone.

◆ **Key Points**

A CSF leak cannot be closed if it cannot be identified. There were five patients in this series in whom a fine cut CT scan and an MRI scan could not identify the site of the leak preoperatively.[6] Intrathecal fluorescein was placed in all elective CSF leak closures including those in whom the radiologic investigations indicated the likely site of the leak. This is an off-label usage of fluorescein so all patients had counselling regarding the potential complications of its usage and signed a separate consent form for its use.[4,5,11,12] In four patients the blue light filter and manipulation of the CSF space was needed before the site of the leak could be identified. Although placement of a lumbar drain and the off-label use of fluorescein are controversial, we have found this to be very useful in some patients in whom there was difficulty identifying the site of the CSF leak. In addition the staining of the fluorescein allows the surgeon to carefully evaluate the security of the seal of the CSF leak by testing the leak by raising the intracranial pressure and looking for any evidence of fluorescein-stained CSF. Finally the lumbar drain is kept in for 24 hours to prevent any sudden increases in CSF pressure from putting excessive pressure on the repair.

The introduction of a fat plug into the intracranial space has the potential risk of damage to intracranial vascular structures. The risk of such vessels being in the region of the CSF leak is higher in patients who have a meningoencephalocele especially if the brain is adherent to the dura around the skull base defect. We have modified our technique in these cases to use a two-layer closure (small defects fascia and mucosa and large defects two layers of fascia) or an underlay fascia lata graft with a nasal pedicled rotated septal flap. If there is concern regarding vessels in the region of the defect, appropriate radiologic investigations should be performed. The advent of radiologic software that is able to reconstruct the vasculature of the skull base without the need to perform an angiogram makes this a relatively simple investigation to perform. If doubt exists about the resection of brain tissue, neurosurgical opinion should be sought. Finally, the manipulation of the fat plug through the defect should be very gentle and the probe should not be introduced more than a few millimeters intracranially with each maneuver. This will minimize the risk of intracranial damage. In this series of patients, no such complication occurred and from postoperative observation of the patients there was no need to perform any postoperative radiologic investigations.

References

1. Marshall AH, Jones NS, Robertson IJA. CSF rhinorrhoea: the place of endoscopic sinus surgery. Br J Neurosurg 2001;15(1):8–12
2. Hughes RGM, Jones NS, Robertson IJ. The endoscopic treatment of cerebrospinal fluid rhinorrhoea: the Nottingham experience. J Laryngol Otol 1997;111(2):125–128
3. Hegazy HM, Carrau RL, Snyderman CH, Kassam A, Zweig J. Transnasal endoscopic repair of cerebrospinal fluid rhinorrhea: a meta-analysis. Laryngoscope 2000;110(7):1166–1172
4. Bolger WE, McLaughlin K. Cranial bone grafts in cerebrospinal fluid leak and encephalocele repair: a preliminary report. Am J Rhinol 2003;17(3):153–158
5. Wormald PJ, McDonogh M. 'Bath-plug' technique for the endoscopic management of cerebrospinal fluid leaks. J Laryngol Otol 1997;111(11):1042–1046
6. Wormald PJ, McDonogh M. The bath-plug closure of anterior skull base cerebro-spinal fluid (CSF) leaks. Am J Rhinol 2003;17(5):299–305
7. Casiano RR, Jassir D. Endoscopic cerebrospinal fluid rhinorrhea repair: is a lumbar drain necessary? Otolaryngol Head Neck Surg 1999;121(6):745–750
8. Badia L, Loughran S, Lund V. Primary spontaneous cerebrospinal fluid rhinorrhea and obesity. Am J Rhinol 2001;15(2):117–119
9. Ommaya AK, Di Chiro G, Baldwin M, Pennybacker JB. Non-traumatic cerebrospinal fluid rhinorrhoea. J Neurol Neurosurg Psychiatry 1968;31(3):214–225
10. Har-El G. What is "spontaneous" cerebrospinal fluid rhinorrhea? Classification of cerebrospinal fluid leaks. Ann Otol Rhinol Laryngol 1999;108(4):323–326
11. Gacek RR. Arachnoid granulation cerebrospinal fluid otorhea. Ann Otol Rhinol Laryngol 1990;99(11):854–862
12. Mattox DE, Kennedy DW. Endoscopic management of cerebrospinal fluid leaks and cephaloceles. Laryngoscope 1990;100(8):857–862
13. Syms CA III, Syms MJ, Murphy TP, Massey SO. Cerebrospinal fluid fistulae in a canine model. Otolaryngol Head Neck Surg 1997;117(5):542–546
14. Mao VH, Keane WM, Atkins JP, et al. Endoscopic repair of cerebrospinal fluid rhinorrhea. Otolaryngol Head Neck Surg 2000;122(1):56–60
15. Zweig JL, Carrau RL, Celin SE, et al. Endoscopic repair of cerebrospinal fluid leaks to the sinonasal tract: predictors of success. Otolaryngol Head Neck Surg 2000;123(3):195–201

13 Endoscopic Resection of Pituitary Tumors

Pituitary tumors are commonly benign pituitary adenomas and only rarely are pituitary carcinomas or posterior pituitary neoplasias diagnosed.[1] Pituitary adenomas present most commonly in the third and fourth decades.[1] Their clinical presentation depends whether the tumor is secreting (less common) or nonsecreting (more common).[1] Secreting adenomas present with the endocrine manifestations of the hormone secreted.[1,2] The most common is a prolactin-secreting tumor, followed by growth hormone, adrenocorticotropic (ACTH), follicle-stimulating hormone, and luteinizing hormone.[1,2] Nonsecreting adenomas usually present due to their mass effects. Symptoms may include headache, hypopituitarism, visual loss, and visual field defects (most commonly bilateral hemianopia) and cranial nerve defects.

Magnetic resonance imaging (MRI) is the radiologic investigation of choice for pathologic tumor evaluation and used to define involvement of surrounding structures. Pituitary adenomas are divided, for clinical purposes, into microadenomas (< 1.0 cm in diameter) and macroadenomas (> 1.0 cm in diameter). Microadenomas are often difficult to see on MRI, but the normal anterior pituitary gland will usually be visible with a gadolinium-enhanced T1-weighted image allowing the microadenoma to be identified. In patients who have macroadenomas, the normal anterior pituitary will usually not be visualized. There are several grading systems available, but the most commonly used (**Table 13.1**) is based on extrasellar extension of the tumor.[3]

In recent years the surgical approach to the pituitary fossa has been either transeptal or transethmoid.[4,5] The transseptal approach is performed through either a sublabial incision or through a hemitransfixion incision. Once the septal flaps have been raised and the anterior face of the sphenoid removed, the Cushing speculum is inserted. The microscope is swung into place and the anterior face of the pituitary fossa visualized. The sphenoid rostrum is removed and the intersinus septum identified and removed. The advantage of this technique is that the surgeon can now use an instrument in each hand to proceed with the surgery. The disadvantages of this technique are the morbidity associated with

a sublabial incision and dissection and the incidence of septal perforations, adhesions, and postoperative sinusitis. In addition, the surgeon cannot visualize lateral or superior extensions of the tumor.

Recently several surgeons have advocated a transnasal approach where the sphenoid sinus and the pituitary fossa are approached transnasally with lateralization of the middle turbinate and resection of the superior turbinate and anterior face of the sphenoid.[5-9] The Cushing speculum is introduced through the nares and into the sphenoidotomy and opened.[6,7] Opening of the speculum tends to further fracture the middle turbinate laterally as well as fracture the septum toward the opposite nasal cavity. Once the speculum is in place the microscope is again brought in by the surgeon and the anterior face of the pituitary fossa resected with the surgeon using an instrument in each hand.[6,7] The advantages of this technique are the lack of any incisions around the face but the disadvantage is the fracture or displacement of the septum and middle turbinate. Additionally, and most importantly, the surgeon cannot visualize tumor extensions laterally or superiorly. When the speculum is opened it fractures the septum laterally. The septum is usually unstable and will often result in a septal deviation postoperatively. The middle turbinate may remain displaced and may cause obstruction of the sinus ostia although this would be unusual.

The major reason for developing endoscopic pituitary tumor resection techniques is to minimize intranasal complications and to provide superior visualization. The endoscopic view is panoramic when compared with the microscopic view and this helps with identification of critical anatomical landmarks within the sphenoid. In addition, angled endoscopes allow tumor that extends outside the sella to be seen and this improves the surgeon's ability to achieve complete tumor resection.[8,9] Tumor remnants in the recesses of the sella which would not have been seen with the microscope may be visualized with an endoscope (**Fig. 13.1**). If complete tumor resection is achieved there is less likelihood of recurrence.

Table 13.1 Wilson Grading System for Pituitary Adenomas Based on Extrasellar Extension

Stage 0 – no suprasellar extension
Stage A – extension into suprasellar cistern only
Stage B – extension into anterior recess of the third ventricle
Stage C – obliteration of anterior recess and deformation of floor of third ventricle
Stage D – intradural extension into anterior, middle, or posterior fossa
Stage E – extradural invasion into cavernous sinus

Source: Data from Wilson CB. A decade of pituitary microsurgery. The Herbert Olivecrona lecture. J Neurosurg 1984;61:814–833.

◆ **Preoperative Assessment**

The standard radiologic evaluation prior to endoscopic resection of a pituitary tumor is a standard computed tomography (CT) scan of the sinuses and MRI scan of the brain. These two modalities allow assessment of both the nose, sinuses, and the pituitary tumor. The MRI scan requested is performed according to the image guidance protocol for our computer-aided surgical (CAS) guidance system.

Image guidance during surgery adds to the safety of the procedure by confirming the positions of the optic nerves and carotid arteries. In addition, during tumor resection, image guidance is used to confirm the limits of the pituitary fossa and the position of the internal carotid arteries within the cavernous sinuses, which may add to the safety of the procedure. In the preoperative evaluation of the radiology special attention needs to be paid to the course of the internal carotid arteries. Normally the carotid arteries enter the base of the sphenoid sinus and turn vertically to ascend to the base of the pituitary gland where they move posteriorly and slightly medially before turning back on themselves, forming the internal carotid siphon lateral to the pituitary gland in the cavernous sinus. They then travel anteriorly and can usually be seen on the lateral nasal wall before turning vertically and posteriorly to run lateral to the optic nerve into the middle cranial fossa (**Fig. 13.2**).

In some patients the carotid may turn medially as it moves anteriorly after the siphon and, in so doing, cover the anterior face of the pituitary fossa limiting the access to the gland (**Fig. 13.3**). In such a patient, care needs to be exercised so that the carotid is not injured as the dura is opened for access to the pituitary tumor.

◆ **Surgical Technique (Videos 39 and 40)**

Macroadenoma

Patients are catheterized prior to surgery. This allows manipulation of fluid balance during surgery and allows the patient's postoperative urine output to be monitored. This is important in identifying and managing diabetes insipidus due to disturbance in antidiuretic hormone (ADH)

Fig. 13.1 The MRI (**A**) is a coronal image showing suprasellar extension of tumor. (**B**) The same tumor is shown in the parasagittal plane in MRI. Angled telescopes can be very helpful to visualize extensions above the sella as shown in these two MRI scans.

regulation. This may result from the manipulation of the pituitary stalk (relatively common and usually transient) or from injury or dysfunction of the posterior pituitary gland during the procedure. Intravenous antibiotic prophylaxis is given—usually cephalosporin, gentamicin, and metronidazole. Standard preparation of the nose is performed with topical vasoconstriction and infiltration. Any significant septal deviation is dealt with via either a Killian or Freer (hemitransfixion) incision. Correction of any septal defect allows both nasal cavities to be used for access to the sphenoid during the surgery. If a significant septal deflection is not dealt with, significant trauma of that nasal cavity may occur. During surgery instruments are often passed through the nasal cavity without endoscopic visualization. Difficulty in passing instruments in such a blinded manner can be due to septal deflection and may slow the surgery significantly.

Fig. 13.2 (A) Cadaveric dissection image taken within the sphenoid sinus, with removal of bone over the lateral sphenoid wall. The paraclival carotid artery (*PCA*) enters the base of the sphenoid sinus and runs in a vertical direction. At approximately the level of the V2 (maxillary division of trigeminal nerve) the carotid artery then enters the cavernous sinus and becomes the intracavernous carotid artery (*CCA*). Once the artery enters the cavernous sinus it continues to ascend for a short distance, called the vertical portion of the CCA (*V. CCA*), before turning anteriorly at the posterior genu of the CCA (*P. Genu CCA*). This posterior genu corresponds to the floor of the sella. The artery then runs horizontally as the horizontal portion of the CCA (*H. CCA*), before reaching the anterior genu of the CCA (*A. Genu CCA*). After the anterior genu of the CCA the artery becomes extracavernous, exiting the roof of the cavernous sinus to briefly become the clinoidal segment of the ICA, and then the cisternal segment of the ICA. The clinoidal ICA is wedge-shaped and at the base of the optic strut (lateral opticocarotid recess), and the cisternal segment courses posterosuperiorly and medially until its bifurcation, where the artery divides into the anterior and middle cerebral arteries. **(B)** The anterior bend of the carotid in the cavernous sinus is seen on the lateral nasal wall (*white oval*) just below the optic nerve (*ON*). The opticocarotid recess is marked with a *black arrow* and the pituitary gland by the *white arrow*.

Fig. 13.3 This picture from our computer-aided surgical system illustrates the course of the internal carotid arteries in all three planes as they approach the midline bilaterally with a small window between them through which the pituitary tumor can be accessed. The *black arrows* indicate on the endoscopic image the medial extent of the right carotid artery. The septation on the anterior face of the pituitary is almost in the midline.

Fig. 13.4 (A) Endoscopic view of the left superior meatus and sphenoid ostium indicated with a *black arrow* and the superior turbinate (*ST*) and middle turbinate (*MT*) clearly visible. **(B)** Cadaveric dissection image of the left superior meatus and sphenoid ostium. The superior turbinate shares a common border with the middle turbinate, with the anterosuperior border of the superior turbinate attaching to the middle turbinate.

The endoscope and microdebrider are passed medial to the middle turbinate and the superior turbinate and often the sphenoid ostium are identified (**Fig. 13.4**).

The next step is to remove bilaterally the lower two-thirds of the superior turbinate and expose the natural ostium of the sphenoid sinus (**Fig. 13.5**). To protect the vascular pedicle of the septal flap, a horizontal incision from the lower edge of the sphenoid ostium is made onto the septum angulating superiorly. This allows a suction Freer to be used to roll this pedicle inferiorly and in this rolled mucosa flap will lie the postnasal artery which is the major blood supply of the septal flap. In patients who end up with large defects in the diaphragm or with exposed carotid arteries, repair with the septal flap is needed. If this pedicle is not raised and a standard opening of the sphenoid performed, the pedicle will be destroyed as the anterior face of the sphenoid is lowered sufficiently to allow adequate endoscopic approach to the pituitary. After preservation of the pedicle, the sphenoid ostium is enlarged inferiorly until a straight instrument is passed easily under the floor of the pituitary fossa. This is done bilaterally. The posterior 1 cm of the septum is removed with the cutting burr and back-biting forceps and the sphenoid sinus septum visualized. This is important as a Kerrison punch will be placed in the left nostril and will be used to remove the bone of the right side of the pituitary fossa and vice versa for the right nostril. The sphenoidotomies are

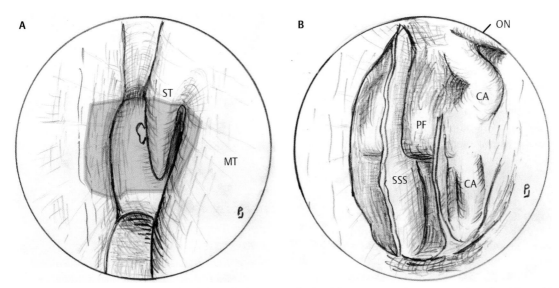

Fig. 13.5 (A) The area to be resected including the lower two-thirds of the superior turbinate, posterior ethmoids, and large sphenoidotomy are shaded. **(B)** After resection the carotid artery (*CA*), optic nerve (*ON*), pituitary fossa (*PF*), and sphenoid sinus septum (*SSS*) are seen.

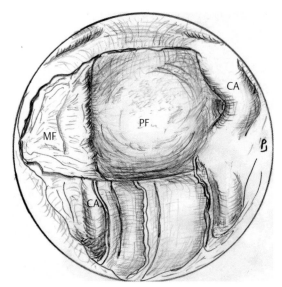

Fig. 13.6 The bone of the anterior face of the pituitary fossa (*PF*) is widely removed. The mucosal flap (*MF*) has been laid aside and the bone of the pituitary fossa exposed from one cavernous sinus to the other. *CA*, carotid artery.

Fig. 13.7 Cadaveric dissection image demonstrating that the sphenoid sinus septum has been removed flush with the pituitary fossa (*PF*). *PCA*, paraclival carotid artery; *A. Genu CCA*, anterior genu of the intracavernous carotid artery.

enlarged up to the lateral wall of the sphenoid. The access provided should allow passage of an instrument below the pituitary fossa and laterally onto the internal carotid artery and optic nerve eminences (**Fig. 13.6**). The next step is to remove the sphenoid mucosa starting on the sphenoid septum in the larger of the two sinuses. The mucosa is removed from medial to lateral over the entire pituitary fossa and left pedicled in the lateral inferior aspect of the sphenoid. This is covered with a strip of Surgicel (Ethicon, Somerville, NJ) to prevent it from been suctioned into the suction during the remainder of the surgery. The sphenoid sinus septum is removed flush with the pituitary fossa (**Fig. 13.7**). If the anterior wall of the pituitary fossa is thick, the drill is used to thin this down until it is soft. Most patients with macroadenomas will have a soft anterior face of the pituitary as the pressure exerted by the expanding tumor thins the bone. However, patients who have a microadenoma may have thick bone forming the anterior face of the pituitary.

The key to endoscopic pituitary surgery is to have full access to the pituitary fossa from both sides of the nose. This allows two surgeons to work off the video monitor at the same time. Our team consists of a neurosurgeon (with endoscopic interest and skill) and a sinus surgeon. The roles of these surgeons are interchangeable with both surgeons able to perform all parts of the procedure. Having two surgeons allows an endoscope with camera attached and two instruments to be used at all times during the procedure. If significant bleeding occurs, a blood-free field can be maintained by one of the surgeons using a high volume suction. The thin bone of the anterior face of the pituitary is fractured and removed with a Kerrison punch (**Fig. 13.8**). Wide opening of the anterior face of the pituitary is achieved with bone removal from one cavernous sinus to the other. Care is taken with the superior bone removal as a fold of dura occurs below the tuberculum sella and in this region it is closely attached to the bone. If the Kerrison punch is not kept solidly

in contact with the undersurface of the bone, this dural fold can be caught by the punch and a cerebrospinal fluid (CSF) leak can result.

In most cases the dura is not cauterized as this tends to shrink the dura. If, however, cautery is felt to be needed for visible blood vessels on the surface of the dura, a suction

Fig. 13.8 Cadaveric dissection of the sphenoid sinus with bone removal over the pituitary fossa exposing the periosteal layer of dura (*POD*).

Fig. 13.9 Cadaveric dissection illustrating the U-shaped incision performed into the dura. In this dissection just the periosteal layer of dura (*POD*) has been reflected, exposing the superior (*SIS*) and inferior intercavernous dural sinus (*IIS*). These sinuses run between the periosteal layer of dura and the meningeal layer of dura (*MD*).

Fig. 13.10 The first surgeon is using the ring curette to remove tumor from the lower half of the pituitary fossa while the second surgeon is holding the endoscope and a second suction to keep the surgical field clear or to retract the dura so that the first surgeon may obtain a better view of the lateral walls and diaphragma region.

bipolar* (Medtronic Xomed, Jacksonville, FL) is used to cauterize the dura before a no. 11 scalpel blade on a no. 7 BP handle is used to create an U-shaped incision into the dura (**Fig. 13.9**). We prefer the U-shaped incision to the cruciate incision as the dural corners of the cruciate incision partially blocks the view into the sella during surgery. The U-shaped incision allows an unobstructed view of the diaphragm and the lateral walls and lateral and superior recesses of the sella where residual tumor may be missed if a clear view is not obtained. In addition the dura can be used to help seal any small leaks on the anterior edge of the diaphragm by rolling the dura into the pituitary fossa over the leak.

In patients with a macroadenoma, tumor under pressure will often ooze through these dural incisions. A Deckers or skull base Blakesley forceps (Medtronic ENT) is used to remove a sample of tumor for histology. Malleable suction ring curettes* (Medtronic ENT skull base set) and standard pituitary ring curettes are used to first clear the tumor along the floor of the pituitary fossa until the posterior wall of the pituitary fossa is seen (**Fig. 13.10**).

Attention is then turned to tumor sited laterally on the cavernous sinuses. The ring curette is gently scraped along the cavernous sinus and tumor removed using the suction on the ring curette. The curette can be felt rolling over the carotid artery. Finally, the tumor on the pituitary fossa diaphragm is removed. Care should be taken to visualize the diaphragm as it descends with the tumor removal. In patients who have a significant suprasellar tumor extension, a 30-degree endoscope can be used to visualize this suprasellar extension and to remove it under direct vision.

This use of angled endoscopes is the great advantage of the endoscopic approach. It allows tumor that can traditionally not be visualized with the standard microscopic approach to be seen and removed under vision. In addition the malleable skull base set* (Medtronic ENT) has malleable suction ring curettes that can be bent so that even a large suprasellar component can be reached from below. **Figure 13.11** shows a patient with a large suprasellar extension. In this patient the tumor was removed from below. As the tumor was debulked from below so the suprasellar component descended into the pituitary fossa. This is especially true for tumors with a broad-based suprasellar extension. Tumors with a dumbbell shaped extension or narrow neck may have ruptured through the diaphragm and be better approached with an extended pituitary approach (**Fig. 13.12**).

The other significant advantage of the two-surgeon approach is the ability of one surgeon to hold the diaphragma up while the other surgeon removes tumor that may otherwise be left unresected in the angle between the diaphragm and cavernous sinus (**Fig. 13.10**). In our experience this is the most common area for residual tumor and this area is not usually visible with the microscope as it sits above the level of the anterior bony opening made in the pituitary fossa. In addition the diaphragm may obliterate this angle as it descends. Gently holding the diaphragm up with a Freer elevator helps to keep this angle open and allows the other surgeon to gently remove any residual tumor (**Fig. 13.13**).

To remove any microscopic or small pieces of tumor that may still be adherent to one of the walls of the sella, a small neuropattie is placed into the sella and wiped around the sella (**Fig. 13.14**). This also absorbs blood clots and allows clear visualization of the diaphragma and lateral

A

B

Fig. 13.11 The large suprasellar extension is seen with extension into the third and lateral ventricles (*white arrow*). Note the broad-based extension in both (**A**) and (**B**) and the superior compression of the pituitary gland in (**B**, *black arrow*).

walls and floor of the sella. The 30-degree endoscope is usually placed within the sella cavity and rotated so that anterosuperior and anterolateral recesses can be clearly seen. In **Fig. 13.14B** the white arrow indicates anterolateral residual tumor that was missed by a solely microscopic hypophysectomy for a growth hormone secreting tumor. This residual tumor could be clearly seen with the angled endoscope and was removed and the growth hormone levels have remained low to normal in the postoperative period. This case illustrates one of the most important advantages of the endoscopic approach to resection of both macro- and microadenomas.

Once the tumor has been completely removed, Gelfoam paste (Gelfoam powder mixed with saline to form a paste [Pharmacia and Upjohn Company, Kalamazoo, MI]) is placed

within the pituitary fossa. The preserved dural flap and sphenoid mucosa are positioned over the anterior face of the sella and fibrin glue applied to the surface (**Fig. 13.15**).

The middle turbinates are repositioned in their correct orientation and the operation is complete. No packing is placed within the sphenoid or the nasal cavity. If the patient has a CSF leak from the diaphragm, then the hole in the diaphragm is identified and a conically shaped fat graft is placed into the defect and gently pushed through the hole with the malleable probe* (Medtronic skull base set) until the leak is completely sealed. This plug forms a dumbbell with some of the fat through the defect but with most of the fat still in the sella. The rest of the sella is filled with fat and a fascia lata graft is placed over the fat with the edges of the graft tucked under the dura of the opening

A

B

Fig. 13.12 Dumbbell suprasellar extension in the (**A**) coronal and (**B**) parasagittal planes. The neck is marked with a white arrow.

Fig. 13.13 The Freer elevator (*FE*) is being held up by one surgeon while the second surgeon visualizes the residual tumor (*arrow*) in the angle between the cavernous sinus and diaphragm and removes it.

into the sella. The dura and sphenoid mucosa is placed over this fascia and fibrin glue applied (**Fig. 13.16**). This region is covered with Gelfoam and the sphenoid sinus is packed with bismuth iodoform paraffin paste (BIPP), impregnated ribbon gauze, or antibiotic-soaked ribbon gauze. The gauze allows pressure to be placed on the fascia during the healing period. The ribbon gauze is trailed into the nasal cavity and is removed after 5 days in the outpatient department. No additional nasal packing is used. If the CSF leak was profuse a lumbar drain is inserted postoperatively for 2 to 3 days to ensure the pressure is taken off the fat plug during healing.

Microadenoma Resection

The image guidance scan for these patients is an MRI scan. This helps with the intraoperative localization of the microadenoma and ensures that the correct portion of the gland is removed. Essentially, the same approach is used for microadenomas as is used for macroadenomas up to the point where the dura is incised. After opening the dura, incisions are made over the region of the microadenoma. Using blunt dissection this region of the gland is explored. Usually the tumor is soft and a different consistency from the rest of the gland and, in most cases, can be dissected from the gland. However, some microadenomas are unable to be differentiated from normal gland and the gland may need to be sliced in multiple places before the tumor is found. Care should be taken to avoid confusing the posterior pituitary gland with tumor as it is softer and often a paler color than the anterior pituitary gland.

Cavernous Sinus Invasion

Pituitary tumors may invade the cavernous sinus to various degrees. The classification of tumor invasion that we use is by Knosp et al. (**Fig. 13.17**).[10]

Grades 1 and 2 are treated no differently to a standard pituitary dissection as described previously. Grade 3 has tumor lateral to the carotid. It is important to plot out the carotid artery and to see where the tumor has entered the cavernous sinus. Normally tumor enters the sinus above the horizontal portion of the intracavernous portion of the carotid (**Fig. 13.18**). If invasion is extensive there may be an inferior component that wraps underneath this part of the carotid. In general, tumor from nonsecreting adenomas that does not come away easily is not extensively looked for or followed into the cavernous sinus. A more conservative

A

B

Fig. 13.14 **(A)** A neuropattie (*black arrow*) placed against the posterior wall of the sella. The diaphragma (*white solid arrow*), cavernous sinus (*white broken arrow*), and floor of the sella can all be clearly seen. **(B)** A hypophysectomy had been performed by a microscopic approach 3 weeks previously and, although the growth hormone levels initially dropped, they rose to high levels in the third week. The patient underwent an endoscopic exploration and residual tumor was seen in the lateral anterior region (*white arrow*) and removal of this has resulted in a cure for the patient. The diaphragma can be clearly seen (*black arrow*).

Fig. 13.15 The inferiorly based dural flap (this can be an alternative to the U-shaped superiorly based flap) is positioned over the Gelfoam paste and then the sphenoid mucosal (*SM*) flap is placed over the dura to cover the anterior face of the sella. Fibrin glue is applied.

Fig. 13.16 Cadaveric dissection with replacement of the dura and sphenoid sinus mucosa at the end of the pituitary procedure.

approach is adopted in these nonsecreting tumors as well as in elderly patients. However, in secreting tumors these extensions are actively chased in an attempt to remove all tumor so that a endocrinological cure can be achieved. Tumor can be followed into the cavernous sinus from the pituitary fossa. In some instances this is broad-based but in other patients it may have a narrow neck and form a dumbbell through this dural opening. The tumor in the cavernous sinus will obliterate the venous sinusoids and following the tumor into the

cavernous sinus does not normally result in a significant increase in bleeding. This dissection is done with a 30-degree scope angled laterally and usually placed within the pituitary fossa for this dissection. Angled and malleable ring curettes are used to remove the tumor. In some instances the third nerve may be visible in the lateral wall of the cavernous sinus. Suction on the third nerve will almost always result

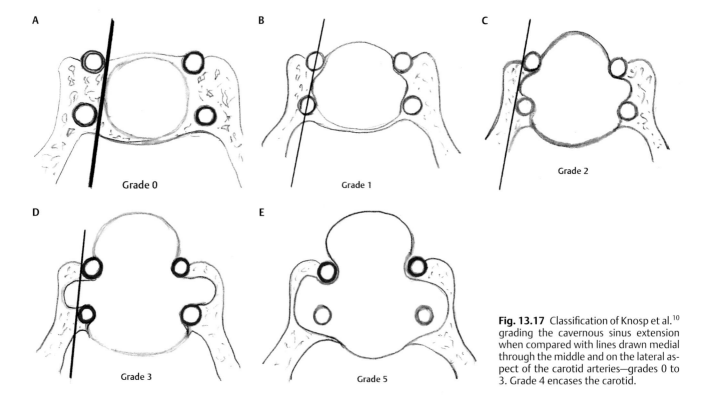

Fig. 13.17 Classification of Knosp et al.[10] grading the cavernous sinus extension when compared with lines drawn medial through the middle and on the lateral aspect of the carotid arteries—grades 0 to 3. Grade 4 encases the carotid.

in a neurapraxia with postoperative palsy. However, where this has happened to us, the palsy has fully recovered after 3 months. Tumor extensions under the carotid artery and into the cavernous can also be followed in this manner and removed. When patients who have secreting tumor lateral and anterior to the carotid, an additional incision is made lateral to the carotid directly into the cavernous sinus. This allows dissection into the cavernous with a direct access into the cavernous sinus from an anterior approach. Remember that the sixth cranial nerve traverses the cavernous sinus and may be at risk if the dissection is taken below the anterior genu of the carotid as this nerve hugs the inferior anterior border of this genu (**Fig. 13.18**).

Extended Pituitary Dissection (Video 56)

This approach is used for pituitary tumors that extend anterior to the tuberculum sella or that extend significantly into the suprasellar region with disruption of the diaphragm. Additionally, this approach is used for tuberculum sella tumors such as meningiomas that push the pituitary inferiorly and ride over the tuberculum sella onto the planum sphenoidale. Pituitary tumors that disrupt the diaphragm are suspected when the tumor has a significant dumbbell shape or if extension occurs into or beyond the third ventricle. The exposure for this approach involves removing the bone above the pituitary fossa and

Fig. 13.19 In this cadaver dissection the anterior genu of the carotid is seen with the optic nerve (*ON*) running above it and creating the lateral opticocarotid recess (*L.OCR*). Between the optic nerve as it exits the sphenoid and the carotid as it enters the anterior cranial fossa is the medial opticocarotid recess (*M. OCR*). *P*, pituitary gland.

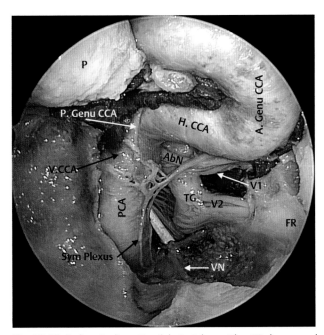

Fig. 13.18 Cadaveric dissection (photo taken with a 70-degree endoscope) of the lateral sphenoid wall demonstrating the different portions of the intracavernous carotid artery (*CCA*). *P*, pituitary; *A. Genu CCA*, anterior genu of the intracavernous carotid artery; *H. CCA*, horizontal portion of the intracavernous carotid artery; *P. Genu CCA*, posterior genu of the intracavernous carotid artery; *V. CCA*, vertical portion of the intracavernous carotid artery; *PCA*, paraclival carotid artery; *Sym. Plexus*, sympathetic plexus; *TG*, trigeminal ganglion; *V2*, Maxillary division of the trigeminal nerve; *FR*, foramen rotundum; *VN*, vidian nerve; *AbN*, abducens nerve.

on the planum sphenoidale. Once dural exposure of the pituitary is achieved, the bone overlying the tuberculum sella is removed. Both optic nerves are identified and the bone removed from between them. The bone between the optic nerve and anterior superior portion of the carotid anterior genu is called the medial opticocarotid recess (medial OCR) (**Fig. 13.19**). Between these two medial OCRs is the narrowest part of the access into the subchiasmatic cistern and care should be taken to remove as much of this bone as possible to widen surgical access. However, be aware that the two structures bordering this bone are the optic nerve and carotid artery so great care should be taken with this bone removal. Should the medial OCRs not be removed then surgeons can have difficulty manipulating instruments through this narrow access and may compromise the resection of the tumor. Once the dura is exposed between the optic nerves the dissection progresses onto the planum sphenoidale (**Fig. 13.20**). Bone is removed up to the anterior face of the sphenoid sinus. The dural exposure widens over this area giving an hour-glass exposure. The dura is incised with a no. 11 blade in the midline and the subchiasmatic cistern inspected (**Fig. 13.21**). The superior hypophyseal artery should be seen with both optic nerves and suprasellar extension of the tumor. In patients with a pre-fixed optic chiasm, displacement of the optic chiasm is limited which severely limits surgical access into the region above the optic chiasm as the optic nerves and chiasm form the anterior limit and the lower they are fixed the more the surgeons are forced to work around them. If this can be detected preoperatively this is a relative contraindication to the extended pituitary approach.

Fig. 13.20 Cadaveric dissection with further bone exposure between the intracavernous carotid arteries (*CCA*) and optic nerves. A portion of the planum sphenoidale (*PS*) has been removed allowing for wider exposure of the periosteal layer of dura (*POD*). *SIS*, superior intercavernous sinus; *IIS*, inferior intercavernous sinus; *MD*, meningeal layer of dura.

Fig. 13.21 Cadaveric dissection with view into the subchiasmatic cistern. *PS*, planum sphenoidale; *ON*, optic nerve; *OC*, optic chiasm; *Oph. A*, ophthalmic artery; *CCA*, intracavernous carotid artery; *SHA*, superior hypophyseal artery; *PS*, pituitary stalk; *P*, pituitary.

All patients who have an extended approach to their pituitary performed required an underlay fascia lata graft with or without fat and an on-lay pedicled vascularized septal flap placed over the defect to ensure solid closure. The subchiasmatic cistern is a high CSF flow region and needs to be managed with best possible closure techniques.

◆ Postoperative Care

Patients are monitored in high dependency overnight with routine neurologic observations and hourly monitoring of urine output. If the urine output is greater than 250 mL per hour for more than 2 hours an endocrinologist should be consulted and desmopressin may be given. Cortisol is usually not given in the perioperative period but levels are monitored by the endocrinologists and augmentation prescribed if necessary. If the procedure was uncomplicated the patient is mobilized the following day and discharged when the endocrinologists are satisfied with their hormone status.

◆ Results[11]

Although we have reported on our first 32 consecutive and unselected patients who underwent an entirely endoscopic resection of their pituitary tumors utilizing the technique described, this number is now in the hundreds. In this report five patients had secretory microadenomas.

In the macroadenoma group there were six patients with extensive suprasellar and/or parasellar extensions. Postoperative imaging showed residual tumor in four patients, with tumor located lateral to the carotid artery in three of these patients.[11] In the microadenoma group all patients have normalized their hormone status. Six CSF leaks were seen during surgery and repaired. Two patients developed CSF leaks postoperatively and one patient who had a very fibrous tumor developed a leak after revision surgery and required two returns to theater before closure of the leak was achieved. No other complications were seen. In the remaining 22 patients, complete removal of the macroadenoma was achieved and verified with postoperative MRI scanning.[11] Five patients have required continued treatment for diabetes insipidus and eight patients have required ongoing hormonal replacement therapy. These results are compatible with the published results of most international centers.[12,13] In an analysis of our most recent case series (unpublished) our CSF leak rate is now less than 5% and the tumor recurrence rate in macroadenomas is less than 15%. The cure rate for hormone-secretory tumors is greater than 85%.

◆ Key Points

The two major advantages of this technique are the minimal trauma involved in accessing the pituitary gland with bilateral sphenoidotomies and, in some cases, septoplasty being the only surgery necessary for the approach to the pituitary. In addition there is considerable advantage in the use of angled telescopes in the pituitary fossa during the resection of the tumor. This allows for tumor that may remain unseen with the traditional microscopic approaches to be resected under direct vision (see **Fig. 13.13**). It also allows the descending diaphragm to be held up so that any residual tumor remaining in the angle between the diaphragm and the cavernous sinus can be visualized with a 30-degree angled telescope and to be removed under vision.

Patients with extensive invasion of the cavernous sinus have their tumors aggressively chased if these tumors are secretory. Nonsecretory tumors in the cavernous sinus are followed as long as the tumor continues to come away easily without putting the patient at risk.

Patients with an anterior or significant superior extension of their tumor may have an extended approach to the pituitary performed. This patient group requires septal flap closure of the defect.

The technique does require two surgeons working together off the video monitor and our team consists of a neurosurgeon and an otolaryngologist. Both surgeons have developed the skills to do all parts of the surgery and this maintains the skill level and enthusiasm for the different aspects of the operation.

References

1. Otori N, Haruna S, Kamio M, Ohashi G, Moriyama H. Endoscopic trans-ethmosphenoidal approach for pituitary tumors with image guidance. Am J Rhinol 2001;15(6):381–386

2. Sawers HA, Robb OJ, Walmsley D, Strachan FM, Shaw J, Bevan JS. An audit of the diagnostic usefulness of PRL and TSH responses to domperidone and high resolution magnetic resonance imaging of the pituitary in the evaluation of hyperprolactinaemia. Clin Endocrinol (Oxf) 1997;46(3):321–326

3. Wilson CB. A decade of pituitary microsurgery. The Herbert Olivecrona lecture. J Neurosurg 1984;61(5):814–833

4. de Divitiis E, Cappabianca P. Microscopic and endoscopic transsphenoidal surgery. Neurosurgery 2002;51(6):1527–1529, author reply 1529–1530

5. Thomas RF, Monacci WT, Mair EA. Endoscopic image-guided trans-ethmoid pituitary surgery. Otolaryngol Head Neck Surg 2002;127(5):409–416

6. Mason RB, Nieman LK, Doppman JL, Oldfield EH. Selective excision of adenomas originating in or extending into the pituitary stalk with preservation of pituitary function. J Neurosurg 1997;87(3):343–351

7. Aust MR, McCaffrey TV, Atkinson J. Transnasal endoscopic approach to the sella turcica. Am J Rhinol 1998;12(4):283–287

8. Shah S, Har-El G. Diabetes insipidus after pituitary surgery: incidence after traditional versus endoscopic transsphenoidal approaches. Am J Rhinol 2001;15(6):377–379

9. Cooke RS, Jones RA. Experience with the direct transnasal transsphenoidal approach to the pituitary fossa. Br J Neurosurg 1994;8(2):193–196

10. Knosp E, Steiner E, Kitz K, Matula C. Pituitary adenomas with invasion of the cavernous sinus space: a magnetic resonance imaging classification compared with surgical findings. Neurosurgery 1993;33(4):610–617, discussion 617–618

11. Uren B, Vrodos N, Wormald PJ. Fully endoscopic transsphenoidal resection of pituitary tumors: technique and results. Am J Rhinol 2007;21(4):510–514

12. Cappabianca P, Cavallo LM, Colao A, et al. Endoscopic endonasal transsphenoidal approach: outcome analysis of 100 consecutive procedures. Minim Invasive Neurosurg 2002;45(4):193–200

13. Kabil MS, Eby JB, Shahinian HK. Fully endoscopic endonasal vs. transseptal transsphenoidal pituitary surgery. Minim Invasive Neurosurg 2005;48(6):348–354

14 Endoscopic Orbital Decompression for Exophthalmos, Acute Orbital Hemorrhage, and Orbital Subperiosteal Abscess

Endoscopic orbital decompression plays an important role in the management of patients with Graves orbitopathy, in patients with acute orbital hemorrhage with proptosis, and for the drainage of orbital subperiosteal abscesses.

◆ Graves Disease

Exophthalmos in Graves disease is thought to result from the deposition of immune complexes in the extraocular muscles and fat, which in turn leads to edema and fibrosis.[1] The resultant increase in intraorbital pressure pushes the globe forward causing proptosis. If this proptosis becomes severe enough, the eyelids cannot close properly and chemosis with or without exposure keratitis of the cornea may occur. In addition, the crowding of the orbital apex by the significantly enlarged extraocular muscles places pressure on the optic nerve. In a small minority of patients stretching of the optic nerve by increasing proptosis may play a role in the development of optic neuropathy and visual loss. Visual loss is uncommon in Graves disease occurring in only 2 to 7% of patients.[2,3] If medical treatment (high-dose steroids with or without low dose radiotherapy) fails, surgical decompression of the eye is indicated.[4] Although this has in the past been performed via external procedures, excellent reduction of proptosis is now possible with endoscopic techniques.[5,6] **Figure 14.1** shows the extraocular muscle enlargement commonly seen in patients with Graves disease and visual loss.

Preoperative diplopia is seen in up to 30% of patients with Graves disease. If **Fig. 14.1** is reviewed it can be seen that the extensive muscle enlargement limits globe movement in the extremes of gaze which in turn will cause diplopia. After decompression significant medial and inferior prolapse of orbital tissue occurs and diplopia can be seen in up to 30% of patients who did not have preoperative diplopia. Decompression of the lateral wall is thought to balance this

intraorbital tissue displacement with resultant less likelihood of postoperative diploplia.[7] Although orbital decompression results in significant reduction in proptosis, the patient's eyes may still have a staring appearance due to fibrosis and shortening of the levator palpebrae muscle. This results in increased sclera show and, although there may have been significant reduction of proptosis, the cosmetic appearance would still not be ideal. A release of the levator muscles can be performed which can reduce or eliminate the scleral show.

◆ Intraorbital Hemorrhage

Intraorbital hemorrhage is fortunately a rare occurrence and usually occurs during endoscopic sinus surgery (ESS) as a result of injury to the anterior ethmoidal artery. The damaged artery retracts into the orbit and continues to bleed within the orbital contents with increasing intraorbital pressure. This pressure results in progressive proptosis with stretching or compression of the optic nerve. This combined with impairment of arterial blood flow to the retina from increasing intraorbital pressure can result in progressive visual loss. Color vision is reduced before visual acuity is lost. If impending visual loss is suspected, the patient should be tested for loss of red color discrimination and tested for a relative afferent pupil defect. Color vision is tested by showing the patient a picture with red in it and asking them to name the colors in the picture. Once visual acuity is lost the time before irreversible blindness occurs is variable but can be as short as 40 minutes if blood flow to the retina is lost. It is therefore important that, if intraorbital hemorrhage occurs, the surgeon immediately takes appropriate steps to reduce intraorbital pressure and restore blood flow to the retina and optic nerve. Other than progressive proptosis, subconjunctival and periorbital hemorrhage may also be visible. If the proptosed globe is palpated, it is hard and resists direct pressure. If the optic fundus can be visualized,

Fig. 14.1 Extraocular muscle enlargement marked with *white arrow* in coronal soft tissue CT scan (**A**) and axial CT scan (**B**). Note the orbital apex crowding.

the retinal arterial circulation may be seen to be intermittent or pulsatile.

If an intraorbital hemorrhage is recognized intraoperatively and the patient is still on the operating table, an orbital decompression should be performed as described in later text. If the patient is in recovery area or on the ward, and significant proptosis and visual loss is noticed then, the following steps should be taken:

- Sit the patient up in bed
- Remove any nasal packing
- Infiltrate the lateral canthus with local anesthetic and perform a lateral canthotomy and cantholysis

These are important steps with which to buy time allowing the patient to be taken back to theater for reexploration and orbital decompression.

Surgical Technique of Lateral Canthotomy and Cantholysis

Local anesthetic (lidocaine 2% with 1:80 000 adrenaline) is placed in the lateral canthal region. A sharp scissors is used to make a horizontal incision through skin and soft tissue at the lateral junction of the eyelids onto the bone of the orbital rim (**Fig. 14.2**).

The eyelid is drawn outward with forceps exposing the tendon attaching the inferior tarsal plate to the bone and the scissors are turned vertically and this tendon cut (**Fig. 14.3**).

Orbital fat should be seen as this tendon is cut and the eyelid should be able to be laid on the cheek without tension (**Fig. 14.4**). This reduces the intraorbital pressure and should allow reperfusion of the optic nerve and retina. However, it may be insufficient and is used only to buy time and allow

Fig. 14.2 (**A**) A horizontal cut is demonstrated on a cadaver. The horizontal cut is made onto the orbital rim through the lateral canthus. (**B**) Pulling the eyelid down reveals the lateral canthal tendon (*white arrow*).

Fig. 14.3 The lateral canthal tendon is held between the forceps with the scissors held vertically to cut the tendon.

Fig. 14.4 The eyelid is laid on the cheek. The cut lateral canthal tendon is marked with a black arrow and the orbital fat with a white arrow.

the patient to return to theater for a formal decompression of the orbit.

No stitches are placed in this wound and a dressing is placed over the wound. The wound and the lateral canthal tendon can be sutured after 24 to 48 hours. The lateral canthal tendon is sutured to the orbital periosteum. As the incision is in the crease formed by the eyelids, scarring is uncommon.

Fig. 14.5 Cadaveric dissection image of a total sphenoethmoidectomy with complete removal of the ethmoid air cells and exposure of the fovea ethmoidalis (*FE*), lamina papyracea (*LP*), sphenoid sinus (*SS*), maxillary sinus (*MS*), and frontal sinus (*FS*). *MT*, middle turbinate.

Surgical Technique for Endoscopic Orbital Decompression[5] (Videos 46 to 48)

After standard preparation and infiltration of the nasal cavity and lateral nasal wall, an uncinectomy is performed. The natural ostium of the maxillary sinus is identified and enlarged into the area of the posterior fontanelle with straight through-biting Blakesley forceps and the microdebrider.[5] It is essential to create the largest possible antrostomy as this gives access to the floor of the orbit and, after the decompression, prevents obstruction of the ostium if significant prolapse of fat occurs. If the antrostomy is small, blockage of the antrostomy and resultant sinusitis may develop.

An axillary flap is performed and the frontal recess cleared of cells with identification of the frontal ostium. A total spheno-ethmoidectomy is performed with identification of the sphenoid sinus ostium.[5] This ostium is enlarged into the posterior ethmoids allowing entry into the sphenoid through the posterior ethmoids. The skull base is identified and cleared so that the entire lamina papyracea is able to be viewed (**Fig. 14.5**).

The hard bone of the frontal process of the maxilla is palpated with a Freer elevator and the soft lacrimal bone identified (in much the same way as is done for endoscopic dacryocystorhinostomy) (**Fig. 14.6**). This soft lacrimal bone may be left and the junction of the lacrimal bone and lamina papyracea identified. If there is doubt about the lacrimal bone, this may be flaked off and the lacrimal sac palpated to accurately identify the lacrimal sac. The blunt end of the Freer elevator is then gently pushed through the lamina papyracea and the thin bone forming the lamina papyracea flaked off.[5] Great care must be taken to preserve the orbital periosteum at this early stage as a tear of the orbital periosteum with prolapse of orbital fat can obscure the remaining lamina papyracea and make its removal more difficult (**Fig. 14.7**). Care should also be taken not to remove the bony lamina papyracea for at least 1.5 cm below the frontal ostium. This bone is left in place to prevent prolapse of orbital fat obstructing the outflow tract of the frontal sinus. If chronic frontal sinusitis results after endoscopic orbital decompression this can be difficult to treat. The remaining bone of the lamina

Fig. 14.6 Cadaveric image of the palpation of the left frontal process with a Freer elevator.

Fig. 14.7 Cadaveric dissection demonstrating the removal of the lamina papyracea and exposure of the periorbita (*PO*). Care has been taken not to tear the periorbita and prevent the prolapse of orbital fat. A 1.5–cm margin of bone below the frontal ostium (*FO*) is preserved to prevent frontal sinus obstruction by fat. *SS*, sphenoid sinus; *FE*, fovea ethmoidalis; *AEA*, anterior ethmoidal artery; *MT*, middle turbinate.

papyracea is removed up to the skull base and posterior as far as the sphenoid sinus. Orbital periosteum is then removed (**Fig. 14.8**). This may be sufficient for orbital decompression for intraorbital hemorrhage or for a small reduction in proptosis from exophthalmos from Graves disease (around 2 mm).[5–11] If a greater amount of decompression and globe retrogression is required further decompression can be achieved by

Fig. 14.8 Cadaveric dissection clearly shows that the orbital periorbita has been removed exposing orbital fat (*OF*). *MT*, middle turbinate; *FE*, fovea ethmoidalis; *SS*, sphenoid sinus; *MS*, maxillary sinus.

removal of the posterior half of the orbital floor.[5,11] The bone thickens at the transition from medial orbital wall to floor of the orbit. Angled curettes and Blakesley forceps are used to fracture this bone and remove it. The infraorbital nerve is identified as it runs along the floor of the orbit (roof of the maxillary sinus). The posterior floor of the orbit is removed up to the infraorbital nerve (**Fig. 14.9**). Only the posterior half of the orbital floor can be accessed through the maxillary antrostomy. This is a technical problem as access to the anterior half of the orbital floor is usually not possible through the antrostomy with currently available instrumentation.[5,11]

The average amount of globe retrogression with the removal of both the medial wall and floor of the orbit is 5 mm.[5–11] The orbital periosteum is either incised in a series of horizontal incisions or removed entirely. Retention of a medial strip of orbital periosteum may reduce the incidence of postoperative diplopia but this is not my practice to retain this strip. If still greater regression of the globe is necessary, then the anterior part of the orbital floor and lateral orbital wall is approached through a subciliary incision. The conjunctiva is incised and further dissection identifies the lower lid fat pads. The orbital rim is identified and orbital periosteum elevated. The remaining anterior floor of the orbit is removed both medial and lateral to the infraorbital nerve. This is done with Kerrison forward- and backward-biting punches. This dissection is continued onto the lateral orbital wall and the lateral orbital wall removed with a diamond drill. This lateral decompression balances to some extent the orbital fat prolapse and may result in less postoperative diplopia. It certainly increases the amount of orbital regression that can be achieved and in our series this three-walled decompression averaged 5 to 7 mm.

Fig. 14.9 Cadaveric dissection image taken with a 70-degree endoscope of the left maxillary sinus (*MS*). The floor of the orbit has been removed up to the infraorbital nerve (*ION*) through an enlarged maxillary antrostomy. *OF*, orbital fat; *LNW*, lateral nasal wall.

Results of Orbital Decompression for Graves Disease

The degree of regression of proptosis in the 16 orbits decompressed was 5.4 mm.[5] If only the medial wall and floor were operated on, the average globe regression was 5.75 mm. In four orbits only the medial orbital wall was removed with an average globe regression of 1.75 mm. In six orbits a three-wall decompression was performed with an average regression of the globe of 6.5 mm. These results are slightly different from those results we published recently as we have added three subsequent patients who underwent bilateral three-wall orbital decompression.[5] Of the 16 orbits done, one patient with complete long-standing visual loss had no improvement in vision. All other patients had normal vision preoperatively and no patient had worsening of vision in the postoperative period.[5] Two patients who did not have preoperative diplopia developed postoperative diplopia. In both of these patients their diplopia was transient, lasting between 1 and 3 months before fully resolving. Four patients had preoperative diplopia which continued postoperatively and required extraocular muscle surgery for correction.

◆ Orbital Decompression for Subperiosteal Abscess (Video 48)

Patients presenting with orbital complications of sinusitis commonly have a degree of cellulitis and edema (chemosis) around the eye with associated proptosis. There may also be some restriction of eye movement. Patients typically give a history of nasal obstruction, purulent rhinorrhea, and

Fig. 14.10 Pus can be seen in the middle meatus. The mucosa is edematous with obliteration of the space between the middle turbinate and lateral nasal wall.

facial pressure or pain. Endoscopy reveals an inflamed and edematous nasal mucosa usually with the presence of pus in the middle meatus (**Fig. 14.10**).

If a subperiosteal abscess is suspected, a CT scan of the sinuses with contrast will reveal the classic presentation of a mass located on the lamina papyracea or in relation to the floor of the frontal sinus. The rim of the mass will enhance with the contrast as seen in **Fig. 14.11**. In addition, the proptosis will be visible on the axial scans.

The surgeon should consider their endoscopy experience and skill level before deciding if a patient with a subperiosteal abscess should be managed endoscopically or through an external approach. The external approach is quick, easy, and the abscess can usually be rapidly and safely drained. If the surgeon is skilled and experienced in ESS, endoscopic drainage of the subperiosteal abscess can be performed. The difficulty with this procedure is the significant vascularity that is associated with acute sinusitis. If a mucosal surface is touched with an instrument or endoscope it will usually bleed and if the surgeon is inexperienced they may lose orientation and complications may occur. Frequent packing with decongestant-soaked neuropatties throughout the procedure helps to minimize the bleeding but will not control it entirely. In a patient with acute sinusitis, the anesthetist needs to optimize the patient's hemodynamic parameters to create the optimal surgical field (Chapter 2). If the anesthetist is inexperienced with creating optimal conditions for sinus surgery patients, as may be the case on an emergency operating surgery list, this may lead to more troublesome bleeding.

The surgical approach is to perform an uncinectomy and enlarge the maxillary ostium to a moderate degree. Uncinectomy alone without antrostomy carries the risk of postoperative closure of the maxillary sinus as the inflammation and edema predisposes to scarring and adhesion formation. Clearance of the frontal recess depends on whether the frontal sinus is

Fig. 14.11 (**A**) Subperiosteal abscess (*white arrow*) associated with the roof of the orbit in coronal CT scan. (**B**) Proptosis (*white arrow*) of left globe visible on the axial soft tissue scan.

thought to be the origin of the subperiosteal abscess. If the abscess is located adjacent to the ethmoidal sinuses (the most common location) then the frontal recess should be left alone and no surgery performed in this region. Clearance of the bulla ethmoidalis and posterior ethmoids is performed with identification of the lamina papyracea. The lamina papyracea over the subperiosteal abscess is widely exposed and removed. If the abscess is related to the floor of the frontal sinus it can still be drained endoscopically. A mini-trephine is usually placed in the frontal sinus before dissection of the frontal recess. This aids in identification of the frontal sinus outflow track (the pathway along which the instruments will be passed to remove the cells of the frontal recess). The frontal recess is cleared and the frontal ostium identified. The lamina papyracea directly behind the lacrimal sac is removed and, using a malleable suction curette, the orbital periosteum (which is mobile) is kept intact and gently pushed laterally while the curette advances into the subperiosteal abscess. The abscess is drained.

A malleable suction Freer elevator or frontal sinus suction* (Medtronic ENT, Jacksonville, FL) is introduced into the cavity and any fibrin within the cavity removed. A narrow triangulated corrugated Penrose drain is slid into the abscess cavity and left in place. This ensures that pus does not reaccumulate in the abscess cavity. It is shortened the next day and removed the second day after surgery. Endoscopic drainage of subperiosteal abscesses remains highly effective but it must be emphasized that the surgeon should be experienced.

◆ Key Points

Orbital decompression for exophthalmos from Graves disease is an effective method for reduction of proptosis for cosmetic proptosis, eye complications from exposure of the cornea, and for visual loss. The amount of regression of proptosis is related to the number of walls decompressed at the time of surgery. Three-walled decompression may give a more balanced decompression with less likelihood of postoperative diplopia. However, this still has to be conclusively demonstrated.

Intraorbital hemorrhage should be managed with lateral canthotomy and cantholysis (if the patient has left the operating suite) followed by orbital decompression with removal of the medial orbital wall. Orbital decompression can be performed without canthotomy and cantholysis if the complication is noticed intraoperatively.

Endoscopic decompression of a subperiosteal abscess should only be performed by very experienced endoscopic sinus surgeons as the surgical field can be very bloody and this can increase the degree of difficulty significantly and complications are more likely. If the surgeon is not experienced then the abscess should be drained via an external incision.

References

1. Konishi J, Herman MM, Kriss JP. Binding of thyroglobulin and thyroglobulin-antithyroglobulin immune complex to extraocular muscle membrane. Endocrinology 1974;95(2):434–446
2. Warren JD, Spector JG, Burde R. Long-term follow-up and recent observations on 305 cases of orbital decompression for dysthyroid orbitopathy. Laryngoscope 1989;99(1):35–40
3. Garrity JA, Fatourechi V, Bergstralh EJ, et al. Results of transantral orbital decompression in 428 patients with severe Graves' ophthalmopathy. Am J Ophthalmol 1993;116(5):533–547
4. Asaria RHY, Koay B, Elston JS, Bates GEM. Endoscopic orbital decompression for thyroid eye disease. Eye (Lond) 1998;12(Pt 6):990–995
5. Wee DTH, Carney AS, Thorpe M, Wormald PJ. Endoscopic orbital decompression for Graves' ophthalmopathy. J Laryngol Otol 2002;116(1):6–9
6. Lund VJ, Larkin G, Fells P, Adams G. Orbital decompression for thyroid eye disease: a comparison of external and endoscopic techniques. J Laryngol Otol 1997;111(11):1051–1055
7. Kennedy DW, Goodstein ML, Miller NR, Zinreich SJ. Endoscopic transnasal orbital decompression. Arch Otolaryngol Head Neck Surg 1990;116(3):275–282
8. Metson R, Dallow RL, Shore JW. Endoscopic orbital decompression. Laryngoscope 1994;104(8 Pt 1):950–957
9. Metson R, Shore JW, Gliklich RE, Dallow RL. Endoscopic orbital decompression under local anesthesia. Otolaryngol Head Neck Surg 1995;113(6):661–667
10. Neugebauer A, Nishino K, Neugebauer P, Konen W, Michel O. Effects of bilateral orbital decompression by an endoscopic endonasal approach in dysthyroid orbitopathy. Br J Ophthalmol 1996;80(1):58–62
11. Koay B, Bates G, Elston J. Endoscopic orbital decompression for dysthyroid eye disease. J Laryngol Otol 1997;111(10):946–949

15 Endoscopic Optic Nerve Decompression

The most common indication for endoscopic optic nerve decompression is traumatic optic neuropathy.[1] Currently it is thought that ~5% of severe head injuries will have a concomitant injury to the optic nerve, optic tract, or optic cortex.[1–3] However, if the literature is reviewed, there are only a limited number of patients who have undergone this procedure.[4] Major brain injury occurs in 40 to 72% of patients with traumatic optic neuropathy[5] and the management of this injury obviously takes precedence. This may result in the optic nerve injury only being diagnosed some time after the original injury. Some authors feel that early diagnosis and treatment of traumatic optic neuropathy may be of greater benefit to the patient[6,7] and advocate diagnosis of the optic nerve deficit by the presence of an absolute or relative afferent pupillary defect supported by disc edema and congestion of the vessels.[6] These findings, in combination with the computed tomography (CT) scan, possibly a magnetic resonance imaging (MRI) scan and visual evoked potentials, may provide sufficient evidence to undertake optic nerve decompression.[6,7] However, the patient management protocol suggested in this chapter is more conservative as there is still considerable debate as to the value of both high-dose steroid treatment and surgical optic nerve decompression.[3–5,7] Currently there are no properly conducted randomized controlled trials comparing high-dose steroid therapy, surgical decompression, and observation.[8] In a meta-analysis of all published cases in the literature, Cook et al. concluded that treatment in the form of high-dose steroids or surgery or both was better than no treatment.[4] Tandon et al. evaluated the role of steroids with and without surgery in a large study of 111 patients who were placed in two groups: one group of patients had high-dose steroids and if they failed to improve underwent an optic nerve decompression whereas the second group had steroids alone.[1] This study showed that the patient group treated with steroids and surgery had significantly better outcome than the patient group treated with steroids alone.[1] Sofferman, in a study on an animal model of traumatic optic neuropathy, showed that injury to the optic nerve results in a progressive loss of myelin but with preservation of axons so that in theory the progression of the injury may be reversed with steroid or surgical decompression.[7]

Traumatic optic neuropathy is thought to result from two distinct injuries to the nerve. The primary injury results from either a direct contusive force on the optic canal and nerve or as a result of elastic deformation of the sphenoid with a transfer of force into the intracanalicular optic nerve disrupting the axons and blood vessels.[5] This primary injury may result in compression of the nerve by bony fragments or in hemorrhage into the nerve sheath. If this injury is not treated a secondary injury may occur. As the nerve swells in its dural sheath and bony canal, compression of the blood supply to the nerve occurs with resultant ischemia and continued axon loss.[5,7] Our department has adopted a conservative approach to traumatic neuropathy with all patients undergoing high-dose steroid treatment first before being offered surgical intervention. The exception is when bony fragments are seen to impinge on the optic nerve.

◆ Medical Therapy for Traumatic Optic Nerve Injury

Currently, mega-dose intravenous methylprednisolone is used following the spinal cord injury management protocol. Methylprednisolone 30 mg/kg intravenous (IV) loading dose is given followed by an infusion of 5.4 mg/kg/hour thereafter.[4] The patient's visual acuity is monitored hourly and surgical intervention is considered if the patient fills any of the criteria listed below:

- Fracture of optic canal on CT scan with vision less than 6/60
- Fracture of the optic canal with vision > 6/60 but the patient's vision deteriorates on steroids
- Vision is < 6/60 (or there is a deterioration of vision) after 48 hours of steroid treatment with probable canal injury

(indicated by the presence of fluid levels in the posterior ethmoids and sphenoid and/or the presence of fractures of the ethmoids, orbital apex, and sphenoid)

◆ Surgical Technique for Traumatic Optic Neuropathy (Video 49)

The standard preparation of the nose is performed with decongestion and infiltration. An uncinectomy with exposure of the maxillary ostium is performed. An axillary flap is performed and the agger nasi cell removed. This improves access to the skull base. The fovea ethmoidalis is exposed in the region above the bulla ethmoidalis. If there is disruption of the cells of the frontal recess or reason to suggest that the frontal recess is obstructed then this will be cleared; otherwise, the cells in the frontal recess are left untouched. In some patients with severe sinus fractures, the entire skull base may be mobile. In the patient presented in **Fig. 15.1**, the entire posterior skull base was mobile.

In most patients the posterior ethmoid cells will be full of blood and, when this is combined with mobility of the lamina papyracea and skull base, the surgeon can become disorientated. Therefore this surgery should only be undertaken by very experienced endoscopic sinus surgeons. A posterior ethmoidectomy and sphenoidotomy should be performed as described in Chapter 8. In the posterior ethmoids, the posterior lamina papyracea and fovea ethmoidalis should be identified (**Fig. 15.2**). If significant disruption of the posterior ethmoids and lamina papyracea has occurred, then a large middle meatal antrostomy provides an extra reference point and lessens the likelihood of surgeon disorientation (**Fig. 15.2**). The natural ostium of the sphenoid sinus should be identified and the anterior face of the sphenoid widely opened. It is important for the surgeon to be fully aware of the anatomy of the lateral wall of the sphenoid (**Fig. 15.3**). If available the computer-aided surgery (CAS) navigation system may help in patients where there has been significant anatomical disruption.

The anterior face of the sphenoid needs to be taken as high as possible so that the roof of the sphenoid and

Fig. 15.1 (**A–D**) Sequential coronal CT scans from (**A**) the posterior ethmoids to (**D**) the sphenoid sinus. The *white arrows* indicate fractures and note the blood in the ethmoids and sphenoids. (**B**) In addition, the *white arrow* indicates the loose segment of skull base. The scans are of relative poor quality due to patient movement from confusion from an associated head injury.

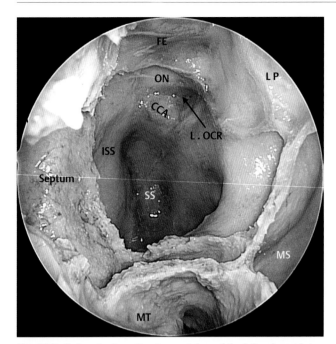

Fig. 15.2 Cadaveric dissection image taken of the left sphenoid sinus demonstrating the fovea ethmoidalis (*FE*) and lamina papyracea (*LP*). *ON*, optic nerve; *CCA*, anterior genu of the intracavernous carotid artery; *L. OCR*, lateral opticocarotid recess; *ISS*, sphenoid intersinus septum; *SS*, sphenoid sinus; *MS*, maxillary sinus; *MT*, middle turbinate.

Fig. 15.3 Cadaveric dissection image taken of the left sphenoid sinus through a maximal sphenoidotomy. The vidian canal (*VC*) and trigeminal impression (*TI*) for the maxillary division of the trigeminal nerve can be clearly seen. If the sphenoid sinus is well pneumatized then the lateral recess (*LR*) can be seen, a depression in the lateral sphenoid wall between the VC and the TI. The lateral opticocarotid recess can be seen. This depression corresponds to pneumatization of the optic strut (the bony bridge that separates the optic canal from the superior orbital fissure). Further pneumatization into the optic strut may result in a pneumatized anterior clinoid process which will place the optic nerve on a mesentery. The optic tubercle (*OT*) is the bone located at the junction of the orbital apex and the sphenoid sinus. *ISS*, intersinus septum; *ON*, optic nerve; *CCA*, anterior genu of the intracavernous carotid artery; *PCA*, paraclival carotid artery.

the posterior ethmoids is continuous.[3,9,10] The sphenoid should be inspected and the optic nerve, carotid artery, and pituitary fossa identified.[9,10] If there has been significant disruption of the orbital apex or the lateral wall of the sphenoid, then identification of these basic structures can be difficult (**Fig. 15.4**). In these cases image guidance may help.

The thick bone overlying the junction of the orbital apex and sphenoid sinus is known as the optic tubercle. This bone is normally too thick to flake off and an irrigated diamond burr (the 15-degree 3.2-mm diamond skull base burr or the 2.5-mm 25-degree dacryocystorhinostomy [DCR] diamond burr from Medtronic ENT [Jacksonville, FL]) is used to thin this bone down until it is almost transparent (**Fig. 15.4**).[9,10]

A blunt Freer elevator is pushed through the lamina papyracea ~1.5 cm anterior to the junction of the posterior ethmoids air cell(s) and the sphenoid (**Fig. 15.4**). Care should be taken to keep the orbital periosteum intact while this is done, otherwise prolapse of orbital fat can severely obstruct the dissection of the optic nerve. The bone of the posterior orbital apex is flaked off the underlying orbital periosteum (**Fig. 15.4**).[9,10]

Once the bone over the orbital apex is removed the bone of the optic canal is approached. This bone is usually quite thin and can, in a large proportion of patients, be simply flaked off the underlying nerve (**Fig. 15.5**). However, in some cases, the bone over the nerve can be too thick and will need to be thinned with a diamond burr prior to removal. Once the bone is thin enough to be flaked off the underlying nerve,

only suitably designed instruments should be used. Any instrument that has a thick working end is unsuitable. If the back of the instrument indents the nerve as the edge of the instrument is used to engage the edge of the optic canal bone, it should not be used. Suitable instruments include the Beale elevator and the House curette, both from the ear tray (**Fig. 15.5**).[9]

Once all the bone has been cleared off the optic canal and the underlying optic nerve sheath is clearly visible, the sheath should be incised (**Fig. 15.6**).[9,10] The location of the ophthalmic artery should be kept in mind. The ophthalmic artery usually runs in the posteroinferior quadrant of the nerve. However, in a small proportion of patients, this artery can migrate around the lower edge of the nerve and potentially into the surgical field (**Fig. 15.7**).[8] However, if the nerve is incised in the upper medial quadrant, the risk to this artery should be minimal.[9,11] A sharp sickle knife* (single use disposable DCR mini-sickle knife [Medtronic ENT] is the most suitable) is used to incise the sheath of the optic nerve. Usually the pressure from the swollen optic nerve will cause the sheath to split as it is incised. The underlying pressure will often cause the nerve to protrude through the incision. This incision is continued onto the

Fig. 15.4 Cadaveric dissection image of the left sphenoid sinus. The anterior face of the sphenoid has been removed so that the roof of the sphenoid and posterior ethmoids is continuous. A diamond burr has been used to allow the removal of bone at the junction of the orbital apex and sphenoid sinus (the optic tubercle). The lamina papyracea (*LP*) has been removed 1.5 cm from the junction of the posterior ethmoids with the sphenoid sinus, exposing periorbita (*PO*).

Fig. 15.5 The thin bone overlying the orbital apex and optic nerve is gently flaked off. *PO*, periorbita; *CCA*, anterior genu of the intracavernous carotid artery; *PCA*, paraclival carotid artery; *ISS*, intersinus septum; *TI*, trigeminal impression.

Fig. 15.6 The optic nerve sheath (*ONS*) is incised to release the optic nerve. *PO*, periorbita; *ISS*, intersinus septum.

Fig. 15.7 Cadaveric dissection image taken of the left optic nerve and ophthalmic artery. The optic sheath has been removed to expose the contents within. The ophthalmic artery (*OA*) can be seen branching from the carotid artery at the lower medial quadrant of the optic nerve (*ON*). Therefore, incision in the upper medial quadrant poses little risk to the artery. *P*, pituitary gland; *PCA*, paraclival carotid artery; *CCA*, anterior genu of the intracavernous carotid artery.

Fig. 15.8 Cadaveric dissection of the lateral wall of the left sphenoid sinus. The optic sheath and periorbita (*PO*) of the orbital apex has been incised. *PS*, planum sphenoidale; *CCA*, anterior genu of the intracavernous carotid artery; *L. OCR*, lateral opticocarotid recess; *OS*, optic sheath.

Fig. 15.9 Cadaveric dissection image demonstrating the medial rectus muscle (*MR*) at the orbital apex. *PO*, periorbita; *OS*, optic sheath.

orbital periosteum of the posterior orbital apex with resultant protrusion of orbital fat (**Fig. 15.8**). The orbital fat covering this area of the medial rectus muscle is thin and care should be taken to avoid injuring this muscle (**Fig. 15.9**). Potentially such an incision can create a CSF leak but to date none has been seen after this incision. This may be due to the fact that the nerve has swollen and any potential CSF space has been obliterated. No packs are placed on the nerve or in the sinuses.

◆ Results of Optic Nerve Decompression for Traumatic Optic Neuropathy

Blunt Injury

Four patients presented with traumatic optic neuropathy after blunt trauma (usually a motor vehicle accident). Visible trauma to the frontal bone was seen with fractures involving the posterior ethmoids and sphenoid. Blood was seen in posterior ethmoids and sphenoid in all patients.

Two patients had an obvious fracture through the bony optic canal (**Fig. 15.10**).

All patients were operated on after failed medical therapy (high-dose IV steroids) for the optic neuropathy and all underwent surgery within 5 days of the original injury. Two patients with hematomas around the orbital apex (**Fig. 15.1**) improved from light perception preoperatively to 6/9 vision. The third patient improved from light perception to 6/60 vision and the fourth patient improved from no light perception to 6/60 vision. Three of these patients were left with limited visual field defects.

Sharp Injury to the Optic Nerve

Two patients suffered optic neuropathy after a penetrating knife-wound and both had no light perception after the initial injury. One patient underwent surgery 8 days after the injury and the second patient 12 days after the injury. Preoperative medical therapy was significantly delayed due to patients presenting to a rural hospital before referral to our hospital. Preoperative CT and MRI suggested the optic nerve was intact and, in one case, an obvious injury to the optic canal was seen. During surgery in one patient a bony fragment was seen to significantly indent the nerve. This was removed and the optic nerve decompressed and sheath was slit but the patient showed no postoperative improvement in vision. The other patient also showed no improvement after surgery. It is not known if the mechanism of injury after such a localized insult is different or whether the delayed presentation may have also contributed to the lack of improvement after surgery.

◆ Results of Optic Nerve Decompression for Pseudotumor of the Orbital Apex and for Tumors Compressing the Optic Canal

Four patients presented with compressive lesions of the orbital apex or optic canal with progressive visual loss. One patient had a pseudotumor of the orbital apex which extended significantly into the bony optic nerve canal. This patient presented with progressive visual loss and

Fig. 15.10 One of the patients who presented with significant fractures through the optic nerve canal, around the carotid artery, and in the lateral aspects of the sphenoid (*white arrows*). (**A–C**) Sequential coronal CT scans through the sphenoid sinus.

underwent decompression of the posterior orbit and optic canal. Postoperatively she regained normal vision which over a period of months slowly deteriorated. The surgery was revised and the annulus of Zinn was divided. This again improved her vision to 6/18 without further deterioration (**Fig. 15.11**).

The second patient presented with an 8-month progressive visual loss and at presentation could only see hand

movements. He had a fairly extensive compressive lesion of his orbital apex and optic canal. After decompression his vision remained stable but did not improve (**Fig. 15.12**). Patients with long-term visual loss may not respond as well as patients who present with more rapid visual loss due to optic nerve decompression.

Two patients with compressive lesions (lateral sphenoid wing meningioma and an encircling fibrous dys-

Fig. 15.11 (**A**) CT scan and (**B**) MRI scan of the patient with a pseudotumor of the orbital apex.

Fig. 15.12 (**A–D**) Sequential coronal CT scans from the posterior ethmoids to the sphenoid. The compressive lesion on the orbital apex and optic canal is indicated by the *white arrows*.

plasia) both had significant visual acuity and visual field loss and both had their vision return to normal after decompression.

◆ Key Points

Optic nerve decompression is a highly complex procedure and should only be undertaken by endoscopic sinus surgeons with significant experience and skill. Potentially, injury to the skull base with a resultant CSF leak may occur and an associated injury to the internal carotid artery may also be present (**Fig. 15.10**).[12] Injudicious manipulation of bony fragments may have catastrophic consequences for the patient. Patients should be given a trial of medical therapy before surgery is contemplated unless there is an obvious bony fragment impinging on the optic nerve.[4] Results from the small case series presented in this chapter and from larger studies in the literature[1–4,10] suggest that patients should be operated on if medical therapy fails to improve the vision within 24

to 48 hours. Significant delays again would seem to lessen the potential for success of the surgery.[5,7] Great care should be taken in exposing the optic nerve especially when flaking the bone from the nerve. Injudicious use of inappropriate instruments has the potential to worsen the vision and this should be kept in mind during the procedure.[12] In the hands of an experienced endoscopic sinus surgeon this procedure is a relatively safe operation with low morbidity and has the potential to improve and in some cases restore lost vision especially after blunt trauma.

References

1. Tandon D, Thakar A, Mahapatra A, Ghosh P. Transethmoidal optic nerve decompression. Clin Otolaryngol 1993;19:98–104
2. Kountakis SE, Maillard AA, El-Harazi SM, Longhini L, Urso RG. Endoscopic optic nerve decompression for traumatic blindness. Otolaryngol Head Neck Surg 2000;123(1 Pt 1):34–37
3. Kuppersmith RB, Alford EL, Patrinely JR, Lee AG, Parke RB, Holds JB. Combined transconjunctival/intranasal endoscopic approach to the

optic canal in traumatic optic neuropathy. Laryngoscope 1997;107(3): 311–315

4. Cook MW, Levin LA, Joseph MP, Pinczower EF. Traumatic optic neuropathy. A meta-analysis. Arch Otolaryngol Head Neck Surg 1996;122(4):389–392

5. Steinsapir KD, Goldberg RA. Traumatic optic neuropathy. Surv Ophthalmol 1994;38(6):487–518

6. Lübben B, Stoll W, Grenzebach U. Optic nerve decompression in the comatose and conscious patients after trauma. Laryngoscope 2001;111(2):320–328

7. Sofferman RA. Harris P. Mosher Award thesis. The recovery potential of the optic nerve. Laryngoscope 1995;105(7 Pt 3, Suppl 72):1–38

8. Steinsapir KD, Seiff SR, Goldberg RA. Traumatic optic neuropathy: where do we stand? Ophthal Plast Reconstr Surg 2002;18(3):232–234

9. Luxenberger W, Stammberger H, Jebeles JA, Walch C. Endoscopic optic nerve decompression: the Graz experience. Laryngoscope 1998;108(6):873–882

10. Chow JM, Stankiewicz JA. Powered instrumentation in orbital and optic nerve decompression. Otolaryngol Clin North Am 1997;30(3):467–478

11. Chou PI, Sadun AA, Lee H. Vasculature and morphometry of the optic canal and intracanalicular optic nerve. J Neuroophthalmol 1995;15(3):186–190

12. Metson R, Pletcher SD. Endoscopic orbital and optic nerve decompression. Otolaryngol Clin North Am 2006;39(3):551–561, ix

16 Endoscopic Resection of Tumors Involving the Maxillary Sinus, Pterygopalatine Fossa, and Infratemporal Fossa

As endoscopic sinus surgery (ESS) has progressed over the last 10 years, new techniques have been introduced to aid with the resection of tumors in regions which traditionally have been difficult to access.[1] In general the approaches described in this chapter are more suitable for benign tumors but, as techniques and adjuvant therapy develop, these techniques will be increasingly applied to the resection of malignant tumors.

To assess the endoscopic resectability of a tumor, both computed tomography (CT) and magnetic resonance imaging (MRI) scans are required.[2–4] Using both these modalities the surgeon can determine if sinuses that are opacified on the CT scan contain retained secretions or tumor.[2,3] By being able to accurately define the extent of the tumor, resection can then be carefully planned. Endoscopic resection of the medial maxilla is useful to access the anterior, posterior, and lateral walls of the maxillary sinus.[3,5,6]

◆ Surgical Techniques for Access to the Maxillary Sinus, Pterygopalatine Fossa, and Infratemporal Fossa

Canine Fossa Trephination for Access to the Maxillary Sinus (Videos 8 and 9)

Tumors that involve the medial wall, anterior floor, or anterior or anterolateral wall of the maxillary sinus cannot be accessed through a maxillary antrostomy irrespective of how large this is made. It is necessary in these patients to provide an alternative route of access. Although this can be achieved through an inferior meatal puncture, placement of a 4–mm microdebrider blade through the inferior meatal antrostomy tends to destabilize the inferior turbinate as the blade is moved within the maxillary sinus. This is because the nasal vestibule provides a fulcrum around which the blade is rotated, causing significant disruption

of the second fulcrum which is the inferior meatal port. In addition, this route of access does not give access to the anterior and medial compartments of the maxillary sinus. The best port is provided by the canine fossa trephine as described in Chapter 5. As there is only a single fulcrum around which the blade rotates, good access is provided to the medial and lateral walls, and the floor of the maxillary sinus (**Fig. 16.1**).

However, canine fossa trephine is not suitable for tumors originating from or with extensive attachment to the anterior wall of the maxillary sinus as the trephine will be placed through tumor attachment.

Endoscopic Medial Maxillectomy for Access to the Anterior Wall of the Maxillary Sinus and Infratemporal Fossa[5,6] (Videos 41 and 42)

The nasal cavity is prepared by placing cocaine- and adrenaline-soaked neuropatties in the nasal cavity. The lateral nasal wall and septum are infiltrated with 2% lidocaine and 1:80 000 adrenaline. A pterygopalatine fossa block is placed via the greater palatine canal using 2 mL of lidocaine and adrenaline (see Chapter 2). This helps to reduce bleeding during the dissection of the medial wall of the maxilla and pterygopalatine fossa.

The first step in endoscopic medial maxillectomy is to remove the uncinate process and perform a large middle meatal antrostomy (**Fig. 16.2**). The maxillary antrum is enlarged posteriorly up to the posterior wall of the maxillary sinus (**Fig. 16.3**). This provides visualization of the medial orbital wall and allows removal of the residual medial maxilla without endangering the orbit. Most large tumors of the maxillary sinus and/or pterygopalatine fossa will involve the posterior ethmoids and sphenoid. In these patients an axillary flap is performed and the frontal recess dissected with exposure of the frontal ostium. The bulla ethmoidalis is removed and a posterior ethmoidectomy and sphenoidotomy

A, B   C

Fig. 16.1 (**A–C**) An axially cut right maxillary sinus of a cadaver illustrating the access that can be achieved within the maxillary sinus (lateral, floor, and medial) through a canine fossa trephine. The *white arrow* indicates the trephination port in the anterior face of the maxillary sinus.

is performed. The skull base is clearly identified. Any tumor extension into the anterior and posterior ethmoids can be assessed and, if necessary, biopsies or frozen sections of the mucosa from these regions can be sent for examination. This helps ensure complete tumor clearance.

To perform the medial maxillectomy, the inferior turbinate is medialized. A Tilley's packing forceps is used to crush the turbinate just distal to the junction of the anterior end of the turbinate and the lateral nasal wall.[5] If there is a

large intranasal component of a soft nonvascular tumor, the tumor is debulked (**Fig. 16.4**). If the tumor is very vascular or firm then it can be pushed superiorly or partially debulked. Because of the posterior location of angiofibroma, debulking is usually not necessary.

Turbinectomy scissors are used to cut along the crushed region of the inferior turbinate up to the point where the turbinate inserts into the lateral nasal wall (**Fig. 16.5**). A scalpel is used to make mucosal incisions from just below

Fig. 16.2 Cadaveric image following a right sided uncinectomy. *BE*, bulla ethmoidalis; *MO*, maxillary ostium.

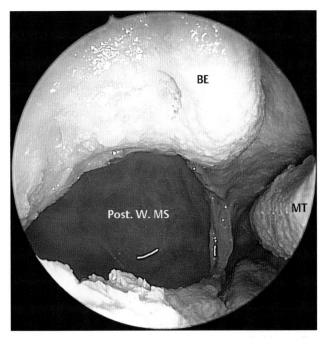

Fig. 16.3 Maxillary ostium enlargement to the posterior wall of the maxillary sinus. *Post. W. MS*, posterior wall of the maxillary sinus; *BE*, bulla ethmoidalis.

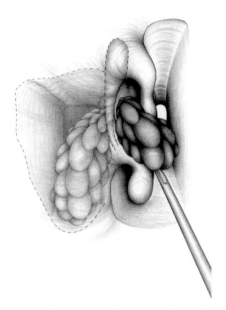

Fig. 16.4 Inverting papilloma originating in the maxillary sinus is partially debulked with a microdebrider to establish the region of origin of the tumor.

the orbit, through the cut inferior turbinate onto the floor of the nasal cavity.[5] This incision is continued along the floor of the nose to the posterior region of the inferior turbinate (**Fig. 16.5**). Here the mucosal incision is turned vertically toward the posterior region of the maxillary sinus antrostomy. A sharp chisel is used to cut the bone under the mucosal incisions following the mucosal incision (**Fig. 16.5**). The posterior vertical cut needs to enter the maxillary sinus adjacent to the posterior wall of the maxillary sinus and into the large antrostomy[5] (**Fig. 16.5**).

Once the bone forming the medial maxillary wall is mobilized, the nasolacrimal duct will tether the bone anteriorly and the duct will be visualized (**Fig. 16.6**). The duct should be transected with a scalpel (**Fig. 16.6**). At the end of the operation, the dacryocystorhinostomy (DCR) spear knife* (Medtronic ENT, Jacksonville, FL) is used to open the lower half of the sac creating anterior and posterior flaps which are then rolled out.[5–7] This prevents postoperative stenosis of the sac.[5,6] The edges of the resected portion of the maxilla are trimmed with the microdebrider. If a 70–degree telescope is used, the entire maxillary sinus should be able to be visualized[5] (**Fig. 16.7**). This includes the anterior wall and floor of

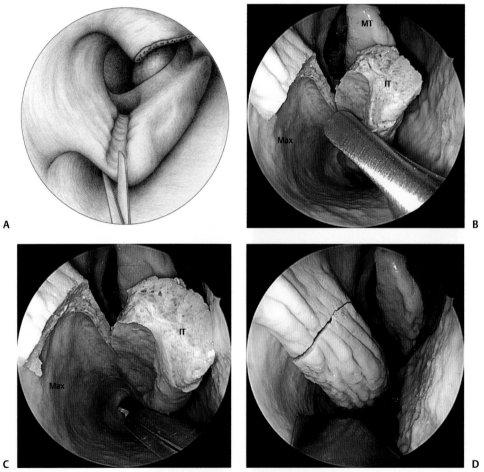

Fig. 16.5 (**A**) The inferior turbinate is crushed and cut up to the insertion of the turbinate on the medial wall of the maxilla. (**B**) Cadaveric image demonstrating the inferior turbinate (*IT*) has been cut up to the insertion on the medial wall of the maxilla (*Max*).

MT, middle turbinate. (**C**) This incision is continued along the floor of the nose to the posterior region of the inferior turbinate. (**D**) A sharp chisel is used to cut the bone under the mucosal incisions following the mucosal incision.

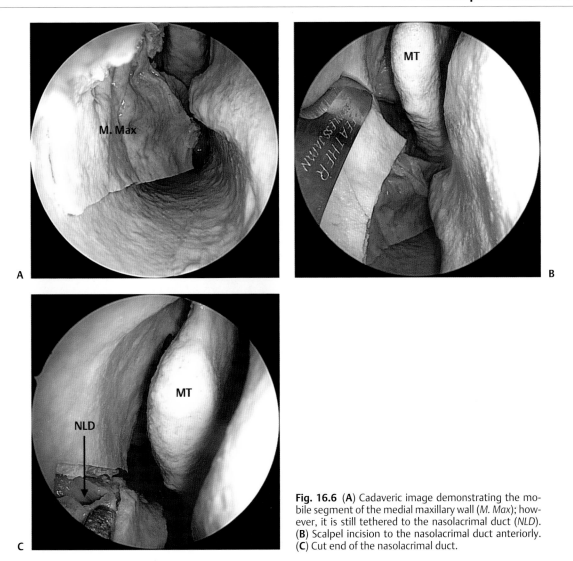

Fig. 16.6 (**A**) Cadaveric image demonstrating the mobile segment of the medial maxillary wall (*M. Max*); however, it is still tethered to the nasolacrimal duct (*NLD*). (**B**) Scalpel incision to the nasolacrimal duct anteriorly. (**C**) Cut end of the nasolacrimal duct.

Fig. 16.7 Cadaveric images demonstrating the exposure following a medial maxillectomy of the maxillary sinus taken with a (**A**) zero-degree and (**B**) 70-degree endoscope. *PW*, posterior wall; *LW*, lateral wall; *AW*, anterior wall; *MT*, middle turbinate.

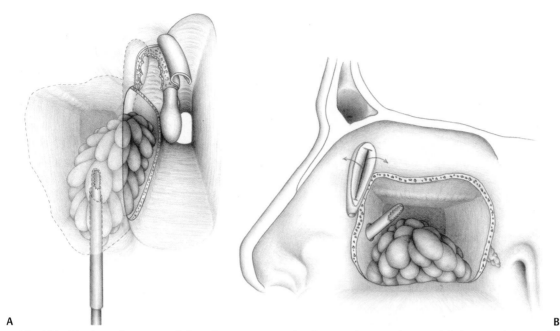

A   B

Fig. 16.8 (**A**) After endoscopic medial maxillectomy as viewed with a zero-degree endoscope. (**B**) The view of the maxillary sinus with a 70-degree endoscope. Note the microdebrider blade that has been placed through the canine fossa trephine.

the maxillary sinus (**Figs. 16.7 and 16.8**). Tumor can now be removed from the maxillary sinus under direct visualization. If additional access is required and the tumor does not attach to the anterior wall of the maxillary sinus, a canine fossa puncture can be performed. This allows instruments or an endoscope to be introduced through the anterior wall of the maxillary sinus which can be useful to access areas within the sinus that may be otherwise difficult to access. Malleable suction dissectors* (both curette and Freer elevator; Medtronic ENT) are also very useful as these instruments can be bent to the required angle for dissection in difficult areas such as the anterior wall or anterolateral region of the maxillary sinus.

If the anterior face of the maxillary sinus cannot be well seen or, if better access to the anterior face is required for a tumor that attaches extensively to the anterior face of the maxillary

sinus, further resection of the anteromedial wall and frontal process of the maxilla can be performed (**Fig. 16.9**). In such cases a canine fossa trephine is not thought to be suitable due to the small risk of seeding the tumor into the soft tissues of the cheek. Although seeding is unlikely to occur, this risk is thought to be greater if the entry point into the maxillary sinus is through tumor rather than through normal mucosa.

If access is still difficult and the anterior wall of the maxillary sinus is not fully accessible, a transseptal route provides a better angle of approach to this region. This access is achieved by performing a hemitransfixion incision in the opposite nasal vestibule (**Fig. 16.10A**) and then removing a small horizontal area of cartilage and/or bone opposite the region of the anterior maxillary sinus (**Fig. 16.10B**). The instrument can then be passed through the hemitransfixion incision, through the

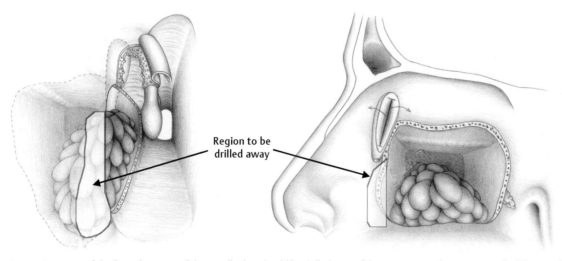

Region to be
drilled away

Fig. 16.9 Region of the frontal process of the maxilla that should be drilled away if direct access to the anterior wall of the maxillary sinus is needed.

Fig. 16.10 (**A**) Cadaveric dissection image demonstrating a hemitransfixion incision anteriorly in the left nostril (contralateral side to the tumor dissection). (**B**) A mucoperichondrial flap is elevated. C, cartilage; F, flap. (**C**) A cartilaginous septal window has been removed and a horizontal incision is performed through the mucoperichondrial flap on the ipsilateral side (*IF*). This allows the passage of a 70-degree diamond tipped drill (*D*). (**D**) The endoscope has been placed within the right nasal cavity demonstrating the working tip of the drill passing into the right maxillary sinus through the left hemitransfixion incision and through the horizontal septal flap incision (*HI*).

cartilage window (**Fig. 16.10C**) and then through the horizontal mucosal incision in the opposite nasal cavity (**Fig. 16.10D**), giving greater access to the anterior wall of the maxillary sinus (**Fig. 16.11B**). This approach significantly improves the angle of approach and usually allows complete access to the entire anterior maxillary wall (**Fig. 16.11A**). This region is best approached using either a 60-degree microdebrider blade or a 70-degree diamond burr (Medtronic ENT).

Access to the Pterygopalatine Fossa (Videos 41 and 42)

Access to the pterygopalatine fossa is achieved by removing the posterior wall of the maxillary sinus. In most cases a medial maxillectomy is unnecessary as most of the pterygopalatine fossa can be accessed through a large middle meatal antrostomy. If necessary this antrostomy can be taken through the inferior turbinate to the floor of the nose by partial inferior turbinate resection. The mucosa from the posterior wall of the maxillary sinus is elevated and preserved. This exposes the bone and removal of this bone is necessary to expose the pterygopalatine fossa. To remove this bone it is necessary to expose the sphenopalatine artery (SPA) as described in Chapter 10. The artery is cauterized with suction bipolar forceps. A Hajek-Kofler punch or 45-degree through-biting Blakesley forceps is used to remove the bone anterior to the SPA. The punch is introduced into the sphenopalatine foramen and the bone anterior to the foramen removed until the posterior wall of the maxillary sinus is reached (**Fig. 16.12**). Further removal of this bone can be done either with the punch or with a 45-degree through-biting Blakesley. Bone is removed until the contents of the pterygopalatine fossa are exposed (**Fig. 16.13**).

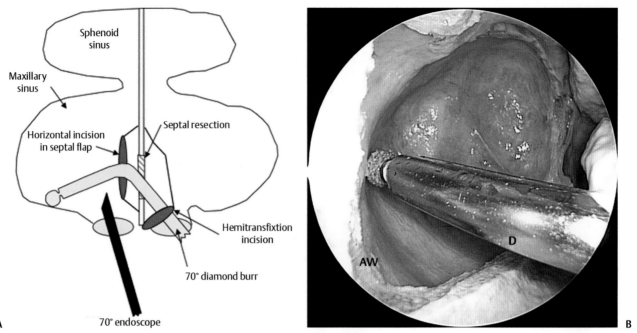

Fig. 16.11 **(A)** Illustration of the septal incisions necessary to achieve good access to the entire anterior wall of the maxillary sinus for tumors either originating from this region or with a significant anterior wall attachment. **(B)** Cadaveric image demonstrating the access to the anterior wall (*AW*) of the maxillary sinus with a 70-degree diamond drill (*D*).

Fig. 16.12 Cadaveric dissection demonstrating the contents of the right pterygopalatine fossa as viewed through a maximal maxillary antrostomy. *PW*, posterior wall of maxillary sinus; *SS*, sphenoid sinus; *MT*, middle turbinate.

Fig. 16.13 Cadaveric dissection image taken from within the maxillary sinus on the right side. This image demonstrates the contents of the pterygomaxillary sinus following fat removal. *PPG*, pterygopalatine ganglion; *GPN*, greater palatine nerve; *VA*, vidian artery; *GPA*, greater palatine artery; *SPA*, sphenopalatine artery; *ZN*, zygomatic nerve; *ION*, infraorbital nerve; *PSAA*, posterior superior alveolar artery; *PSAN*, posterior superior alveolar nerve; *3rd MA*, third division of the maxillary artery.

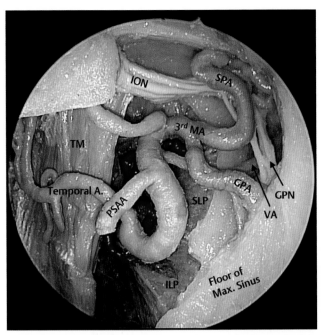

Fig. 16.14 Cadaveric dissection image following the removal of the lateral wall, floor, and posterior wall of the right maxillary sinus. This image reveals the temporalis muscle (*TM*) located superficial to the lateral wall of the maxillary sinus. The superior (*SLP*) and inferior (*ILP*) heads of the lateral pterygoid muscle can be seen where they attach and cover the superficial surface of the lateral pterygoid plates. *GPN*, greater palatine nerve; *VA*, vidian artery; *GPA*, greater palatine artery; *SPA*, sphenopalatine artery; *ION*, infraorbital nerve; *PSAA*, posterior superior alveolar artery; *3rd MA*, third division of the maxillary artery.

Access to the Infratemporal Fossa (Videos 41 and 42)

To access the infratemporal fossa, all of the bone of the posterior and lateral wall of the maxillary sinus needs to be removed. Most of the bone can be removed through the same nostril as the tumor using either the Hajek-Kofler punch or through-biting Blakesley. For complete access the bone should be removed from the roof to the floor of the maxillary sinus (**Fig. 16.14**).

Bone removal can continue until the anterior wall of the maxillary sinus is reached by inserting the punch or Blakesley forceps through the opposite nostril via a septal port. The septal port for the infratemporal fossa is very similar to that used to access the front wall of the maxillary sinus. This angle of approach allows the instruments to be advanced up to the anterior maxillary sinus wall as described under "Maxillary Sinus Access."

◆ Endoscopic Anatomy

Endoscopic Anatomy of the Greater Palatine Canal and the Pterygopalatine Fossa

The greater palatine canal and the pterygopalatine fossa are continuous (**Figs. 16.15 and 16.16**). The pterygopalatine fossa is similar to an inverted cone and the bottom

of this cone forms the greater palatine canal. The pterygopalatine fossa contains the distal branches of the maxillary artery, namely the SPA and the greater palatine artery (**Fig. 16.13**). In addition the vidian nerve enters the posterior aspect of the fossa before moving laterally to end in the pterygopalatine ganglion which is suspended from the maxillary nerve (**Fig. 16.13**). The pterygopalatine fossa narrows gradually as it opens laterally into the region of the infraorbital fissure and pterygomaxillary fissure before widening into the infratemporal fossa (**Figs. 16.14, 16.15, and 16.16**).

The roof of the pterygopalatine fossa is formed by the greater wing of the sphenoid bone and the infraorbital fissure, foramen rotundum, and the maxillary nerve coursing from the foramen rotundum from medial to lateral across the roof of the fossa just below the orbital apex (**Figs. 16.15 and 16.16**). The medial wall is formed by the palatine bone, sphenopalatine foramen, and SPA (**Fig. 16.17**), whereas the floor is formed by the greater palatine canal and the lateral wall is formed by the pterygomaxillary fissure (**Figs. 16.13 and 16.16**). In **Fig. 16.18** the relationships between the foramina that enter the posterior wall of the pterygopalatine fossa—namely, the palatovaginal canal, the vidian canal, and the foramen rotundum—are demonstrated. In addition the infraorbital fissure and pterygomaxillary fissure are seen (**Fig. 16.16**).

If the anatomy of this region is viewed endoscopically and each layer removed so that the underlying layer can be appreciated, a good understanding of the anatomy can be achieved. The first fact to be appreciated is that the pterygopalatine fossa forms a relatively small part of the total area behind the posterior wall of the maxillary sinus (**Fig. 16.12**). Second the first structures to be encountered when entering the fossa are the blood vessels (**Fig. 16.13**). The neural structures all lie deep to this plexus of arteries (**Fig. 16.13**).

Further dissection in the roof to the fossa allows the maxillary nerve to be seen just below the orbit in the roof of the fossa. If this nerve is followed posteromedially the foramen rotundum can be seen (**Fig. 16.19**). If we now remove the major blood vessels from the fossa we can identify the vidian nerve entering the fossa posteriorly.

The Endoscopic Anatomy of the Infraorbital Fissure

The other relationship that is important to understand is how the pterygopalatine fossa and infratemporal fossa relate to the infraorbital fissure. It is through this fissure that tumors can extend from the infratemporal fossa and pterygopalatine fossa up toward the orbital apex. Additionally, tumors may follow the infraorbital nerve and maxillary nerve to enter the pterygopalatine fossa and move posteriorly toward the cavernous sinus and carotid artery.

As the orbital apex and sphenoid is approached, the inferior portion of the lamina papyracea thickens. The lateral wall of the fissure is formed by the medial wall of the middle cranial fossa. The infraorbital nerve can consistently be seen in the infraorbital fissure and it is around this structure that tumor can insinuate to reach the orbital apex and then expand into

Fig. 16.15 (A) Parasagittal CT scan showing the pterygopalatine fossa is cone shaped (*white arrow*). The vidian canal can be seen entering the posterior wall of the pterygopalatine fossa (*black arrow*). **(B)** The pterygopalatine fossa (*white arrow*) is seen to sit between the maxillary sinus (*MS*) and the sphenoid sinus (*SS*). The pterygopalatine fossa is continuous with the greater palatine canal (*black arrow*). Note it narrowing as it becomes the pterygomaxillary fissure before it expands into the infratemporal fossa.

(C) Coronal scan where the cone shape of the fossa is outlined by a *broken white line* and the sphenopalatine foramina are indicated with the *white arrows*. **(D)** The cadaver picture demonstrates the contents of the pterygopalatine fossa on the right side following removal of the posterior wall of the maxillary sinus. *GPN*, greater palatine nerve; *VA*, vidian artery; *GPA*, greater palatine artery; *SPA*, sphenopalatine artery; *ION*, infraorbital nerve; *PSAA*, posterior superior alveolar artery; *3rd MA*, 3rd division of the maxillary artery.

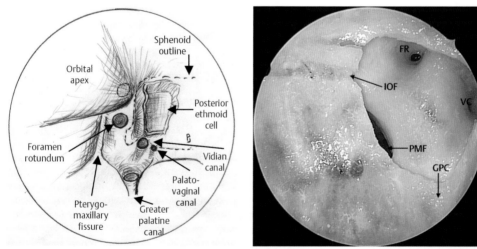

Fig. 16.16 (A) The relationships of the structures entering the posterior region, roof, and floor of the pterygopalatine fossa. The medial wall with the sphenopalatine foramen is not depicted. **(B)** This dry bone image has been taken with a zero-degree endoscope placed within the maxillary sinus. The posterior wall of the maxillary sinus has been removed in the region of the pterygopalatine fossa and we can

visualize the pterygoid process and several important surrounding structures. The foramen rotundum (*FR*), vidian canal (*VC*), and the infraorbital fissure (*IOF*) can be appreciated, along with the pterygomaxillary fissure (*PMF*). Note how the pterygomaxillary fissure and the infraorbital fissure are continuous with each other. *GPC*, greater palatine canal.

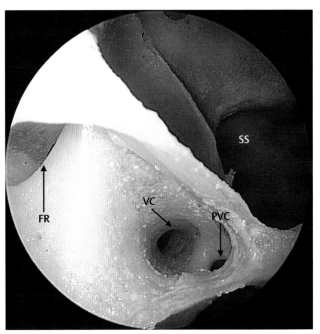

Fig. 16.17 Dry bone specimen image of the right sphenopalatine foramen (*SPF*). The vertical portion of the palatine bone (*VPB*) divides into two processes—the orbital process (*OP*) and the sphenoidal process (*SP*)—and the SPF is located in between. *MT*, middle turbinate; *IT*, inferior turbinate.

Fig. 16.18 Close-up image of a dry bone specimen following the widening of the right sphenopalatine foramen, and removal of the sphenoidal process of the palatine bone. The vidian canal (*VC*) can be seen clearly with the palatovaginal canal (*PVC*) located more medially. *SS*, sphenoid sinus; *FR*, foramen rotundum.

A   B

Fig. 16.19 (**A**) Endoscopic cadaveric image taken of the right pterygopalatine fossa. The maxillary division of the trigeminal nerve (*V2*) can be seen exiting the foramen rotundum before it divides into the infraorbital nerve (*ION*) and zygomatic nerve. *LPM*, lateral pterygoid muscle; *SPA*, sphenopalatine artery. (**B**) Closer image of V2 exiting the foramen rotundum, with the middle cranial fossa laterally, maxillary strut superiorly, and the supraorbital fissure posteriorly. Note how the maxillary strut (*MS*) is the strut of bone that separates the foramen rotundum and its contents (*V2*) from the supraorbital fissure. The supraorbital fissure (*SOF*) forms the anterior wall of the cavernous sinus, and as such the intracavernous carotid artery (*CCA*) can be seen in the distance. The medial pole of the SOF has been outlined. *LSW*, lateral sphenoid wall.

the space between the lateral sphenoid wall and middle cranial fossa (**Fig. 16.19**). Significant expansion can occur so that the tumor may reach the cavernous sinus and even the carotid artery.

To understand how the medial aspect of the infraorbital fissure can be surgically accessed, **Figs. 16.20, 16.21, 16.22, and 16.23** demonstrate the anatomy as it would be seen if this region were to be approached endoscopically. **Figure 16.22** shows the infraorbital fissure with the infraorbital nerve and zygomatic nerve running through it. Note how the medial part of the fissure communicates with the pterygopalatine fossa whereas the lateral part of the fissure communicates with the orbit. In **Fig. 16.24** note that the posterior wall of the maxillary sinus has been removed and a complete sphenoethmoidectomy has been performed on the right side. In **Fig. 16.20** we can see the lateral wall of the sphenoid sinus. Note the landmarks of the lateral wall including the optic nerve, the anterior genu of the intracavernous carotid artery, the maxillary impression for the maxillary division of the trigeminal nerve, and the vidian nerve in the floor of the sphenoid sinus. The optic nerve and the lateral opticocarotid recess can be seen. **Figure 16.21** is following the removal of the bone of the

Fig. 16.21 Cadaveric dissection image of the lateral sphenoid wall following bone removal. *P*, pituitary gland; *CCA*, intracavernous carotid artery; *V2*, maxillary division of the trigeminal nerve; *TG*, trigeminal ganglion; *VN*, vidian nerve; *PCA*, paraclival carotid artery; *P. CCA*, posterior genu of the intracavernous carotid artery; *SS*, sphenoid sinus.

Fig. 16.20 Cadaveric dissection image taken of the right sphenoid sinus through a maximal sphenoidotomy. The vidian canal (*VC*) and trigeminal impression (*TI*) for the maxillary division of the trigeminal nerve can be clearly seen. If the sphenoid sinus is well pneumatized then the lateral recess (*LR*) can be seen as a depression in the lateral sphenoid wall between the VC and the TI. The lateral opticocarotid recess can be seen. This depression corresponds to pneumatization of the optic strut (the bony bridge that separates the optic canal from the superior orbital fissure). Further pneumatization into the optic strut may result in a pneumatized anterior clinoid process which will place the optic nerve on a mesentery. *ISS*, intersinus septum; *ON*, optic nerve; *CCA*, anterior genu of the intracavernous carotid artery; *PCA*, paraclival carotid artery.

lateral sphenoid wall. The blue silicone shows the anterior genu of the intracavernous carotid is completely within the cavernous sinus. The anterior limit of this marks the beginning of the orbital apex, the supraorbital fissure. The occulomotor, trochlea, and ophthalmic division of the trigeminal nerve can be seen in **Fig. 16.22** leaving the lateral wall of the cavernous sinus to enter the orbital apex periorbita. In the **Fig. 16.23** the space between the lateral wall of the sphenoid and the medial wall of the temporal fossa has been dissected, with the dura of the temporal fossa excised to reveal the medial side of the temporal lobe. In this image the periorbita of the orbital apex has been retracted with a Freer dissector. Analysis of the maxillary nerve can clearly show the path which tumors in this region may take. Heading posteriorly they may enter the cavernous sinus and invade the intracavernous structures such as the intracavernous carotid artery. Moving medially they will expand into the lateral wall of the sphenoid sinus. If a tumor pushed laterally then it will enter the middle cranial fossa.

Endoscopic Anatomy of the Region of the Middle Cranial Fossa

To access the region of the middle cranial fossa and foramen ovale, further removal of the lateral wall of the sphenoid is necessary (**Fig. 16.25**). To achieve this both the vidian nerve in the floor of the sphenoid sinus and the maxillary nerve in the lateral wall of the sphenoid are exposed and the bone around these nerves removed with a diamond burr

Fig. 16.22 Cadaveric dissection image of the right lateral wall of the sphenoid sinus. The bone has been removed and the anterior genu of the intracavernous carotid artery (*CCA*) retracted medially. This allows clear visualization of the nerves within the dural layers of the lateral wall of the cavernous sinus. The abducens nerve (*CN VI*) can be visualized medially, running within the cavernous sinus. Note the periorbita of the orbital apex. The bone of the anterior clinoid (*AC*) process has been left in place, positioned within the lateral opticocarotid recess. *ON*, optic nerve; *Oph. A*, ophthalmic artery; *CN III*, occulomotor nerve; *CN IV*, trochlear nerve; *V1*, ophthalmic division of the trigeminal nerve; *V2*, maxillary division of the trigeminal nerve; *V3*, mandibular division of the trigeminal nerve.

Fig. 16.23 Cadaveric dissection of the right lateral sphenoid wall following removal of the lateral sphenoid wall. Dissection has continued anteriorly to the pterygopalatine fossa inferiorly and the orbital apex superiorly. In this image the periorbita has been retracted superiorly. Note the remnant of the maxillary strut (*MS*), the strut of bone that separates the foramen rotundum from the superior orbital fissure/orbital apex. The vidian nerve (*VN*) can be seen moving into the posterior aspect of the pterygopalatine fossa and enters the pterygopalatine ganglion (*PPG*). The relationship between the foramen rotundum (*FR*) and the temporal lobe (*TL*) can be seen clearly. *V2*, maxillary division of the trigeminal nerve; *PN*, pharyngeal nerve; *PCA*, paraclival carotid artery; *CCA*, intracavernous carotid artery; *SS*, sphenoid sinus; *TG*, trigeminal ganglion.

Fig. 16.24 This diagram illustrates the important relationships between the right maxillary nerve and the infraorbital fissure and the pterygopalatine fossa as viewed from an anterosuperior aspect. The maxillary nerve exits the foramen rotundum and crosses the roof of the pterygopalatine fossa and occupies the gap created by the infraorbital fissure. Note that the medial aspect of the fissure connects to the pterygopalatine fossa whereas the lateral (more anterior) part of the fissure connects to the infratemporal fossa. This relationship is important as it helps one to understand how tumors spread from one fossa to another and on occasions into orbital apex. *OA*, orbital apex; *VN*, vidian nerve; *PPG*, pterygopalatine ganglion; *GPC*, greater palatine canal; *GPA*, greater palatine artery; *GPN*, greater palatine nerve; *SPA*, sphenopalatine artery; *ION*, infraorbital nerve; *ZN*, zygomatic nerve; *PSAA*, posterior superior alveolar artery; *PSAN*, posterior superior alveolar nerve; *3rd MA*, third division of maxillary artery.

Fig. 16.25 Cadaveric dissection of the right lateral sphenoid sinus wall. Bone has been removed at the lateral recess (between the vidian nerve and the maxillary division of the trigeminal nerve). This allows identification of foramen ovale (*FO*), with the mandibular division (*V3*) moving through this canal almost immediately after leaving the semilunar shaped trigeminal ganglion (*TG*). Note that the dura between V1 and V2, and V2 and V3 has been removed. *VN*, vidian canal; *V2*, maxillary division of trigeminal nerve; *V1*, ophthalmic division of trigeminal nerve; *AN*, abducens nerve.

remove the bone overlying the medial middle temporal fossa and expose the underlying dura. Although dura covers the cavernous sinus as it is approached from the sphenoid sinus, this covering is very thin and tenuous with multiple small veins joining or leaving the cavernous sinus so that such a dissection can be quite bloody and the bleeding difficult to control. The relationship of the vidian nerve (VN), carotid artery (CA), cavernous sinus (CS), V2, V3, foramen ovale, and middle cranial fossa (MCF) can be appreciated in **Figs. 16.21, 16.22, 16.23, and 16.25**.

Endoscopic Anatomy of the Infratemporal Fossa

Once the bone overlying the posterior wall of the maxillary sinus has been removed, the pterygopalatine fossa and infratemporal fossa are seen (**Fig. 16.26**). The infraorbtial nerve (MN) can be seen at the junction of the infratemporal fossa and orbit. These fossae are covered by periosteum and the contents are exposed by removing the periosteum. Both fossae contain fat, blood vessels, and nerves. The fat and blood vessels usually lie anteromedial to the neural structures. Once the fat has been removed the underlying maxillary artery and muscles of the infratemporal fossa can be seen. The superior and inferior heads of the lateral pterygoid muscle (LP) can be seen originating directly behind

(**Fig. 16.25**). The vidian canal leads directly to the second genu of the internal carotid artery as it turns vertically and runs up the lateral wall of the sphenoid toward the pituitary fossa. **Figure 16.25** shows the relationship between the vidian canal and the maxillary nerve as the bone is removed between these structures. This bone removal exposes the space between the middle cranial fossa plate and the lateral wall of the sphenoid both below and above the maxillary nerve. As the bone removal continues posteriorly the foramen ovale and the mandibular branch of the trigeminal nerve are seen which are lateral and anterior to the carotid artery (**Fig. 16.25**). The vidian nerve is medial and marks the position of the carotid at the junction of the floor and posterior wall of the sphenoid. Directly above the foramen ovale in the lateral wall is the cavernous sinus (CS) and above the cavernous sinus is the orbital apex (OA). The space above the maxillary nerve is just below the orbital apex, and tumors expanding into this region will cause compression of the orbital apex. The relationship of the orbital apex, lateral wall of sphenoid, and medial wall of the middle cranial fossa is demonstrated in **Figs. 16.22 and 16.23**.

The final dissection of the lateral wall of the sphenoid exposes the cavernous sinus anterior to the paraclival carotid artery and the posterior genu of the intracavernous carotid artery. If the remaining bone of the lateral wall of the sphenoid is removed, the cavernous sinus and mandibular branch of the trigeminal nerve (V3) will be exposed above the foramen ovale (**Fig. 16.21**). Further bone removal laterally will

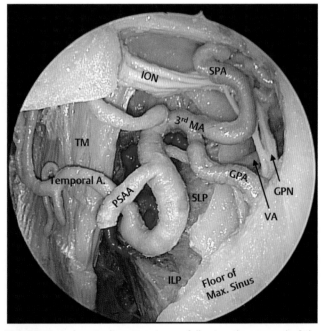

Fig. 16.26 Cadaveric dissection image following the removal of the lateral wall, floor, and posterior wall of the right maxillary sinus. This image reveals the temporalis muscle (*TM*) located superficial to the lateral wall of the maxillary sinus. The superior (*SLP*) and inferior (*ILP*) heads of the lateral pterygoid muscle can be seen, where they attach and cover the superficial surface of the lateral pterygoid plates. *GPN*, greater palatine nerve; *VA*, vidian artery; *GPA*, greater palatine artery; *SPA*, sphenopalatine artery; *ION*, infraorbital nerve; *PSAA*, posterior superior alveolar artery; *3rd MA*, third division of the maxillary artery.

Fig. 16.27 Cadaveric dissection of the right infratemporal fossa following removal of the temporalis muscle revealing the ramus of the mandible (*RM*). With an angled endoscope the superficial head of the medial pterygoid muscle (*SMP*) can also be visualized. Note that the medial pterygoid muscle has both a superficial head and a deep head. The superficial head lies just superficial to the inferior head of the lateral pterygoid muscle (*ILP*). The maxillary artery enters the infratemporal fossa between the superior and inferior head of the lateral pterygoid muscles. *GPN*, greater palatine nerve; *GPA*, greater palatine artery; *SPA*, sphenopalatine artery; *ION*, infraorbital nerve; *3rd MA*, third division of the maxillary artery.

the greater palatine canal with the maxillary artery entering the infratemporal fossa between the two heads of the lateral pterygoid muscle. As one moves further laterally, the temporalis muscle (TM) comes into view. Removing the temporalis muscle reveals the ramus of the mandible (**Fig. 16.27**). With the use of an angled endoscope looking inferiorly the superficial head of the medial pterygoid muscle can be appreciated.

◆ Tumors Involving the Maxillary Sinus, Pterygopalatine, and Infratemporal Fossae

Antrochoanal Polyp

Antrochoanal polyps commonly form from the posterior wall of the maxillary sinus. These tumors need to have the site of origin resected to prevent recurrence. The first step is to perform a large middle meatal antrostomy and to expose the site of origin of the tumor. If the entire site can be easily accessed through the middle meatal antrostomy then the tumor and the site of origin are resected with a margin of normal mucosa around the attachment. If the site of origin

is not easily accessible through a middle meatal antrostomy, a canine fossa trephination should be performed and the microdebrider or Freer elevator placed through the trephine site and the origin of the polyp resected with the margin of normal tissue.

Inverting Papillomas (Video 43)

The other most common benign tumor involving the maxillary sinus is inverting papilloma (IP). Small IP tumors of the maxillary sinus that do not arise from the anterior wall of the maxillary sinus can be resected by creating a large middle meatal antrostomy and a canine fossa trephine (described in Chapter 5). The endoscope can be placed into the maxillary antrostomy while the dissecting instrument is placed through the canine fossa puncture. This can be reversed with the endoscope being placed through the canine fossa puncture and instrument through the maxillary antrostomy. Using this technique, almost the entire maxillary sinus can be accessed. The only area where access may not be adequate is the anterior face of the maxillary sinus. Tumors located on the anterior face may require an endoscopic medial maxillectomy for adequate access and complete resection. All other small or localized tumors can be resected using this two-site approach.

◆ Large or Anterior Wall Maxillary Sinus Tumors (Videos 44 and 45)

If a tumor cannot be accessed with the canine fossa trephination or it originates from a large area or from the anterior wall of the maxillary sinus, endoscopic medial maxillectomy should be performed. If additional access is required, the frontal process of the maxilla can be drilled away. This can be combined with a transseptal access to improve the angulation to the anterior wall as described previously in this chapter. All walls of the maxillary sinus should be able to be accessed and the tumor and underlying mucosa should be removed. In **Fig. 16.28** the patient has a large inverting papilloma extending laterally beyond the limits of the maxillary sinus.

This inverting papilloma was based on the inferior turbinate. Resection of the medial maxilla removed a large part of the tumor origin. In addition the tumor took origin from the adjacent floor and posterior wall of the maxillary sinus. This could be easily accessed after endoscopic medial maxillectomy. The bone in the region of origin of the tumor was able to be drilled with a diamond burr to ensure no tumor had infiltrated into bony crevices seen in the region of new bone formation classically associated with the tumor origin.

The following patient presented with an inverting papilloma that took origin around a region of new bone formation on the lateral and anterior wall of the maxillary sinus. This anterior and lateral area was able to be accessed (after an endoscopic medial maxillectomy) with a 70-degree diamond burr and the origin of the tumor completely cleared with drilling of the underlying

Fig. 16.28 A large inverting papilloma eroding the lateral wall of the maxillary sinus (*white arrow*). The CT (**A**) and the MRI (**B**, **D**, T2 weighting; **C**, T1 weighting) show the tumor's extent. (**D**) MRI shows an obstructed frontal sinus with mucus lighting up in the frontal sinus.

bone (**Fig. 16.29**). It is common for inverting papilloma to originate from a region of new bone formation and therefore it is important to drill away this new bone as mucosa may invaginate into the bony crevices associated with new bone and failure to remove this may result in tumor recurrence.[8]

◆ Results of the Endoscopic Resection of Inverted Papillomas

Patients with inverting papilloma were classified according to the classification of Krouse[4] presented in **Table 16.1**.

The published series of patients who have undergone endoscopic resection of inverting papillomas, including those patients with large and extensive lesions that have had an endoscopic medial maxillectomy as part of the tumor resection, are presented in **Table 16.2**. As can be seen from these results and from recent publications by Krouse[9] and a review article by Melroy and Senior,[10] the results obtained by endoscopic

removal of inverting papillomas are better than those achieved in the past using an open approach. The figures of recurrence rates of inverting papilloma with open procedures average 18% whereas those performed endoscopically average 12%.[10]

Juvenile Nasopharyngeal Angiofibroma (Video 42)

There is currently widespread acceptance that small juvenile nasopharyngeal angiofibromas (JNAs) occupying the nasal cavity alone or with minimal extension into the pterygopalatine fossa or adjacent sinuses can be managed endoscopically.[6,10] The first step is to embolize the tumor within 24 hours of the surgery to reduce its vascularity. If the embolization is done prior to 24 hours, significant collateral blood supply may open and the tumor may regain a degree of its vascularity. The second step is to perform a large middle meatal antrostomy with removal of the posterior fontanelle and a sphenoethmoidectomy to provide access over the top of the tumor into the sphenoid sinus. Thereafter the intranasal component of the

Fig. 16.29 Inverting papilloma originating around the neo-osteogenesis seen on the lateral wall of the maxillary sinus (*black arrow*).

tumor is mobilized with a malleable suction Freer* (Medtronic ENT). Often it is stuck to the septum and posterior bony choana but there is always a surgical plane directly on the tumor surface. If there is sufficient room in the nose, the tumor does not need to be debulked but if the nasal component is very large this may need to be resected before any extension of the tumor

Table 16.1 Staging System for Inverted Papilloma as Proposed by Krouse

Stage	Extent of Tumor
I	Tumor confined to nasal cavity; no malignancy
II	Tumor involving the ostiomeatal complex, and ethmoids and/or medial wall of maxillary sinus; no malignancy
III	Tumor involving the inferior, superior, lateral, or anterior wall of maxillary sinus, sphenoid, and/or frontal sinus; no malignancy
IV	All extranasal/extrasinus tumors; all tumors associated with malignancy

Source: Data from Krouse JH. Development of a staging system for inverted papilloma. Laryngoscope 2000;110:965–968.

is dealt with. After mobilization of the nasal component, the tumor is divided at its entry into the sphenopalatine foramen using a Coblation wand (ArthroCare, Sunnyvale, CA). The concomitant tissue removal and hemostasis achieved with the Coblation wand reduces bleeding from the cut surface of the tumor. The nasal component is then delivered via the nasopharynx through the mouth. Next the extension of tumor into the pterygopalatine fossa needs to be exposed. The posterior wall of the maxillary sinus is removed, starting at the pterygopalatine foramen and moving laterally until the tumor in the pterygopalatine fossa and the attached maxillary artery is exposed (**Fig. 16.30**). Large tumor extensions into the pterygopalatine fossa need to be dealt with as described in the following section.

◆ Large Juvenile Nasopharyngeal Angiofibromas[11] (Video 42)

The most common benign tumor involving the pterygopalatine fossa (and infratemporal fossa) is the JNA. These tumors normally originate in the region of the sphenopalatine foramen

Table 16.2 Presentation, Origin, Stage, Procedure, and Outcome for Endoscopic Removal of Inverting Papilloma Including Patients who Underwent Medial Maxillectomy for Removal of the Inverting Papilloma

Case	Age and Sex	Symptoms	Origin	Stage	Endoscopic Procedure	Current Status and Follow-up
1[a]	51M	Left nasal obstruction, rhinorrhea	Left maxillary antrum, lamina papyracea, sphenoid sinus	IV	Medial maxillectomy, canine fossa puncture, ethmoidectomy, sphenoidotomy, and clearance of the frontal recess	Had recurrence of tumor after 4 months in left infratemporal fossa—surgically cleared and now disease free after 3 years
2	54M	Left nasal obstruction, epistaxis	Left maxillary sinus and inferior turbinate	II	Medial maxillectomy, canine fossa puncture, and DCR	Disease free
3	71M	Right nasal obstruction, rhinorrhea	Right uncinate process	II	MMA	Disease free
4	41M	Left nasal obstruction (previous lateral rhinotomy for IP)	Left lamina papyracea, frontal sinus	III	MMA, ethmoidectomy, sphenoidotomy, and endoscopic Lothrop procedure	Disease free
5	74M	Left nasal obstruction	Left nasal septum	I	Middle meatal antrostomy, ethmoidectomy	Disease free
6	72M	Asymptomatic	Left middle turbinate	I	Resection of middle turbinate, ethmoidectomy, sphenoidotomy	Disease free
7	46M	Left nasal obstruction	Left maxillary sinus	II	MMA, ethmoidectomy, and sphenoidotomy	Disease free
8	53M	Right frontal sinusitis (previous lateral rhinotomy for IP)	Right maxillary sinus floor	III	Medial maxillectomy and canine fossa puncture	Disease free
9	60F	Right nasal obstruction, rhinorrhea	Right maxillary sinus floor	III	MMA, and canine fossa puncture	Disease free
10	78F	Right epistaxis and nasal obstruction	Right maxillary sinus floor	III	Medial maxillectomy, ethmoidectomy, DCR, and canine fossa puncture	Disease free
11	53M	Left nasal obstruction (previous Caldwell Luc)	Left maxillary sinus floor	III	MMA, ethmoidectomy, and frontal recess clearance	Disease free
12	44M	Right nasal obstruction	Left middle meatus	I	MMA, ethmoidectomy, middle turbinectomy	Disease free
13	67M	Left nasal obstruction	Sphenoid and posterior ethmoids	III	MMA, ethmoidectomy, superior turbinectomy, and extended sphenoidotomy	Disease free
14	58F	Right nasal obstruction and blood stained discharge	Posterior septum	I	Sphenoethmoidectomy, septal and middle and superior turbinate resection	Disease free
15	71M	Right nasal obstruction	Right middle meatus and medial wall maxillary sinus	II	Ethmoidectomy, frontal recess clearance, middle turbinectomy, medial maxillectomy, and canine fossa puncture	Disease free
16	50F	Left nasal obstruction, epistaxis and discharge	Left superior rim of maxillary sinus ostium	II	Anterior ethmoidectomy, MMA, and canine fossa puncture	Disease free
17	56M	Right nasal obstruction	Middle meatus on posterior rim of maxillary ostium	II	Ethmoidectomy and MMA	Disease free

[a]Recurrence found associated with squamous cell carcinoma deposits.

Abbreviations: DCR, dacryocystorhinostomy; IP, inverting papilloma; MMA, middle meatal antrostomy.

Source: Used with permission from Wormald PJ, Ooi E, van Hasselt A, Nair S. Endoscopic removal of sinonasal inverted papilloma including endoscopic medial maxillectomy. Laryngoscope 2003;113:867–873.

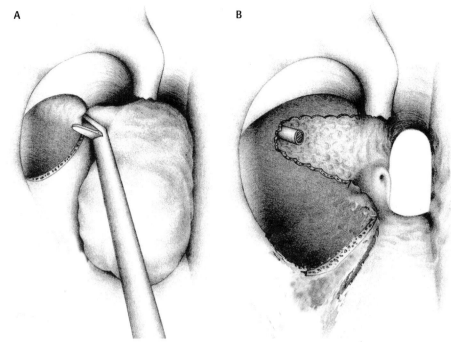

Fig. 16.30 (**A**) The nasal component of the tumor has been mobilized and the large middle meatal antrostomy performed. A 45-degree through-biting Blakesley is used to remove the posterior wall of the maxillary sinus. (**B**) The tumor has been removed and the pterygopalatine fossa exposed. The maxillary artery is seen in the tumor bed.

and expand into the pterygopalatine fossa. Large tumors that extend into the infratemporal fossa will usually have a large intranasal component that may extend into nearby sinuses, especially the sphenoid sinus. Other benign tumors seen in this region are rare but may include inverting papillomas extending from the nasal cavity or tumors originating from the nerve sheath (schwannomas), cartilage, or muscle. The reason why there has been debate about the most appropriate method for removing these tumors is the significant vascularity that is associated with these tumors. Massive bleeding can occur during tumor resection and, if the surgeon is not prepared or unable to manage such hemorrhage, complications can result.

There are two significant steps that are now possible to allow these large JNAs to be tackled endoscopically. The first step is to preoperatively embolize the tumor thereby significantly reducing the vascularity and improving visualization during resection[6,11] (**Fig. 16.31**).

The second step is the two-surgeon approach which allows the second surgeon to place a high volume suction in the operative field when bleeding is problematic and alternatively to place traction on the tumor facilitating the dissection.[6,11]

Before surgery is performed, a large JNA needs careful assessment to decide if it is endoscopically resectable. Large JNAs tend to expand into potential spaces and to follow pathways

Fig. 16.31 (**A**) The significant vascular blush of the tumor can be seen and (**B**) this blush has been removed by embolization of the maxillary artery feeding the tumor.

of least resistance. In the pterygopalatine fossa and infratemporal fossa several areas need to be critically evaluated before the surgeon decides if the tumor is endoscopically resectable.[11] In the pterygopalatine fossa the infraorbital fissure needs to be closely evaluated. There is a potential space between the lateral wall of the sphenoid and the middle cranial fossa as seen in the previous anatomical review of this region. The tumor can infiltrate around the infraorbital nerve and enter the potential space

above the nerve and expand this space. Further growth will cause the tumor to push posteriorly toward the cavernous sinus and second genu of the carotid artery. Such a case is illustrated in **Fig. 16.32** where the tumor abuts the cavernous sinus and carotid and compresses the orbital apex within this potential space above the infraorbital fissure.

In this case (**Fig. 16.32**) the maxillary nerve would be completely surrounded by tumor and it would be unlikely that

Fig. 16.32 (**A**) Coronal MRI shows the tumor extends around the infraorbital nerve into the space between the lateral wall of the sphenoid sinus and the temporal lobe and significantly compresses the orbital apex (*white arrow*). (**B**) Axial MRI shows the tumor can be seen extending posteriorly into this space and abutting the cavernous sinus and carotid artery (*white arrow*). (**C**) In the intra-operative image guidance picture, the suction probe is placed in this space between the lateral wall of the sphenoid and temporal lobe after tumor resection as can be seen by the cross hairs on the adjacent CT scans.

Fig. 16.33 (**A**) Coronal MRI shows the tumor fills the nasopharynx, and expands the vidian canal posteriorly until it abuts the internal carotid artery (*white arrow*). (**B**) This abutment of the carotid artery (*white arrow*) is seen in the axial MRI. (**C**) After endoscopic removal of the tumor, it is placed on a ruler for evaluation of its size.

the tumor could be separated from the nerve and indeed the nerve needed to be sacrificed during the dissection. In most cases where the tumor does not expand through the infraorbital fissure, the nerve is pushed upward by the tumor and can usually be dissected free from the tumor. The nerve should be identified both distally and proximally early in the dissection and preserved. The suction dissection instruments are used to separate the nerve from the tumor. Fibrous tissue that will not dissect away is divided with endoscopic soft tissue scissors from the Medtronic skull base set* (Medtronic ENT). These scissors come in 3- and 5-mm blade lengths with a left-curved, right-curved, upturned, and straight blades in both sizes.

The other region that is often involved in the spread of large JNAs is the vidian canal.[11] The tumor grows in this region in close proximity to the mouth of the vidian canal. This funnel shaped opening allows the tumor to grow down the canal and expand the canal. This region and particularly the vidian canal should always be assessed on both CT and MRI imaging. It is vitally important to understand the anatomy and relationships of the vidian canal and to be able to assess tumor spread in this region. As was demonstrated earlier in this chapter, the vidian

canal runs in the floor of the sphenoid in an anteroposterior direction toward the carotid artery as it moves from its lacerum segment into its cavernous segment. Tumor may expand this canal and erode the floor of the sphenoid and in some cases (**Fig. 16.33**) abut the carotid artery. It is our belief that failure to fully evaluate the vidian canal at the time of removal of the JNA is one of the biggest causes of tumor recurrence. Small pieces of tumor lying within the canal can easily be missed and may grow progressively over time after tumor removal.

◆ Endoscopic Two-Surgeon Technique for Tumors of the Pterygopalatine and Infratemporal Fossae[6,11] (Video 41)

Although excellent access is provided by an endoscopic medial maxillectomy, the key to successful endoscopic removal of large JNAs is having two surgeons operating at the same time.[6,11] This is achieved by providing access to the tumor bed for the second surgeon through the septum. At the beginning of the procedure a Freer (hemitransfixion) incision is made on the opposite side to that of the tumor. Using standard septoplasty techniques the mucosa is elevated off the cartilage of the septum. The cartilage of the septum is preserved but most of the posterior bony septum is resected. At the point where access is required a horizontal incision is made in the opposite septal mucosa to allow instruments placed through the opposite nostril and into the Freer incision to cross the septum and access the tumor region on the opposite side of the nose (**Fig. 16.34**).

During removal of the tumor, the second surgeon can provide significant traction on the tumor. This traction is vital to help the primary surgeon keep the dissection progressing around the posterior region of the tumor. This rotation of the tumor will also allow the feeding vessel (usually the maxillary artery) to be identified and clipped or cauterized before it is divided. If significant bleeding occurs, then a large volume suction can be placed in the field that allows the skull base angled vascular clamps (Medtronic ENT) to be placed on the bleeding vessels and the vessel to be either clipped or cauterized with the suction bipolar forceps. Once the tumor is removed the tumor bed can be closely inspected to ensure no tumor remnant remains, especially in the region of the vidian canal. If remnants are seen they are carefully removed. Once hemostasis is achieved with the suction bipolar forceps, the preserved mucosa from the posterior wall of the maxillary sinus is replaced. Surgicel (Ethicon, Somerville, NJ) or Gelfoam powder (Pharmacia and Upjohn Company, Kalamazoo, MI) can be placed in the cavity if required and the horizontal incision in the septal mucosa is sutured. This stitch is continued anteriorly as a through and through plication suture of the septum until it is brought out at the base of the Freer incision and used as a continuous suture to close this incision.

The final step is to ensure that the lacrimal sac is adequately exposed to prevent postoperative stenosis and epiphora.

Without intraoperative management of the lacrimal sac the incidence of postoperative epiphora has been described to be as high as 30%.[7]

◆ Results of Endoscopic Removal of Juvenile Nasopharyngeal Angiofibromas

In a series of 14 consecutive patients with angiofibroma managed endoscopically, eight patients had extensive disease requiring endoscopic medial maxillectomy.[6,11] The classification of Radkowski et al.[12] was used to classify the patients and the distribution of the patients in each category is presented in **Table 16.3**. Only patients classified as either IIC or IIIA required endoscopic medial maxillectomy for an entirely endoscopic removal of their tumor.

All patients described in this series have had regular postoperative MRI scans. In two patients there is residual tissue enhancement with contrast in the region of the vidian canal. Both of these patients have had repeated MRI scans over several years without any enlargement of this enhancing area and are monitored every 6 months for any change. Whether this enhancement reflects disease recurrence or increased tissue vascularity is unclear but revision surgery will only be offered if this tissue shows growth on repeated MRI scans. The rest of the patients are currently disease free with an average follow-up time of 4.1 years. The patient numbers have increased from the recently published series[6,11] to include all patients operated on over the last 5 years.

Schwannoma Involving the Pterygopalatine and Infratemporal Fossae (Video 41)

Medial maxillectomy also provides access to other tumors that may involve the pterygopalatine and infratemporal fossae. In **Fig. 16.35** a schwannoma of the maxillary nerve involves the entire pterygopalatine fossa and extends

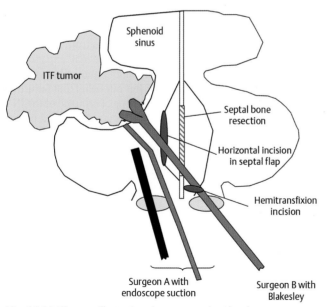

Fig. 16.34 Diagram illustrating the access points for the two-surgeon technique.

Table 16.3 Radkowski Classification of Juvenile Angiofibromas

Stage	Description	n = 14
IA	Limited to nose and nasopharyngeal area	1
IB	Extension into one or more sinus	0
IIA	Minimal extension into pterygopalatine fossa	2
IIB	Occupation of the pterygopalatine fossa without orbital erosion	3
IIC	Infratemporal fossa extension without cheek or pterygoid plate involvement	3
IIIA	Erosion of the skull base (middle cranial fossa or pterygoids)	5
IIIB	Erosion of skull base with intracranial extension with or without cavernous sinus involvement	0

Source: Data from Radowski D, McGill T, Healy GB, et al. Angiofibroma. Changes in staging and treatment. Arch Orolaryngol Head Neck Surg 1996;122:122–129.

Fig. 16.35 The CT (**A**) corresponds to the MRI (**C**) as does the CT and MRI marked (**B**) and (**D**). (**A**) The erosion of the middle cranial fossa is marked with a *black arrow*. (**D**) The extension of the tumor into the infratemporal fossa is marked with a *white arrow*.

significantly into the infratemporal fossa. Medial maxillectomy allows access to the entire posterior wall of the maxillary sinus and after its removal to the tumor.

Figure 16.36 illustrates the tumor seen in **Fig. 16.35** after endoscopic medial maxillectomy and tumor removal. It was confirmed histologically to be a schwannoma.

Malignant Tumors Involving the Pterygopalatine and Infratemporal Fossae

Currently the role of endoscopic resection for the management of malignant tumors is unclear.[13,14] Recently there have been some studies published utilizing endoscopic resection for malignant tumors but the authors have stressed that long-term follow-up is not available for these patients and that radical resection with open approaches remains the gold standard.[13,14] In our practice patients are offered standard external approaches and radical resection if the tumor involves the orbit or does not have a well defined margin. This is especially true for squamous carcinoma. If the tumor margin is well defined on

Fig. 16.36 Resected schwannoma from patient shown in **Fig. 16.28**.

radiology then endoscopic tumor removal with postoperative radiotherapy with or without chemotherapy is offered. Most malignancies in the nose and sinuses have a pushing front and do not infiltrate through the orbital periosteum or dura. These tumors are usually soft and there is usually a surgical plane between the tumor and the natural boundaries of the nose and sinuses. In some instances where there is localized infiltration of the tumor into the dura or orbital periosteum, this can be endoscopically resected and, in the case of the dura, repaired.

The principle of tumor removal is to first debulk the tumor to create space in the nose in which to operate. This is easily done with a Blakesley forceps (to allow tumor to be sent for histology) and a microdebrider blade. No attempt is made to remove tumor from surrounding structures. Once there is space to operate then a surgical plane is established between the tumor and the lamina papyracea or, if absent, the orbital periosteum. In the region of the skull base this plane is established between the skull base or, if absent, the dura. To start the dissection the junction of the tumor and lateral nasal wall is found anteriorly and a malleable suction Freer is used to elevate the mucosa anterior to the tumor establishing the plane between mucosa and bone. This allows the surgical plane to be established around the margins of the tumor. If this plane is followed either onto the exposed orbital periosteum or dura, tumor can be dissected off the periosteum or dura without its disruption. In this way it is usually possible to remove all macroscopic tumor that does not invade these structures and allows preservation of the underlying periosteum and dura. If, however, the tumor invades the periosteum or dura then the dura/periosteum is resected. In the following case example the patient presented with a sinonasal undifferentiated carcinoma (SNUC) (**Fig. 16.37**). The surgical plan was to attempt endoscopic tumor removal but if necessary to combine endoscopic resection with a craniotomy. At the time of surgery, complete macroscopic resection was achieved endoscopically and we felt that there would be no additional benefit in performing a craniotomy. The patient underwent postoperative radiotherapy and to date is still disease free (4+ years of follow-up).

In the following case example a patient presents with a chondrosarcoma with significant proptosis, diplopia, and nasal obstruction (**Fig. 16.38**). He was elderly (85 years) and

Fig. 16.37 (**A**) CT scan shows erosion of the lateral wall of the sphenoid, erosion of the upper pterygoid plates, and widening of the infraorbital fissure. (**B**) MRI scan shows extension of the tumor into the infratemporal fossa (*white arrow*) and (**C**) extension of tumor through the infraorbital fissure into the potential space between the lateral wall of the sphenoid and the temporal lobe (*black arrow*). The sphenoid is filled with mucus (*white arrow*).

Fig. 16.38 (**A**) CT scan shows the skull base has been eroded (*white arrow*) and there is significant compression of the orbit. (**B**) MRI scan shows compression rather than invasion of the orbit, as illustrated by the medial rectus (*white arrow*) being pushed up against the optic nerve. (**C**) The postoperative picture clearly shows the sphenoid sinus (*SS*) and orbit (*O*) with the posterior ethmoid artery (*black arrow*) and maxillary sinus (*white arrow*) and frontal ostium visible (*broken white arrow*).

in poor general health and the Combined Oncology Head and Neck Clinic felt that he would not be suitable for craniofacial resection and so he was offered endoscopic resection and radiotherapy. The tumor was debulked and, after space was created, a good surgical plane was able to be established anterior to the tumor origin. The tumor was then able to be dissected off the dura and the orbital periosteum. There was no invasion into the dura or orbital periosteum. An endoscopic medial maxillectomy was performed to improve lateral access. Complete macroscopic tumor removal was achieved and the patient offered postoperative radiotherapy.

◆ Postoperative Care

Broad-spectrum antibiotics are continued for 5 days after surgery. Douching of the nose with saline is started immediately postoperatively. Crusting will usually continue for a few months and may worsen during and immediately

after radiotherapy. In most patients crusting is not problematic in the long-term although some patients (who have had radiotherapy) can continue to have significant crusting if mucociliary drainage is not reestablished after some months. Topical douches with an ampule (2 mL of 1 mg/mL) of budesonide diluted in 240 mL of saline is used to wash the nasal cavity and sinuses once daily. This is highly effective and if successful can be used for months or even years to keep the patient symptom free.

◆ Conclusion

Knowledge of the anatomy of the pterygopalatine and infratemporal fossae, infraorbital fissure, and adjacent parasphenoid region including the vidian canal is essential if tumors in these areas are to be endoscopically addressed. This chapter presents a detailed overview of this anatomy and the various endoscopic surgical techniques used to address this region.

References

1. Hyams VJ. Papillomas of the nasal cavity and paranasal sinuses. A clinicopathological study of 315 cases. Ann Otol Rhinol Laryngol 1971;80(2):192–206

2. Keleş N, Değer K. Endonasal endoscopic surgical treatment of paranasal sinus inverted papilloma—first experiences. Rhinology 2001;39(3):156–159

3. Sukenik MA, Casiano R. Endoscopic medial maxillectomy for inverted papillomas of the paranasal sinuses: value of the intraoperative endoscopic examination. Laryngoscope 2000;110(1):39–42

4. Krouse JH. Development of a staging system for inverted papilloma. Laryngoscope 2000;110(6):965–968

5. Wormald PJ, Ooi E, van Hasselt CA, Nair S. Endoscopic removal of sinonasal inverted papilloma including endoscopic medial maxillectomy. Laryngoscope 2003;113(5):867–873

6. Wormald PJ, Van Hasselt A. Endoscopic removal of juvenile angiofibromas. Otolaryngol Head Neck Surg 2003;129(6):684–691

7. Vrabec DP. The inverted Schneiderian papilloma: a 25-year study. Laryngoscope 1994;104(5 Pt 1):582–605

8. Chiu AG, Jackman AH, Antunes MB, Feldman MD, Palmer JN. Radiographic and histologic analysis of the bone underlying inverted papillomas. Laryngoscope 2006;116(9):1617–1620

9. Krouse JH. Endoscopic treatment of inverted papilloma: safety and efficacy. Am J Otolaryngol 2001;22(2):87–99

10. Melroy CT, Senior BA. Benign sinonasal neoplasms: a focus on inverting papilloma. Otolaryngol Clin North Am 2006;39(3):601–617, x

11. Douglas R, Wormald PJ. Endoscopic surgery for juvenile nasopharyngeal angiofibroma: where are the limits? Curr Opin Otolaryngol Head Neck Surg 2006;14(1):1–5

12. Radkowski D, McGill T, Healy GB, Ohlms L, Jones DT. Angiofibroma. Changes in staging and treatment. Arch Otolaryngol Head Neck Surg 1996;122(2):122–129

13. Batra PS, Citardi MJ. Endoscopic management of sinonasal malignancy. Otolaryngol Clin North Am 2006;39(3):619–637, x–xi

14. Stamm AC, Pignatari SS, Vellutini E. Transnasal endoscopic surgical approaches to the clivus. Otolaryngol Clin North Am 2006;39(3):639–656, xi

17 Endoscopic Resection of the Eustachian Tube and Postnasal Space

The most common tumor of the postnasal space is nasopharyngeal carcinoma. Fortunately, these tumors are radiosensitive and there is seldom a need for surgical excision. In rare cases nasopharyngeal carcinoma that has recurred despite repeated radiotherapy may need surgical excision. In these cases recurrent tumor is best managed by external procedures such as the maxillary swing technique, transmaxillary approach, facial translocation, transcervical-mandibulo-palatal, infratemporal fossa, and lateral infratemporal middle fossa.[1–7] These recurrent carcinomas are usually only suitable for endoscopic excision if the tumor has not extensively infiltrated the surrounding structures.[8,9] When a patient has previously undergone radiotherapy there is usually significant fibrosis which will often obliterate surgical planes making surgical dissection very difficult. If the tumor significantly infiltrates the surrounding tissue, they are removed by traditional techniques with appropriate vascular control. However, there are a small number of rare benign and malignant tumors that occur in the postnasal space and Eustachian tube (ET) that are nonresponsive to radiotherapy and are best treated by primary surgical excision. Examples of these are the minor salivary gland tumors (benign and malignant), malignant melanomas, and juvenile angiofibromas. These tumors usually have an identifiable plane and a pushing front which will allow identification of the surgical plane and can be excised endoscopically even if there is limited extension into the parapharyngeal space. Endoscopic resection is appealing as it allows a complete resection of the tumor with minimal morbidity in contrast to the external approaches that have significant associated morbidity. To perform endoscopic resections in this region, a detailed knowledge of the anatomy is necessary.

◆ Anatomy

The key anatomical landmark is the medial pterygoid plate. The relationship of the medial pterygoid plate, medial pterygoid muscle, tensor palatini, levator palatini, and ET needs to be understood. If the postnasal space is viewed endoscopically the medial pterygoid plate, ET, and fossa of Rosenmüller can be clearly seen (**Fig. 17.1**).

To access the ET, the medial pterygoid plate needs to be removed and the underlying medial pterygoid muscle exposed (**Figs. 17.2** and **17.3**). Note how the tensor palatine muscle forms a natural surgical plane as it attaches to the anterior aspect of the ET (**Fig. 17.4**). Inferiorly, the ET lies on the levator palatini muscle as it moves laterally to its attachment to the skull base (**Fig. 17.4**). The lateral pterygoid muscle attaches to the lateral aspect of the lateral pterygoid plate and is usually not seen in the dissection unless there is significant infratemporal fossa extension of the tumor. Just anterior to where the ET attaches to the skull base, the mandibular branch (V3) of the trigeminal nerve is seen (**Fig. 17.5**). Directly posterior to V3, in the apex of the fossa of Rosenmüller, the internal carotid artery can be seen (**Figs. 17.2** and **17.5**).

◆ Surgical Approach (Video 50)

The nose is prepared in the standard fashion. A pterygopalatine fossa block is placed through the mouth and greater palatine canal into the pterygopalatine fossa. The first step for this surgery is to remove the posterior half of the inferior turbinate. A large middle meatal antrostomy is done with exposure of the posterior wall of the maxillary sinus (**Fig. 17.6**). The middle meatal antrostomy is taken down to the floor of the nose and the mucosa over the medial pterygoid plate is elevated (**Fig. 17.7**).

To access this region a two-surgeon approach is advocated. The use of both nostrils allows greater angulation and, if significant bleeding occurs, clearance of blood, so that surgery can continue. The first step is to raise a Hadad pedicled septal flap on the contralateral side (see Chapter 20) to the tumor. The posterior aspect of the tumor side of the septum is mobilized by making

Fig. 17.1 Cadaveric image taken of the right postnasal space showing the posterior attachment of the inferior turbinate (*IT*) to the vertical portion of the palatine bone. The right medial pterygoid plate (*MPP*) can be seen as a mucosal prominence directly anterior to the eustachian tube (*ET*). The fossa of Rosenmüller can be seen behind the ET.

superior and inferior horizontal incisions then by joining them with a posterior vertical incision creating an anterior pedicled flap. This flap is now rotated anteriorly and fixed with a 30 Vicryl plication suture (Ethicon, Somerville, NJ). Additionally, to help the passage of instruments in and out of the nose during the two-surgeon approach, a 5–6 × 1.5

cm piece of thin silastic can be placed across the columella and the limbs pushed down each nostril and sutured with silk plication suture placed in the same manner as the septal suture. This results in the removal of the posterior half of the septum and gives great access to both sides of the postnasal space for the two-surgeon approach. This access allows the ET and tumor to be placed on traction when dissection is being performed in the lateral regions of the postnasal space which increases the safety by pulling the ET and tumor medially lessening the risk to the carotid artery (**Fig. 17.8**).

The next step is to remove the bone of the medial pterygoid plate using a Stylus skull base curved diamond burr (Medtronic ENT, Jacksonville, FL; **Fig. 17.3**). As the bone is removed the descending palatine artery is exposed. This needs to be cauterized using the suction bipolar then divided. This gives the surgeon access to the medial pterygoid muscle and the lateral pterygoid plate. The medial pterygoid muscle is surrounded by a dense venous plexus and sharp dissection of this muscle can result in significant venous bleeding. We prefer to use the coblation wand to remove this muscle as this can be done without significant bleeding.

There is a natural surgical plane anterior to the ET. This is formed by the cartilaginous anterior aspect of the ET and the attached fibrous aponeurosis of the tensor palatini. If the aponeurosis is followed inferiorly the tensor palatini muscle fibers can be seen (**Fig. 17.9**). The surgical removal of the medial pterygoid plate and partial removal of the medial pterygoid muscle with establishment of the anterior surgical plane can also be appreciated (**Fig. 17.10**).

The next step is to release the ET inferiorly and posteriorly (**Fig. 17.11**). These horizontal and posterior incisions are made with the coblation wand to minimize bleeding. The horizontal incision cuts through the tensor and levator palatini muscles and further dissection enters the parapharyngeal

Fig. 17.2 In diagram (**A**) and axial CT scan (**B**), the medial pterygoid plate (*MPP*) and lateral pterygoid plate (*LPP*) are identified. The medial pterygoid muscle (*MPM*) is seen between these two plates. The lateral pterygoid muscle (*LPM*) is seen lateral to the LPP. The levator palatini (*LP*) attaches to the medial aspect of the Eustachian tube (ET) while the tensor palatini (*TP*) lies below the ET. The fossa of Rosenmüller (*FR*) forms most of the posterior boundary of the ET. Note the relationship of the mandibular nerve (*V3*) and the carotid artery (*CA*) to the apex of the fossa of Rosenmüller and V3.

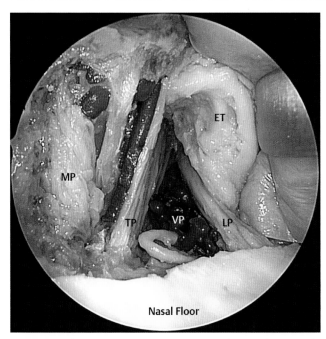

Fig. 17.3 Cadaveric dissection image taken with a 70-degree endoscope of the right Eustachian tube (*ET*). A mucosal flap has been elevated revealing the cartilaginous ET. The right medial pterygoid plate has been drilled away, revealing the deep head of the medial pterygoid muscle (*MP*), along with the tensor palatini (*TP*) and levator palatini (*LP*) muscles. The fibrofatty tissue located between the TP and LP has been removed to reveal a vascular plexus (*VP*).

Fig. 17.4 Cadaveric dissection image of the right side demonstrating tensor palatini (*TP*) attaching to the anterior aspect of the cartilaginous Eustachian tube (*ET*). *LP*, levator palatini; *MP*, medial pterygoid muscle.

Fig. 17.5 Cadaveric dissection image taken with a 30-degree endoscope following resection of the majority of the cartilaginous Eustachian tube (*ET*), and only a remnant stump can be seen which attaches to the skull base. Directly anterolateral to this remnant is the mandibular branch of the trigeminal nerve (*V3*). Directly posterior is the carotid artery (*CA*), seen directly posterior to the attachment of the levator palatini muscle (*LP*). This muscle is a good landmark to the point that the artery enters the carotid canal. *LPP*, lateral pterygoid plate; *DLP*, deep lobe of the parotid gland; *CT*, chorda tympani; *APA*, ascending pharyngeal artery; *LC*, longus capitis.

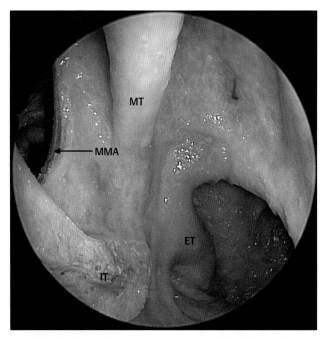

Fig. 17.6 Cadaveric dissection image taken of the right nasal cavity. A large middle meatal antrostomy has been performed. The posterior attachment of the middle turbinate (*MT*) and inferior turbinate (*IT*) to the lateral nasal wall is clearly visualized. The inferior turbinate has been excised.

Fig. 17.7 Cadaveric dissection image shows the mucosal flap (*MF*) over the medial pterygoid plate (*MPP*) has been elevated and the cartilaginous Eustachian tube (*ET*) and levator palatini (*LP*) muscle have been exposed. The conchal crest (posterior attachment of the inferior turbinate to the palatine bone) can be clearly seen. The fibrofatty tissue between the tensor palatini muscle (*TP*) and levator palatini muscles has been excised to reveal a rich vascular plexus (*VP*). The inferior turbinate (*ITA*) branch from the sphenopalatine artery can be visualized.

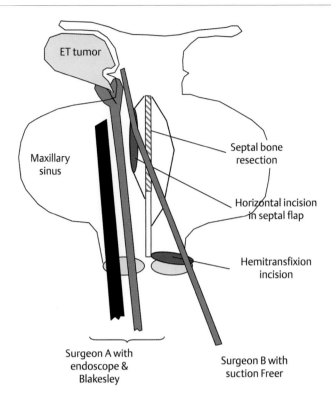

Fig. 17.8 The resection of septal bone is more posterior as is the horizontal incision in the elevated septal mucosal flap. The two-surgeon technique allows greater flexibility in instrument placement and better angulation to the region of the tumor.

space. The dissection is continued laterally directly under the ET thereby mobilizing the ET from the parapharyngeal space. If the fossa of Rosenmüller is to be included in the resection the posterior incision is made onto the longus capitis muscle. The surgical plane is anterior to the fascia of this muscle. If

the plane is deep to these muscles the carotid artery and jugular vein are at increased risk in the most lateral extent of the fossa (**Fig. 17.5**).

The ET complex is relatively immobile until the fibrous attachment of the ET to the skull base is cut. As this tissue is

Fig. 17.9 (**A**) The right Eustachian tube (*ET*) orifice defines the medial extent of the dissection. The medial pterygoid muscle (*MPM*) is being swept laterally with the dissector exposing the anterior cartilage of the ET (*ETC*). Attached to this cartilage is the tensor palatini (*TP*) fibrous aponeurosis

(*solid white line*) with its muscle fibers seen below (*broken white line*). (**B**) The resection of the inferior turbinate, posterior medial maxilla, medial pterygoid plate, and medial pterygoid muscle can be appreciated. The *solid black arrow* indicates the surgical plane anterior to the ET but medial to V3.

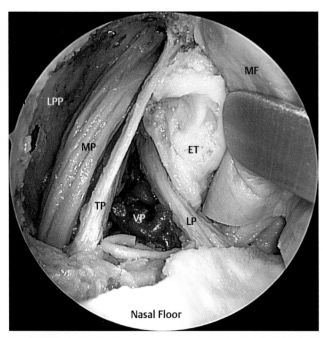

Fig. 17.10 Cadaveric dissection image of the right side, taken with a 30-degree endoscope. The medial pterygoid plate has been drilled away revealing the lateral pterygoid plate (*LPP*) once some fibers of the deep head of the medial pterygoid muscle (*MP*) have been resected. *TP*, tensor palatini; *VP*, vascular plexus; *LP*, levator palatini; *ET*, eustachian tube; *MF*, mucosal flap.

Fig. 17.11 Cadaveric dissection demonstrating the inferior horizontal incision taken through the tensor palatini (*TP*) and levator palatini (*LP*) muscles. The attachment of the TP muscle to the anterior cartilaginous Eustachian tube (*ET*) can be clearly seen with a surgical plane directly anterior to this. The ET has been retracted medially and posteriorly. *MP*, deep head of the medial pterygoid muscle.

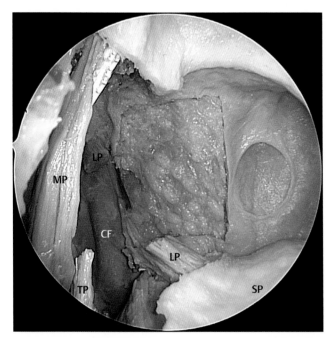

Fig. 17.12 Cadaveric dissection image taken following removal of the cartilaginous Eustachian tube. The carotid fascia (*CF*) can be seen overlying the carotid artery just behind the stump of the levator palatini (*LP*) muscle. This muscle is a good landmark for entry of the carotid artery into the carotid canal, which is directly posterior to the attachment of the levator palatini muscle to the skull base. *TP*, tensor palatini muscle; *MP*, deep head of the medial pterygoid muscle; *SP*, soft palate.

tough, these incisions need to be done with sharp instruments such as the angled scissors from the skull base set* (Medtronic ENT). It is not advisable to use a scalpel to perform this step as the internal carotid artery is at risk during this maneuver. It is better to use the natural curve of the scissors angled anteriorly (away from the carotid). In addition, the second surgeon should place the ET under traction thereby allowing each cut made with the scissors to be more effective and less likely to damage the internal carotid.

Once the ET has been removed the surrounding anatomical structures can be clearly identified (**Fig. 17.12**). Further dissection in **Fig. 17.13** demonstrates the lateral pterygoid plate, mandibular branch of the trigeminal nerve, ascending pharyngeal artery, a portion of the deep lobe of the parotid gland, the cervical carotid artery entering the petrous temporal bone, and also the longus capitis muscle. Above and lateral to the attachment of the ET to the skull base is the mandibular branch (V3) of the trigeminal nerve. The internal carotid artery is usually posterior and in some patients more lateral than V3.

◆ Postoperative Care

Hemostasis is achieved with the suction bipolar forceps. The pedicled septal flap is rotated into place to cover the dissection bed and edges are secured with Surgicel (Ethicon). The area is covered using a fibrin glue sealant. No packing is

Fig. 17.13 Cadaveric dissection image taken with a 30-degree endoscope, with the removal of the carotid fascia and deep lobe of the medial pterygoid muscle on the right side. This reveals the lateral pterygoid plate (*LPP*) and the mandibular branch of the trigeminal nerve (*V3*) just anterior to the attachment of the Eustachian tube (*ET*) to the skull base. *LC*, longus capitis muscle; *LP*, levator palatini muscle; *TP*, tensor palatini muscle; *SP*, soft palate; *CA*, carotid artery; *APA*, ascending pharyngeal artery; *CT*, chorda tympani; *DLP*, deep lobe of parotid gland.

placed. Broad-spectrum antibiotics are given for 5 days. To decrease postoperative crusting the patient performs regular nasal douches using the squeeze bottle nasal wash method. Nasal toilet is performed at 2 weeks postoperatively and as necessary thereafter. A repeat magnetic resonance imaging (MRI) scan is performed to ensure that there is no tumor recurrence at 6 and 12 months and yearly thereafter.

◆ Case Examples

We have had three patients in recent years in whom we have performed this surgery. The first patient had a malignant melanoma of the mucosa within the ET and the second patient had a low-grade mucoepidermoid carcinoma originating within the ET lumen and protruding through the wall of the ET into the parapharyngeal space. A component of this tumor prolapsed into the nasopharynx and caused nasal obstruction. The third patient had a recurrent juvenile angiofibroma lateral and inferior to the ET.

The patient with the mucoepidermoid carcinoma presented with nasal obstruction and the following MRI demonstrated a postnasal space mass (**Fig. 17.14**). The patient was taken to theater and the tumor prolapsing out of the ET orifice was removed and sent for histology and the diagnosis confirmed.

The surgeon who performed the biopsy confirmed tumor remained within the ET orifice and the patient was sent to the tumor board where it was decided that endoscopic excision was the best option for the patient. Computer-aided surgery (CAS) is an important part of the surgical plan. In these cases both computed tomography (CT) and MRI should be loaded and a "merge" performed. This tool allows the surgeon to move between CT and MRI and to adjust the image to have any percentage blend of CT and MRI. In this case the tumor could not be visualized on CT scanning but could be visualized on MRI scanning. "Merge" allowed the blend between CT and MRI to be adjusted so that the bony landmarks (pterygoid plates) and the tumor were clearly visible (**Fig. 17.15**). In addition, if contrast is used, the internal carotid arteries can also be clearly seen.

This tumor, the melanoma, and angiofibroma were removed using the technique described. Biopsies of tissue remaining in the surgical bed after excision revealed no residual tumor. No additional treatment modalities were given to these patients and they have remained free of locoregional recurrence of disease. The melanoma patient has, however, developed distant metastasis.

Fig. 17.14 The tumor is indicated by a *black arrow* in the coronal T1-weighted MRI scan (**A**) and in the axial CT scan (**B**).

Fig. 17.15 In axial CT scan (**A**) the tumor is not clearly seen but the bony landmarks are visible. In MRI scan (**B**) the tumor is clearly seen (*white arrow*) but the bony landmarks are absent. In the merged (CT and MRI) scan (**C**) both the bony landmarks (*broken white arrow*) and tumor (*white arrow*) are clearly seen. (**D**) The intraoperative image guidance–merged scan with the tumor (*white arrow*) and bony landmarks seen in all three planes. In addition, the resected Eustachian tube and tumor can be seen.

◆ Key Points

If endoscopic surgery is to be contemplated in this area it is vitally important that the surgeon is familiar with the endoscopic anatomy of this region. The surgeon needs to create a mental three-dimensional image of the anatomy and be able to place the dissection at all times within the three-dimensional picture. The new CAS guidance systems help significantly and the ability to merge the CT and MRI scan allows both bony and soft tissues to be accurately identified. Using the two-surgeon approach also adds significantly to the safety of the procedure as the second surgeon can keep the surgical field clear of blood and provide traction on the tumor at vital stages of the dissection. The biggest risk of this surgery is injury to the internal carotid artery and both the anesthetist and surgeon should have a surgical plan ready to put into action should this complication occur.

References

1. Fee WE Jr, Gilmer PA, Goffinet DR. Surgical management of recurrent nasopharyngeal carcinoma after radiation failure at the primary site. Laryngoscope 1988;98(11):1220–1226

2. Hsu MM, Ko JY, Sheen TS, Chang YL. Salvage surgery for recurrent nasopharyngeal carcinoma. Arch Otolaryngol Head Neck Surg 1997;123(3): 305–309

3. Wei WI, Lam KH, Sham JS. New approach to the nasopharynx: the maxillary swing approach. Head Neck 1991;13(3):200–207

4. Hao SP, Tsang NM, Chang CN. Salvage surgery for recurrent nasopharyngeal carcinoma. Arch Otolaryngol Head Neck Surg 2002;128(1):63–67

5. Morton RP, Liavaag PG, McLean M, Freeman JL. Transcervico-mandibulo-palatal approach for surgical salvage of recurrent nasopharyngeal cancer. Head Neck 1996;18(4):352–358

6. Fisch U. The infratemporal fossa approach for nasopharyngeal tumors. Laryngoscope 1983;93(1):36–44

7. Schramm VL Jr, Imola MJ. Management of nasopharyngeal salivary gland malignancy. Laryngoscope 2001;111(9):1533–1544

8. Yoshizaki T, Wakisaka N, Murono S, Shimizu Y, Furukawa M. Endoscopic nasopharyngectomy for patients with recurrent nasopharyngeal carcinoma at the primary site. Laryngoscope 2005;115(8): 1517–1519

9. Roh JL, Park CI. Transseptal laser resection of recurrent carcinoma confined to the nasopharynx. Laryngoscope 2006;116(5):839–841

18 Anatomy of the Sphenoid and Adjacent Structures of Importance during Skull Base Surgery

When the sphenoid sinus is opened and entered with an endoscope the surgeon should be able to identify whether the dominant sinus is entered. If the intersinus septum attaches to the lateral wall of the sphenoid, usually in the region of the carotid artery on the opposite side to the side entered, then the pituitary fossa should be visible and the surgeon is in the dominant sinus (**Fig. 18.1**). If the sinus is small and the septum implants on the lateral wall directly in front of the surgeon and the pituitary fossa is not seen, the surgeon should be in the nondominant sinus. This should be correlated to the computed tomography (CT) scans. Once the intersinus septum is removed (usually with a through-biting Blakesley or diamond burr—twisting should be avoided to avoid possible damage to the carotid artery by fracturing bone), the normal structures should be identifiable. The pituitary fossa is seen in the midline with the anterior genu of the cavernous carotid seen on either side. As the carotids are followed superiorly, the optic nerves are seen at the junction of the side wall and roof. There is often a depression between the optic nerve and carotid in a well pneumatized sphenoid which represents a pneumatization of the optic strut and is termed the opticocarotid recess (OCR) (**Fig. 18.2**). Between the medial aspect of the optic nerve at the point where it leaves the sphenoid and the anteriosuperior medial region of the carotid, is a slight thickening of bone termed the medial OCR and it corresponds to pneumatization into the medial clinoid process. On the lateral wall the V2 branch of the trigeminal nerve can be seen as well as the vidian nerve in the floor of the sinus. Posterior in the midline below the pituitary fossa the clivus is visible. Depending on the sphenoid pneumatization this bone may be either thick or quite thin. On either side of the clivus are the vertical paraclival portions of the carotid (**Fig. 18.2**). These are important landmarks for any surgical approach to the clivus.

Above the pituitary fossa is the tuberculum sella; this is a thickened area of bone that forms the junction between the anterior face of the pituitary fossa and the roof of the sphenoid (termed the planum sphenoidale).

◆ Anatomy of the Pituitary Fossa

Bone is removed from cavernous sinus to cavernous sinus, onto the floor of the fossa and up to the tuberculum sella. Care must be taken as the tuberculum sella is approached as there is a fold of dura that comes down with the tuberculum sella and, if this is grabbed with the Kerrison punch, a cerebrospinal fluid (CSF) leak will result. Once the bone over the pituitary fossa has been removed, the underlying periosteum is exposed. Between the periosteum and the dura is a potential space. This space is occupied by venous channels that connect the cavernous sinuses in the upper and lower regions of the pituitary (**Fig. 18.3**). In most macroadenomas these venous channels are obliterated by the pressure from the enlarging tumor. However, in microadenomas and tuberculum sella meningiomas, these venous plexuses remain and can bleed significantly when opened. Bipolar cautery may seal the channels but often the most effective way is to open the dura and then attempt to seal the two layers with bipolar cautery. If this fails then Gelfoam (Pharmacia and Upjohn Company, Kalamazoo, MI) paste (or Surgiflo [Ethicon, Somerville, NJ]) can be used. This is injected into the region and pressure is applied with a neuropattie. If bleeding persists, Ligar clips can be applied (Medtronic ENT skull base instrument set Ligar clip applicator [Jacksonville, FL]) to the two layers to seal them together.

◆ Lateral Wall of the Pituitary Fossa

The lateral wall of the pituitary fossa is formed by the cavernous sinus and the cavernous portion of the carotid artery. It is important for the surgeon to have a clear understanding of the carotid artery in the lateral wall. Tumor is routinely removed from the lateral wall with suction and standard pituitary curettes so knowing where to expect the carotid is important for the surgeon so that care is taken not to

Fig. 18.1 The suction rests on the pituitary sella with a clear view of the carotid artery (*ICA*) and the optic nerve (*ON*), indicating that the surgeon is in the dominant sphenoid sinus.

Fig. 18.2 Cadaveric dissection image taken of the left sphenoid sinus through a maximal sphenoidotomy. The vidian canal (*VC*) and trigeminal impression (*TI*) for the maxillary division of the trigeminal nerve can be clearly seen. If the sphenoid sinus is well pneumatized then the lateral recess (*LR*) can be seen, a depression in the lateral sphenoid wall between the VC and the TI. The lateral opticocarotid recess can be seen. This depression corresponds to pneumatization of the optic strut (the bony bridge that separates the optic canal from the superior orbital fissure). Further pneumatization into the optic strut may result in a pneumatized anterior clinoid process which will place the optic nerve on a mesentery. The optic tubercle (*OT*) is the bone located at the junction of the orbital apex and the sphenoid sinus. *ISS*, intersinus septum; *ON*, optic nerve; *CCA*, anterior genu of the intracavernous carotid artery; *PCA*, paraclival carotid artery.

apply any pressure over the carotid. Tumor may also need to be followed into the cavernous sinus so this anatomical understanding is crucial for the surgeon to understand so the tumor may be followed. **Figure 18.4** shows the normal course of the carotid in the lateral wall and the areas where extra care needs to be taken.

◆ Anatomy of the Cavernous Sinus

It is important to understand the anatomy of the cavernous sinus in patients in whom tumor extends into this area. If the surgeon enters the cavernous sinus from the pituitary fossa this is usually following a tumor extension through the dura above the horizontal portion of the cavernous carotid and posterior to the anterior genu (**Fig. 18.4**). If tumor is chased in the carotid the lateral wall may be exposed. The third nerve can be seen running horizontally in the lateral wall. As the cavernous carotid forms the anterior genu and becomes the clinoid carotid, the tumor may envelop this as well. It is usually not possible to chase tumor above and lateral to the clinoid carotid. If tumor grows anterior and lateral to the anterior genu of the cavernous carotid, the cavernous sinus may be entered via a separate incision through the dura lateral to the anterior genu. Great care should be taken with this incision and the surgeon should confirm the position of the carotid with image guidance as well as an intranasal Doppler. Gentle suction clearance of tumor in this region will often reveal the third nerve lateral and superiorly in the cavernous sinus (**Figs. 18.5 and 18.6**). If inferior dissection is performed around the anterior genu the sixth nerve may be seen hugging its anterolateral border and traversing the cavernous sinus from medial to lateral (**Fig. 18.6**). Sympathetic

Fig. 18.3 Cadaveric dissection illustrating the exposure of the sella. In this dissection just the periosteal layer of dura (*POD*) has been reflected, exposing the superior (*SIS*) and inferior intercavernous dural sinus (*IIS*). These sinuses run between the periosteal layer of dura and the meningeal layer of dura (*MD*).

Fig. 18.4 Cadaveric dissection image of the lateral sphenoid wall following bone removal. *P,* pituitary gland; *CCA,* intracavernous carotid artery; *V2,* maxillary division of the trigeminal nerve; *TG,* trigeminal ganglion; *VN,* vidian nerve; *PCA,* paraclival carotid artery; *P. CCA,* posterior genu of the intracavernous carotid artery; *SS,* sphenoid sinus.

Fig. 18.5 Cadaveric dissection image of the right lateral wall of the sphenoid sinus. The bone has been removed and the anterior genu of the intracavernous carotid artery (*CCA*) retracted medially. This allows clear visualization of the nerves within the dural layers of the lateral wall of the cavernous sinus. The abducens nerve (*CN VI*) can be visualized medially, running within the cavernous sinus. Note the periorbita of the orbital apex. The bone of the anterior clinoid (*AC*) process has been left in place, positioned within the lateral opticocarotid recess. *ON,* optic nerve; *Oph. A,* ophthalmic artery; *CN III,* occulomotor nerve; *CN IV,* trochlear nerve; *V1,* ophthalmic division of the trigeminal nerve; *V2,* maxillary division of the trigeminal nerve; *V3,* mandibular division of the trigeminal nerve.

Fig. 18.6 Cadaveric dissection of the right lateral sphenoid wall following removal of the lateral sphenoid wall. Dissection has continued anteriorly to the pterygopalatine fossa inferiorly and the orbital apex superiorly. In this image the periorbita has been retracted superiorly. Note the remnant of the maxillary strut (*MS*)—the strut of bone that separates the foramen rotundum from the superior orbital fissure/orbital apex. The vidian nerve (*VN*) can be seen moving into the posterior aspect of the pterygopalatine fossa and enters the pterygopalatine ganglion (*PPG*). The relationship between the foramen rotundum (*FR*) and the temporal lobe (*TL*) can be seen clearly. *V2,* maxillary division of the trigeminal nerve; *PN,* pharyngeal nerve; *PCA,* paraclival carotid artery; *CCA,* intracavernous carotid artery; *SS,* sphenoid sinus; *TG,* trigeminal ganglion.

branches from the carotid are often picked up by the sixth nerve as it passes the carotid. Inferiorly in the lateral wall of the cavernous sinus, the Gasserian ganglion and its branches V1, V2, and V3 can be seen (**Fig. 18.6**). Note the cavernous sinus is always above V2 which does leave an anatomical pathway under V2 into the middle cranial fossa (**Fig. 18.6**).

◆ Anatomy of the Vidian Nerve (Video 32)

Clinically the vidian nerve is always followed from the pterygopalatine fossa posteriorly into the floor of the sphenoid. It can often be seen in a well pneumatized sphenoid as it forms an inferior ridge in the floor of the sphenoid (**Fig. 18.2**). It forms an important lateral boundary when surgeons remove the floor of the sphenoid in preparation for approaching the clivus (**Fig. 18.7**). If the vidian nerve is followed posteriorly it initially approaches the supralacerum genu of the carotid artery at its medial aspect but then moves laterally and over the top of the petrous portion of the carotid (**Fig. 18.6**). If the vidian nerve is being followed to the petroclival genu this anatomical relationship needs to be clearly understood otherwise the carotid may be inadvertently damaged during this dissection. In the petrous region of the carotid the deep petrosal nerve (sympathetic fibers) joins with the greater superficial petrosal nerve (parasympathetic fibers) to form the vidian nerve.

Fig. 18.7 A dry bone image of the sphenoid sinus within the body of the sphenoid. It clearly demonstrates how the vidian canal (*VC*) communicates with the pterygopalatine fossa (*PPF*) anteriorly, and the foramen lacerum posteriorly. The vidian canal runs in the floor of the sphenoid sinus, and frequently has a sphenoid sinus septation (*S*) attaching to the roof of the canal. The foramen lacerum is the location of the supralacerum genu of the carotid artery, where the horizontal petrous carotid artery turns upward to become the paraclival carotid artery (*PCA*). The vidian canal and nerve is a vital landmark in surgical dissection in this area. *PF*, pituitary fossa; *FR*, foramen rotundum; *CCA*, anterior genu of the cavernous carotid artery.

Fig. 18.8 Cadaveric dissection of the left middle clivus (taken with a 30-degree endoscope) demonstrating the different segments of the abducens nerve. The abducens nerve moves through the posterior cranial fossa (cisternal segment) before perforating through the meningeal layer of dura (marked by *). Then the nerve enters a channel between the meningeal layer of dura and the periosteal layer of dura (*POD*). This segment is called the interdural segment (*IDS*), also known as Dorello's canal. In this dissection a "leaf" of periosteal dura has been incised and reflexed to clearly visualize the abducens nerve running within. The nerve then enters the confluence of dural sinus, made up of the superior and inferior petrosal sinuses, the basilar plexus, and the cavernous sinus. Here it is called the gulfar segment (*GS*). *PCA*, paraclival carotid artery.

◆ Anatomy of the Clivus (Videos 51 to 53)

The clivus is flanked by the paraclival carotids and extends from the floor of the sphenoid up to the floor of the pituitary fossa. The thickness of the bone of the clivus varies depending on the pneumatization of the sphenoid. The first step in transclival approaches to the posterior fossa is to accurately identify both paraclival carotids. This prevents inadvertent injury. Then the bone of the clivus is removed to expose the periosteum. Between the periosteum and the dura are a collection of venous lakes. These can bleed extensively and often require the dura to be opened, rolled, and bipolared to stem the bleeding. Additionally, Gelfoam paste or Surgiflo is used with neuropatties in an attempt to fill these venous lakes and stem the bleeding. One of the most important structures encountered in this region is the sixth nerve. The sixth nerve leaves the pons just lateral to the vertebrobasilar junction, and moves laterally, traversing the post fossa (termed the cisternal segment) until it enters the dura (at Dorello's point) and runs between the dura and the clival periosteum in the space between the layers called Dorello's canal (**Figs. 18.8 and 18.9**). Dorello's point can usually be found just behind the carotid about

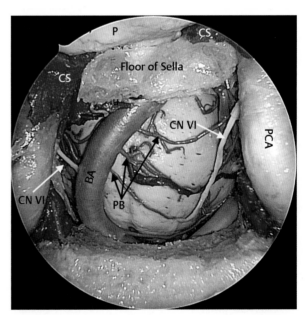

Fig. 18.9 Cadaveric dissection following removal of the middle one-third of the clivus and dura. The basilar artery (*BA*) can be seen very tortuous. Its pontine branches (*PB*) can be clearly seen. *CN VI*, abducens nerve; *CS*, cavernous sinus; *P*, pituitary gland; *PCA*, paraclival carotid artery.

midway between the sphenoid floor and pituitary fossa. A good landmark is the dorsal meningeal artery found just medial to the entry of the nerve into Dorello's canal. Another landmark includes the distance from the posterior clinoid, which averages 20 mm and usually 10 mm from the midline. Dorello's canal runs just below the gulfar venous plexus. This venous plexus is formed between dura and periosteum and is made up from the inferior petrosal venous sinus, the posterior part of the cavernous sinus, and the basilar venous plexus. These all join in this region and the nerve runs in the floor of this so-called gulfar segment. Another landmark in this area is the sphenopetrosal ligament (Gruber's) that is formed from the posterior clinoid process and lateral aspect of the dorsum sella to the petrous apex. After the nerve enters the back of the cavernous sinus below the horizontal portion of the cavernous carotid, it travels forward and hugs the inferior aspect of the anterior genu of the carotid before traversing the cavernous sinus on the lateral wall of the cavernous sinus.

From here it enters the superior orbital fissure and into the orbit.

◆ Anatomy of V2

The mandibular branch of the trigeminal nerve leaves the cavernous sinus from the Gasserian ganglion and proceeds horizontally toward the foramen rotundum and the pterygopalatine fossa. In a well-pneumatized sphenoid it forms a well-defined ridge in the lateral wall called the trigeminal impression (**Fig. 18.2**). The sphenoid may also pneumatize under the nerve thinning the bone between the sphenoid and the middle cranial fossa. This pneumatization may also develop into the upper root of the pterygoid plates. This thin plate between the middle cranial fossa and a laterally pneumatized sphenoid is a common site for prolapse of dura and the development of spontaneous CSF leaks.

19 Endoscopic Resection of Clival and Posterior Cranial Fossa Tumors

Tumors of the clivus and posterior cranial fossa are very difficult to access via traditional neurosurgical approaches. In the past skull base teams would approach the petroclival region either by a lateral or anterior route. The lateral route was via an extended middle cranial fossa approach[1] whereas the anterior route could be transmaxillary, transoral, or trancervical.[2,3] All of these approaches involve significant resection of normal structures with inevitable associated morbidity.[1-4] Even after such a resection the final surgical access was usually limited. The operating microscope did not allow a view around the corner and, if the tumor extended beyond the exposed area, resection under direct vision was not possible.

The advantages of the endoscopic transsphenoidal approach is that it allows access to the entire clivus down to the atlas of the cervical spine. It also allows early identification of the vital vascular structures with clear visualization of both carotid arteries and the cavernous sinuses and associated neurologic structures.[4] The most common tumor presenting in the clival region is a chordoma. Although complete resection of the tumor and the surrounding bone is optimal, this is often not possible due to the location and surrounding vital structures.[2,5] It is accepted that as complete a resection as is possible should be performed.[5] In most cases clival chordomas are slow growing and if surgery can be combined with radiotherapy (especially proton beam radiotherapy), this gives the patient the best possible chance of prolonged survival.[2,5] Because curative surgery is often not possible, the morbidity associated with tumor debulking should be as limited as possible. These factors make an endoscopic approach to these tumors attractive as it provides the best possible chance of complete surgical removal with the least surgical morbidity.[4,5] To remove the clival tumor and any associated intracranial extension, a clear understanding of the anatomy of this region is essential.

◆ Anatomy

The Clivus

The clivus extends from the dorsum sella to the foramen magnum (**Figs. 19.1** and **19.2**). The thickness of the clivus depends on the pneumatization of the sphenoid and can vary significantly. When this bone is thick it may hold significant venous channels (**Fig. 19.3**). This makes removal of the bone a slow process as significant bleeding can occur as the cancellous bone is opened. This is generally quickly controlled by packing the area with Gelfoam paste (Pharmacia and Upjohn Company, Kalamazoo, MI). Further drilling will provoke more bleeding which requires repacking and this process can make bone removal tedious. However, there is no quick and easy solution to the control of the bleeding in this area. The lateral borders of the dissection of the clivus are the paraclival carotid arteries and these need to be exposed at the beginning of the dissection to avoid inadvertent damage (**Fig. 19.4**). The inferior limit of the dissection is usually the floor of the sphenoid but should access be required to the basiocciput, foramen magnum, or even lower to the first cervical vertebra, the entire sphenoid floor can be removed (**Fig. 19.4**).

Complete removal of the clivus exposes the dura of the posterior fossa. Bone behind the inferior portion of the paraclival carotid arteries can be removed so that the arteries stand proud of the lateral margins (**Fig. 19.5**). The limit to which this bone can be removed is determined by the 45-degree angle that the carotid arteries make as they run in their canals through the petrous temporal bone. This region where the petrous portion of the carotid artery turns vertically in the floor of the sphenoid is where bone should be removed to access the petrous apex. In some patients a large cholesterol granuloma may thin down the bone separating the granuloma from the sphenoid allowing the granuloma to be drained through the sphenoid.

Fig. 19.1 Dry skull dissection with the floor of the sphenoid sinus drilled away revealing the middle and lower thirds of the clivus. The vidian canals (*VC*) can be seen bilaterally at the level of the floor of the sphenoid sinus. *PS*, planum sphenoidale; *PF*, pituitary fossa; *ON*, optic nerve; *CCA*, anterior genu of the intracavernous carotid artery; *FR*, foramen rotundum; *PCA*, paraclival carotid artery; *MPP*, medial pterygoid plate; *FR*, foramen rotundum; *A. Arch Atlas*, anterior arch of atlas; *ITF*, infratemporal fossa.

Fig. 19.2 Dry bone specimen demonstrating the middle and lower thirds of the clivus. The middle third (*M. 1/3rd*) begins at the sella floor (*SF*) and extends to the floor of the sphenoid sinus (*SSF*), and the lower third (*L. 1/3rd*) extends from the floor of the sphenoid sinus to the foramen magnum (*FM*). The upper third corresponds to the dorsum sella, and visualization is obstructed by the pituitary gland. A pituitary transposition allows visualization of the upper third of the clivus. *VC*, vidian canal; *HC*, hypoglossal canal; *PCA*, paraclival carotid artery; *PF*, pituitary fossa; *PS*, planum sphenoidale; *CCA*, anterior genu of the intracavernous carotid artery.

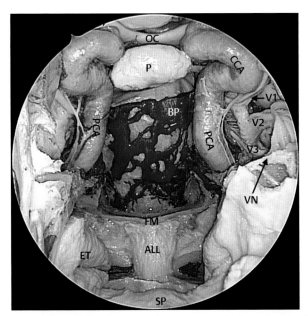

Fig. 19.3 Cadaveric dissection demonstrating the large venous channels within the clivus that constitute the basilar plexus (*BP*) that can cause significant bleeding during surgery. *OC*, optic chiasm; *P*, pituitary gland; *CCA*, anterior genu of the intracavernous carotid artery; *PCA*, paraclival carotid artery; *VN*, vidian nerve; *FM*, foramen magnum; *ET*, Eustachian tube; *ALL*, anterior longitudinal ligament; *SP*, soft palate; *V1*, ophthalmic division of the trigeminal nerve; *V2*, maxillary division of the trigeminal nerve; *V3*, mandibular division of the trigeminal nerve.

Fig. 19.4 Cadaveric dissection demonstrating the identification of the paraclival carotid arteries (*PCA*), the lateral borders of the dissection. If dissection is to continue to the lower clivus then the entire floor of the sphenoid sinus can be removed. The longus capitis muscle (*LC*) attaches firmly to the floor of the sphenoid sinus (*FSS*). *CS*, cavernous sinus; *P*, pituitary gland.

Fig. 19.5 Cadaveric dissection image taken with a 30-degree endoscope. Bone has been removed behind the paraclival carotid artery (*PCA*) so that the arteries stand proud of the lateral margins. *BP*, basilar plexus; *PCA*, paraclival carotid arteries; *CN VI*, abducens nerve; *, gulfar segment of the abducens nerve.

Fig. 19.6 Cadaveric dissection of the left middle clivus (taken with a 30-degree endoscope) demonstrating the different segments of the abducens nerve. The abducens nerve moves through the posterior cranial fossa (cisternal segment) before perforating through the meningeal layer of dura (marked by *). Then the nerve enters a channel between the meningeal layer of dura and the periosteal layer of dura (*POD*). This segment is called the interdural segment (*IDS*). In this dissection a "leaf" of periosteal dura has been incised and reflexed to clearly visualize the abducens nerve running within. The nerve then enters the confluence of dural sinus, made up of the superior and inferior petrosal sinuses, the basilar plexus, and the cavernous sinus. Here it is called the gulfar segment (*GS*). *PCA*, paraclival carotid artery.

Posterior Cranial Fossa

The dura has two layers: a periosteal layer and a meningeal layer. The extensive and rich venous plexus—the basilar plexus—runs between the periosteal and meningeal layers of the dura. Exposure of the clival periosteum can result in significant bleeding. In a patient with a recurrent meningioma previously removed through external approach, bleeding of 3 L was encountered. One of the ways to seal off these venous sinuses is to open the dura and bipolar the two layers together. This was done but it was felt that the patient had lost too much blood to proceed and surgery was stopped and rescheduled for 2 weeks later. At this operation there was minimal bleeding and the tumor was successfully addressed. Before the dura is opened the surgeon needs to have a clear understanding of where the sixth nerve is likely to be. As seen in Chapter 18, the sixth nerve enters Dorello's canal (canal formed by the periosteal and dural layers about midway up the middle third of the clivus just below the posterior meningeal artery) and then progresses to the gulfar region behind the carotid artery (**Figs. 19.5** and **19.6**). The gulfar region is formed by the junction of the inferior and superior petrosal sinus, basilar plexus, and posterior region of the cavernous sinus. All of these sinuses are between the periosteal and meningeal layers of dura. A general landmark for this region is the junction of the floor of the pituitary with the vertical paraclival section of the carotid. Once the dura of the posterior cranial fossa has been opened, the contents of the posterior cranial fossa can be seen (**Figs. 19.7** and **19.8**). The first and most notable structure seen is the basilar artery which is usually covered with arachnoid (**Fig. 19.8**). **Figs. 19.9**, **19.10**, **19.11**, **19.12**, **19.13**, and **19.14** demonstrate the structures that are easily visualized. In most patients the segments of the brainstem that can be easily vi-

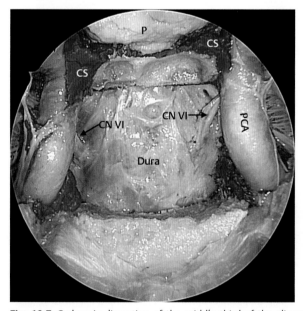

Fig. 19.7 Cadaveric dissection of the middle third of the clivus with removal of the basilar plexus and exposing the dura. The abducens nerves (*CN VI*) can be seen bilaterally as they perforate the meningeal dura and become the interdural segments of CN VI. *CS*, cavernous sinus; *PCA*, paraclival carotid arteries; *P*, pituitary gland.

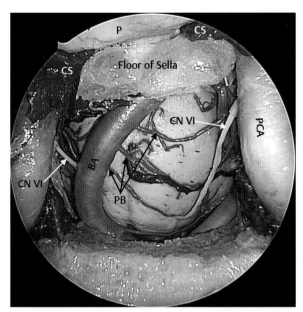

Fig. 19.8 Cadaveric dissection following removal of the middle third of the clivus and dura. The basilar artery (*BA*) can be seen very tortuous. Its pontine branches (*PB*) can be clearly seen. *CN VI*, abducens nerve; *CS*, cavernous sinus; *P*, pituitary gland; *PCA*, paraclival carotid artery.

Fig. 19.9 Cadaveric dissection with removal of the upper third and middle third of the clivus with visualization of the posterior cerebral arteries (*PCA*), superior cerebellar arteries (*SCA*), and the occulomotor nerve in between (*CNIII*). *3rd Vent*, third ventricle; *MB*, mamillary bodies; *PCA*, posterior cerebral arteries; *SCA*, superior cerebellar arteries; *CN III*, occulomotor nerve; *PCA*, paraclival arteries; *BA*, basilar artery; *PB*, pontine branches; *CN VI*, abducens nerve, *CN V*, trigeminal nerve; *AICA*, anterior inferior cerebellar artery.

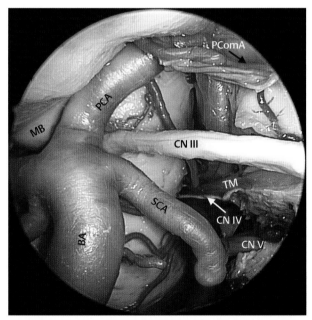

Fig. 19.10 Cadaveric dissection image taken with a 30-degree endoscope following removal of the superior third of the clivus, visualizing the small trochlear nerve seen running along the tentorial membrane edge. *BA*, basilar artery; *PCA*, posterior cerebral artery; *SCA*, superior cerebellar artery; *CN III*, occulomotor nerve; *CN IV*, trochlear nerve; *CN V*, trigeminal nerve; *TM*, tentorial membrane; *PComA*, posterior communicating artery; *MB*, mamillary body.

Fig. 19.11 Cadaveric dissection image demonstrating structures seen following dissection of the lower third of the clivus. Note how the basilar arteries and vertebral arteries can be extremely tortuous in their course. *ALL*, anterior longitudinal ligament; *A. AOM*, anterior atlantooccipital membrane; *FM*, foramen magnum; *HC*, hypoglossal canal; *VA*, vertebral arteries; *BA*, basilar artery; *CN VI*, abducens nerve; *PCA*, paraclival carotid artery.

Fig. 19.12 Cadaveric dissection with image taken just above the skeletonized hypoglossal canal (*HC*) at the cerebellopontine angle. The anterior inferior cerebellar artery (*AICA*) can be seen intimately associated with the vestibulocochlear nerve (*CN VIII*), facial nerve (*CN VII*), and the nervus intermedius (*NI*). The posterior inferior cerebellar artery (*PICA*) can be seen running between the vagus (*CN X*) and spinal and cranial portions of the accessory nerves (*CN XI – S, CN XI – C*).

Fig. 19.13 Cadaveric dissection image taken following dissection of the right lower third of the clivus. As the posterior inferior cerebellar artery (*PICA*) courses from the vertebral artery (*VA*) it frequently runs through the rootlets that make up the hypoglossal nerve (*CN XII*). It may tent these rootlets as it courses to the cerebellomedullary fissure to run intimately with the cranial nerves IX – XI. *CN X*, vagus nerve; *HC*, hypoglossal canal; *IPS*, inferior petrosal sinus; *BA*, basilar artery; *FM*, foramen magnum; *A. AOM*, anterior atlanto-occipital membrane.

Fig. 19.14 Cadaveric dissection image showing the hypoglossal nerve exiting the hypoglossal foramen with its corresponding vein that communicates the internal jugular vein with the basilar plexus. *HC*, hypoglossal canal; *CN XII*, hypoglossal nerve and rootlets; *FM*, foramen magnum; *VA*, vertebral artery; *PICA*, posterior inferior cerebellar artery; *BA*, basilar artery; *CN X*, vagus nerve.

sualized are the upper part of the medulla, the pons, and the lower edge of the midbrain. The vessels that are seen are the basilar, posterior cerebral, superior cerebellar, and anterior inferior cerebellar arteries. Depending on the state of the brain, a variable number of the cranial nerves can be seen. Dehydration of the brain by the administration of mannitol may enlarge the space around the brainstem and allow easier visualization of the nerves.

Pituitary Translocation for Access to the Upper Third of the Clivus

Tumors extending behind the pituitary gland are usually unresectable unless the upper third of the clivus is removed. To do this the pituitary gland must either be translocated anteriorly or, in patients who are hypopit with a nonfunctional gland, removed. Before the gland can be translocated, space needs to be created for the gland to be positioned in the planum sphenoidale. The first step is to remove all the bone over the pituitary fossa onto the carotid arteries. The next step is to remove the bone overlying the tuberculum sella and over the posterior half of the planum sphenoidale (**Fig. 19.15**). This bone is removed from optic nerve to optic nerve and wider on the planum sphenoidale. The dura is incised and the subchiasmatic cistern inspected (**Fig. 19.16**). The diaphragm of the pituitary should be visualized and divided with skull base scissors up to the pituitary stalk (**Fig. 19.17**). Next, to translocate the gland, the periosteum and dura layers over the anterior aspect of the gland need to be separately identified and the plane between these lay-

Fig. 19.15 Cadaveric dissection of the sphenoid sinus demonstrating the removal of bone over the anterior genu of the intracavernous carotid arteries, sella, tuberculum sella, and the posterior half of the planum sphenoidale (*PS*). *CCA*, anterior genu of the intracavernous carotid artery; *IIS*, inferior intercavernous sinus; *SIS*, superior intercavernous sinus; *P*, pituitary gland.

Fig. 19.16 Cadaveric dissection allowing visualization into the subchiasmatic cistern. The superior hypophyseal artery (*SHA*) can be seen giving off its chiasmatic (*C*) and infundibular (*I*) branches. *ON*, optic nerve; *OC*, optic chiasm; *CCA*, cavernous carotid artery.

ers clearly established. As the gland is mobilized the dentate ligaments that hold the pituitary gland in place are identified and divided (**Fig. 19.18**). The inferior hypophysial artery will need to be divided to allow mobilization of the gland (**Figs. 19.19** and **19.20**). Dissection needs to proceed

carefully (**Fig. 19.21**), otherwise the thin layer covering the cavernous sinus can be easily penetrated resulting in substantial venous bleeding. This can be controlled by Gelfoam paste and pressure with a neuropattie but this should be avoided if possible. Once the gland is fully mobile it can be translocated into the region of the planum sphenoidale

Fig. 19.17 Cadaveric dissection image demonstrating the incised diaphragma (*D*) to the pituitary stalk (*PS*). *ON*, optic nerve; *OC*, optic chiasm; *CCA*, cavernous carotid artery.

Fig. 19.18 Cadaveric dissection in the plane between the periosteal layer of dura and the meningeal layer of dura (*MD*) covering the right side of the pituitary gland. The pituitary dentate ligaments (*DL*) can be clearly visualized. *CS*, cavernous sinus.

Fig. 19.19 Cadaveric dissection image of the right side of the pituitary gland. Dissection has occurred between the periosteal layer of dura and the meningeal layer of dura (*MD*) as far posteriorly as the dorsum sella. The inferior hypophyseal artery (*IHA*) is visualized as the base of the posterior clinoid (*PC*).

Fig. 19.20 Cadaveric dissection image of the pituitary gland tethered from its transposed position by the inferior hypophyseal artery (*IHA*). In this image the meningeal and periosteal layers of dura have been removed. The IHA needs to be ligated and cut to allow complete transposition between the carotid arteries. The dorsum sella (*DS*) can be visualized. *P*, pituitary gland; *CS*, cavernous sinus.

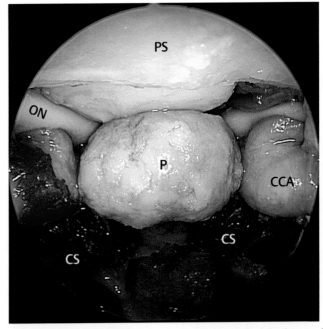

Fig. 19.21 Cadaveric dissection with preservation of the meningeal (*MD*) and periosteal layers (*POD*) of dura, and the pituitary gland (*P*) transposed between the carotid arteries.

Fig. 19.22 Cadaveric dissection image with removal of the layers of dura. The pituitary gland (*P*) lies in its transposed position against the planum sphenoidale (*PS*), and between the cavernous carotid arteries (*CCA*). *ON*, optic nerve; *CS*, cavernous sinus.

Fig. 19.23 Cadaveric dissection demonstrating the osteotomies at the base of the posterior clinoids (*PC*) for separation with the body of the dorsum sella (*DS*). *P. CCA*, posterior genu of the intracavernous carotid artery; *PCA*, paraclival carotid artery; *ICCA*, intracranial carotid artery; *BA*, basilar artery; *PL*, posterior lobe of the pituitary gland; *AL*, anterior lobe of the pituitary gland.

(**Fig. 19.22**). The upper third of the clivus is now visible and can be removed (**Fig. 19.23**). A inverted Y-shaped osteotomy is made with the stem in the midline. A 1- to 2-mm high speed stylus diamond burr (Medtronic ENT, Jacksonville, FL) is used to perform these osteotomies (**Fig. 19.24**). Once the

posterior clinoids are fully mobile a combination of a blunt hook and dissector is used to gently peal the clinoids out of their periosteal layer. Remember that the posterior clinoid abuts both the intracranial carotid artery and the posterior genu of the intracavernous carotid artery simultaneously, and is at risk during this maneuver (**Figs. 19.23** and **19.24**). Now the dura can be opened and the suprasellar anatomy fully visualized. The first structure encountered is the Liliequist membrane, which is a condensation of arachnoid that attaches to the posterior clinoids and third nerves and has a semicircular aperture through which the basilar artery can pass (**Fig. 19.25**).

Once the pituitary has been translocated or removed, a better perspective of the cranial nerves in the posterior fossa can be achieved. In **Fig. 19.26** if the telescope is turned laterally the sixth cranial nerve can be seen just below the carotid artery and again in the cavernous sinus behind the carotid artery. The third cranial nerve can be seen exiting the brainstem between the posterior cerebral artery and the superior cerebellar artery (**Fig. 19.10**). The thin fourth cranial nerve can also be seen in the edge of the tentorium (**Fig. 19.10**).

If the 30-degree endoscope is advanced further into the posterior cranial fossa the rest of the cranial nerves can be seen (**Fig. 19.4**). The trigeminal nerve (V) exits the lateral aspect of the pons with the thin sixth cranial nerve below it (**Fig. 19.10**). The fifth cranial nerve enters Meckel's cave before passing into the cavernous sinus. To evaluate the seventh and eighth nerves, the lateral end of the pontomedullary sulcus is inspected and the facial and vestibulocochlear nerves can be seen emerging from the brainstem, with nervus intermedius located between these nerves, and intimately related to the AICA vessels (**Figs. 19.12** and **19.27**). Below the fifth cranial

Fig. 19.24 Cadaveric dissection image demonstrating the close anatomical relationship of the posterior clinoid (*PC*) with both the intracranial carotid artery (*ICCA*) and the posterior genu of the intracavernous carotid artery (*P. CCA*). *AL*, anterior lobe of the pituitary gland; *PL*, posterior lobe of the pituitary gland; *BA*, basilar artery.

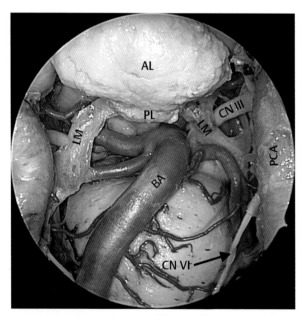

Fig. 19.25 Cadaveric dissection following the removal of the dorsum sella allowing visualization of Liliequist membrane (*LM*), a condensation of arachnoid membrane with a semicircular hole through which the basilar artery (*BA*) passes before dividing into its terminal branches. *AL*, anterior lobe of the pituitary gland; *PL*, posterior lobe of the pituitary gland; *CN III*, occulomotor nerve; *CN VI*, abducens nerve; *PCA*, paraclival carotid artery.

Fig. 19.26 Cadaveric dissection image taken with a 70-degree endoscope. The abducens nerve (*CN VI*) can be seen passing behind the paraclival carotid artery (*PCA*) to run parallel with the horizontal portion of the intracavernous carotid artery (*H. CCA*). Here the nerve is located between the carotid artery medially, and the ophthalmic division of the trigeminal nerve laterally. *P*, pituitary gland; *V2*, maxillary division of the trigeminal nerve; *PN*, pharyngeal nerve; *VN*, vidian nerve; *PPG*, pterygopalatine ganglion; *SPA*, sphenopalatine artery; *ET*, eustachian tube; *IT*, inferior turbinate; *LC*, longus capitis; *PR*, pharyngeal raphe.

Fig. 19.27 Cadaveric dissection image taken with a 70-degree endoscope. The right internal auditory canal (*IAC*) can be clearly visualized with the meatal segment of the anterior inferior cerebellar artery (*AICA*) entering the meatus. This vessel then loops between the facial (*CN VII*) and vestibulocochlear nerves. *CN*, cochlear nerve; *CN V*, trigeminal nerve.

nerve the seventh, eighth, and the nervus intermedius can be seen exiting the brainstem and entering the internal auditory meatus (**Figs. 19.12** and **19.28**). Although in this cadaver there seems to be space between the brainstem and the skull base, this is not always the case in patients and therefore caution should be exercised when contemplating removing tumors from the lateral regions of the posterior cranial fossa. The nervus intermedius mostly arises as a single trunk between the vestibulocochlear and the facial nerve, but may arise from as many as four rootlets. In **Fig. 19.12** we can visualize three rootlets. In most cases the anterior inferior cerebellar artery (AICA) passes just below the facial and vestibulocochlear nerves on its way around the brainstem, but it may also pass through or above as seen in this example as it passes through the facial and vestibulocochlear nerves (**Fig. 19.12**). The AICA gives off a labyrinthine artery, subarcuate arteries, and the recurrent perforating branches to the brainstem. The facial nerve enjoys a consistent relationship to the junction of the glossopharyngeal/vagus/spinal accessory nerves within the medulla. The facial nerve arises 2 to 3 mm above the most rostral rootlet.

Inferior to the seventh and eighth cranial nerves the ninth and tenth cranial nerves can be seen entering the jugular foramen (**Fig. 19.12**). The AICA can in some patients (54%) loop a variable distance into the internal auditory meatus before giving of its labyrinthine branch (**Fig. 19.27**). The glossopharyngeal nerve, the vagus, and the accessory nerve arise from rootlets lined along the postolivary sulcus (a shallow groove between the olive, and the posterolateral surface of the medulla). The glossopharyngeal and vagus nerves arise at the

level of the superior third of the olive, whereas the spinal accessory rootlets arise along the posterior margin of the inferior two-thirds of the olive and from the lower medulla and upper segments of the spinal cord. The glossopharyngeal nerve arises as a line of one or two rootlets from the upper medulla, just below the facial nerve. The posterior inferior cerebellar artery (PICA) arises from the vertebral artery at the level of the medulla and typically travels dorsally between the vagus and the accessory nerves as seen in **Fig. 19.28**. It then continues to reach the surface of the inferior cerebellar peduncle, where it dips to supply the cerebellomedullary fissure and terminates by supplying the suboccipital surface of the cerebellum. The choroid plexus is located directly behind these nerves as it spills out of the foramen of Luschka, located at the lateral margin of the pontomedullary sulcus (**Fig. 19.29**). The folliculus is visible just behind the facial and the vestibulocochlear nerves (**Fig. 19.29**). The hypoglossal nerve arises from a series of rootlets originating from the preolivary sulcus at the medulla, a groove between the olive and the medullary pyramid. The rootlets of the hypoglossal nerve may stretch over the posterior surface of the vertebral artery (**Fig. 19.14**). The PICA may traverse either around or between these rootlets before they enter the hypoglossal canal. The hypoglossal nerve then exits this canal often with a venous lake that joins the internal jugular vein (**Fig. 19.14**).

Cavernous Sinus

The cavernous sinus may be involved in clival tumors, particularly chordomas, and it is therefore important to understand the relationship of the cranial nerves within the

Fig. 19.28 Cadaveric dissection image demonstrating the posterior inferior cerebellar artery (*PICA*) running between the vagus (*CN X*) and the cranial accessory nerve rootlets (*CN XI-C*) at the position where the nerves exit the brainstem. *CN VII*, facial nerve; *CN VIII*, vestibulocochlear nerve; *NI*, nervus intermedius; *CN IX*, glossopharyngeal nerve; *CN XI-S*, spinal accessory nerve

Fig. 19.29 Cadaveric dissection image on the right side with retraction inferiorly of the glossopharyngeal and vagus nerves to reveal the choroid plexus (*CP*) as it spills out of the foramen of Luschka. The folliculus (*F*) can also be visualized laterally, just behind the facial (*CN VII*) and vestibulocochlear nerves (*CN VIII*). AICA, anterior inferior cerebellar artery; *PICA*, posterior inferior cerebellar artery.

cavernous sinus as discussed in Chapter 18. The most important relationship in clival tumors is the sixth nerve as it is the most vulnerable. Its cisternal segment is easily engulfed with intradural tumor extension and its cavernous segment is often involved in the gulfar regions and in Dorello's canal where it lies between layers of dura and periosteum (**Figs. 19.6**, **19.9**, and **19.26**).

The other cranial nerves that may be involved in tumor extension into the cavernous sinus are the third, fourth, and fifth cranial nerves. **Figure 19.30** is a diagrammatic representation of the contents of the cavernous sinus adjacent to the pituitary gland, and **Fig. 19.31** shows these nerves as they run in the lateral wall of the cavernous sinus on their way to

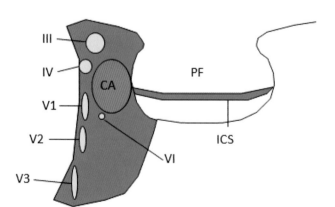

Fig. 19.30 This diagrammatic representation of the right cavernous sinus shows the carotid artery (*CA*) within the cavernous sinus. The sixth nerve is the most medial nerve whereas the third, fourth, and fifth tend to run against the lateral wall of the cavernous sinus. The intercavernous venous sinus (*ICS*), which connects one sinus to the other, is demonstrated.

Fig. 19.31 Cadaveric dissection image of the left lateral wall of the sphenoid sinus. The bone has been removed and the anterior genu of the intracavernous carotid artery (*CCA*) retracted medially. This allows clear visualization of the nerves within the dural layers of the lateral wall of the cavernous sinus. The abducens nerve (*CN VI*) can be visualized medially, running within the cavernous sinus. ON, optic nerve; *Oph. A*, ophthalmic artery; *CN III*, occulomotor nerve; *CN IV*, trochlear nerve; *V1*, ophthalmic division of the trigeminal nerve; *V2*, maxillary division of the trigeminal nerve; *V3*, mandibular division of the trigeminal nerve.

the orbital apex and superior orbital fissure (the cavernous carotid artery has been retracted medially).

The contents of the cavernous sinus are seldom seen during surgery as it is only possible to open the cavernous sinus if tumor has infiltrated it and obliterated the venous sinusoids. However, in such cases, it is important to know the anatomy of the cavernous sinus so that these important structures are not damaged during resection of such tumors. In **Fig. 19.31** the carotid artery is swung medially to expose the contents of the cavernous sinus. Note how the third cranial nerve is a large nerve in the roof of the sinus with the smaller less easily visible fourth cranial nerve directly below it. The sixth cranial nerve is seen to enter the sinus lower down and from the posterior inferior aspect then to traverse from inferior to superior abutting the carotid artery. If this nerve is moved medially the V1 and V2 branches of the fifth cranial nerve can be seen. V3 is in the same surgical plane but lies more inferior.

◆ Surgical Technique (Videos 51 to 53)

The first step is to raise a Hadad pedicled septal flap and place in the maxillary sinus which had been widely opened. The opposite septum is mobilized, as in Chapter 20, to cover the donor site of the pedicled septal flap, thereby removing the posterior half of the septum and creating enough space for a two-surgeon approach. This anteriorly based flap is secured with a 30 Vicryl suture (Ethicon, Somerville,

NJ). Silastic may again be placed over the columella, as in Chapter 17, to facilitate bilateral passing of instruments. Next the superior turbinate is removed and bilateral large sphenoidotomies are created. The floor of the sphenoid is resected with a curved stylus high diamond burr (Medtronic ENT). The landmarks for this resection are the vidian nerves. These are identified at the beginning of the resection and all bone between these nerves is removed. As the supralacerum genu of the carotid is approached remember that the vidian nerve is on the medial side of the genu but as it progresses onto the carotid it travels lateral and over the top of the carotid (**Fig. 19.32**). It is important to resect all of the floor because failure to do so will result in the anterior sill of the floor of the sphenoid driving the instruments upward toward the pituitary (**Fig. 19.33**).

The next step is to identify the vertical portions of both carotid arteries thereby delineating the lateral limits of the dissection (**Fig. 19.3**). Usually this is done with an angled high speed stylus skull base diamond burr (Medtronic ENT) which allows the walls of the carotids to be exposed with minimal risk of injury. Image guidance plays an important role in correctly identifying the arteries so that the bone overlying the arteries can be thinned until transparent and the arteries clearly identified. If the drill inadvertently contacts the adventitia of the wall of the carotid it will usually not damage the wall as long as the artery is immediately recognized. Prolonged contact between the burr and wall is dangerous and may lead to a lesion of the artery. If the tumor extends inferolaterally to the carotid canals it can be followed as long as it is kept in mind that the petrous temporal portion of the carotid runs at ~45 degrees to the vertical portion of the carotids. In a patient with a chordoma such an extension can be removed with a curved diamond burr. In certain

Fig. 19.32 Cadaveric dissection image of the lateral sphenoid wall on the left side demonstrating the vidian nerve coursing laterally toward the supralacerum genu (*SLG*), located at the junction of the vertical paraclival carotid artery (*PCA*) with the horizontal petrous carotid artery. *PCA*, paraclival carotid artery; *CCA*, anterior genu of the intracavernous carotid artery; *V2*, maxillary division of the trigeminal nerve; *VN*, vidian nerve; *PN*, pharyngeal nerve; *PPG*, pterygopalatine ganglion.

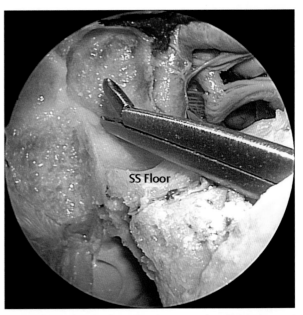

Fig. 19.33 Cadaveric dissection demonstrating that instrumentation without adequate removal of the floor of the sphenoid sinus results in a straight instrument being driven high into the middle third of the clivus beneath the pituitary fossa. Removal of the floor of the sphenoid sinus (*SS*) will allow access to the junction of the posterior sphenoid floor and adjacent clivus.

Fig. 19.34 (**A**) The vertical portions of the carotid arteries have been exposed (*solid black arrows*). Superiorly, the dura overlying the pituitary fossa (*PFD*) has been exposed and the cavernous sinus (*CS*) on both sides can be clearly seen. Note the intercavernous venous sinus connecting the two sinuses. Inferiorly the floor of the sphenoid has been drilled away until almost adjacent to the clival dura (*broken black arrow*). (**B**) The vertical portions of the carotid arteries are seen in an axial CT (*white arrows*) with the clivus between the carotids. (**C,D**) Axial CTs in which the petrous portions of the carotid arteries and foramen lacerum are marked with *black arrows* and the posterolateral portions of the clivus behind the arteries are marked with *white arrows*. Note how the petrous portion of the carotid runs at a 45-degree angle to the vertical portions of the arteries.

situations the 70-degree reverse cut diamond burr (Medtronic ENT) may be useful for very laterally based lesions (**Fig. 19.34**).

If the tumor breaches the clival dura and protrudes intracranially then this portion of the tumor may be separated from the clival component by sharp dissection using the endoscopic skull base scissors* (Medtronic ENT). The residual tumor protruding from the clivus into the posterior cranial fossa is now accessible without the surgeons having to work around the often bulky clival component. The dural opening should be visualized and can be further enlarged with the scissors to allow an endoscopic view of the intracranial tumor component. Clival chordomas are usually soft and amenable to debulking with gentle suction. Care must be taken to ensure that the tumor is not entangled with the sixth nerve or any of the vascular structures of the brainstem. Traction on a tumor wrapped around a brainstem perforator may

cause catastrophic bleeding and hemorrhage into the brainstem and intraoperative death. In this situation it is vitally important for the otolaryngologist and neurosurgeon to work closely as a team. The malleable skull base blunt hook and probe* (Medtronic ENT skull base set) are used to mobilize the tumor while gentle traction is applied and the tumor is gently delivered through the dural defect into the sphenoid. Angled endoscopes and malleable suctions* (Medtronic ENT skull base set) are used to visualize the intracranial cavity to ensure no residual tumor remains. If residual tumor is seen a suction regulator is placed in the suction line to reduce the amount of suction. The malleable skull base suction* (Medtronic ENT) is then placed through the dural defect onto the residual tumor. The suction control port of this instrument is very wide so that if a vessel or nerve is inadvertently sucked into the end of the instrument, removal of the finger

Fig. 19.35 (**A,B**) On axial MRI, the chordoma (*black arrow*) can be seen between the carotid arteries (*broken white arrows*) and abutting the basilar artery (*solid white arrow*). (**C**) On parasagittal MRI, the lesion can be seen in the clivus below the pituitary and abutting the pons.

from the suction port will remove all suction at the tip and the vascular structure or nerve will be released uninjured.

◆ Case Examples and Results (Videos 51 and 52)

A middle-aged woman presented with a large clival chordoma that protruded into the sphenoid sinus, abutted both internal carotid arteries, and extended intracranially where it abutted the basilar artery (**Fig. 19.35**).

This patient was managed with a two-surgeon approach with bilateral large sphenoidotomies, removal of the posterior septum, and removal of the floor of the sphenoid. Once access had been achieved, both vertical portions of the carotids were exposed with a rough diamond burr. The remaining bony clivus was removed with exposure of the clival dura with a central deficit through which the chordoma entered the posterior cranial fossa. Utilizing the two-surgeon approach the intracranial portion of the tumor was slowly mobilized under direct vision. A 30-degree endoscope was used to visualize the inferior intracranial extension of the tumor. The malleable blunt tip and curved probes were used to gently dissect the arachnoid from the tumor and the tumor was delivered

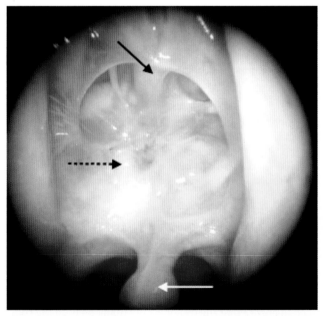

Fig. 19.36 This endoscopic image of the sphenoid indicates the residual septum (*white arrow*), intersinus septum of the sphenoid (*black arrow*), and the region of the reconstruction of the posterior fossa wall (*broken black arrow*).

Fig. 19.37 (**A–C**) MRI T2-weighted axial scans in which the tumor (*white arrow*) is seen between the two vertical portions of the carotids (*broken white arrows*). It is also evident how the tumor indents the pons and displaces the basilar artery (*black arrow*) laterally. (**D,E**) In the coronal T1-weighted scans, the tumor can be seen indenting the pons (*white arrow*). This indentation can be fully appreciated on the parasagittal MRI T1-weighted scan (**F**). Note the significant posterior indentation of the tumor into the pons (*white arrow*).

into the sphenoid and removed. Reconstruction of the skull base was achieved initially with fat alone but the patient developed a cerebrospinal fluid (CSF) leak about 1 month after surgery and the repair was then augmented with fascia lata. This repair remains intact after 4 years follow-up

(**Fig. 19.36**). To date there is no evidence of a recurrent disease on magnetic resonance imaging (MRI) scanning.

The second case example is a middle-aged man who presented with a partial sixth cranial nerve palsy. MRI scans showed a lesion extending from internal carotid to internal

Fig. 19.38 (**A,B**) Axial CT scans and (**C**) a T1-weighted MRI illustrate the horizontal portions of the internal carotid (*black arrow*) and the bony erosion immediately posterior to the carotid in the base of the clivus (*white arrow*).

carotid and extending inferior and lateral to the vertical portions of the carotids. The intracranial extension indents the anterior surface of the pons and displaces the basilar artery laterally (**Fig. 19.37**).

The other area that should always be assessed is the possible inferior bony extension of these tumors. If the CT scans of this case are reviewed, the inferolateral extension behind the petrous temporal portions of the internal carotids can be seen (**Fig. 19.38**). There is significant bony erosion of this part of the clivus down toward the foramen magnum. In this patient more bony erosion is seen on the right side (white arrow) in the petrous apex.

This patient was approached with a two-surgeon standard pituitary exposure with wide sphenoidotomies, septal resection, and floor of sphenoid resection. Once the tumor was fully on view, the vertical portion of the internal carotid arteries was exposed from the base of the sphenoid to the floor of the pituitary fossa using a rough diamond burr. The dura of the entire floor of the pituitary was then exposed. This delineates the superior and lateral margins of the dissection. Next the floor of the sphenoid was drilled away and the tumor followed laterally behind the vertical portions of the

internal carotids and posteriorly until the posterior cranial fossa dura was exposed. Once dura was exposed inferiorly (at the base of the clivus), laterally (behind the carotids), and superiorly at the pituitary-clivus junction the tumor was felt to be fully mobile. The tumor was placed under slight traction and a gush of CSF was seen as the intracranial component was displaced in the posterior fossa dural defect. Using the skull base endoscopic scissors* (Medtronic ENT), the sphenoid/clival component of the tumor was divided from the intracranial extension at the level of the posterior fossa dura. Once the sphenoid component was removed, enough space was created so that the two surgeons could work comfortably on the remaining intracranial tumor. The dural defect was enlarged with the endoscopic skull base scissors and a view of the posterior cranial fossa obtained. Using the malleable right angled hook and blunt tip probe (skull base instrument set, Medtronic ENT), the intracranial component was gently mobilized and delivered through the dural defect. The endoscope was switched to a 30-degree endoscope and the posterior cranial fossa reexplored. Residual tumor was seen superiorly on the anterior face of the pons. A suction regulator was placed in the suction line limiting the amount of suction and the malleable frontal sinus suction was bent so it could be placed through the dural defect superiorly and the residual tumor indenting the pons was gently removed. Complete macroscopic tumor resection was achieved. The skull base defect was repaired with two layers of fascia lata. One layer was placed intracranially and the other on the dura from the sphenoid. Fibrin glue and a nasal pack were put in place. Unfortunately, the patient developed a CSF leak after the pack was removed. On reexploration the dural repair was solid with a very thin stream of CSF seen coming from the junction between the pituitary dura and the repair. This region was opened and repaired with a bath-plug type fat plug and fibrin glue.

To date we have endoscopically removed 13 clival chordomas. Four of the six primary cases had radiotherapy with one patient having proton beam irradiation. Four of the seven revisions had undergone radiotherapy prior to presentation to us. In five of the six primary cases complete macroscopic tumor resection was possible and in this group there has been no recurrence of tumor since resection with a mean follow-up of 3.5 years. In the partially resected patient the residual tumor is growing very slowly and this is being monitored with sequential MRI scans. Further surgery will be offered if the tumor grows significantly or produces symptoms. In the seven revision cases, all had their primary surgery at other institutions. Five still have radiological residual disease with two patients deceased.

◆ Conclusion

Endoscopic resection of clival and posterior cranial fossa tumors presents a challenge to the skull base team. Successful management of these patients requires a detailed knowledge of the anatomy and a high level of endoscopic skill. The endoscopic skull base team, normally consisting of a rhinologist and neurosurgeon, needs to build their endoscopic expertise on less challenging cases, such as with pituitary tumor resection, and once they have sufficient expertise to then progress to clival and posterior cranial fossa tumors.

References

1. Brackmann DE, Arriaga MA. Surgery of the posterior cranial fossa. In: Cummings CW, ed. Otolaryngology Head and Neck Surgery, 4th ed. St. Louis: Mosby; 2005
2. Lanzino G, Dumont AS, Lopes MB, Laws ER Jr. Skull base chordomas: overview of disease, management options, and outcome. Neurosurg Focus 2001;10(3):E12
3. DeMonte F, Diaz E Jr, Callender D, Suk I. Transmandibular, circumglossal, retropharyngeal approach for chordomas of the clivus and upper cervical spine. Technical note. Neurosurg Focus 2001;10(3):E10
4. Solares CA, Fakhri S, Batra PS, Lee J, Lanza DC. Transnasal endoscopic resection of lesions of the clivus: a preliminary report. Laryngoscope 2005;115(11):1917–1922
5. Giorgio F, Vittorio S, Fabio C, Giovanni F, Diego M, Ernesto P. The endoscopic transnasal transphenoidal approach for the treatment of cranial base chordomas and chondrosarcomas. Op Neurosurg Suppl 2006;1:50–57

20 Endoscopic Resection of Anterior Cranial Fossa Tumors

Endoscopic techniques for transnasal resection of anterior cranial fossa tumors were developed for tumors involving the nasal cavity, sinuses, and the anterior cranial fossa. However, experience with these tumors has led to the refinement of these techniques to address tumors of the anterior cranial fossa that do not have a nasal or sinus component. Although most of this experience has been with meningiomas, these techniques can also be used to address malignant nasal tumors that are primary intracranial or that extend intracranially. The first step toward a wholly endoscopic resection of malignant sinonasal tumors was the experience gained with endoscopic management of the sinonasal component of the tumor during a standard craniofacial resection. We found that the endoscopic resection of the sinonasal component could be as effectively dealt with endoscopically as it can with external traditional approaches. In the case of large tumors involving both nasal cavities, the endoscopic approach was more effective as it dealt with both sides as opposed to most of the external approaches which limited access to one side of the nose. A significant number of these malignant tumors attach to the skull base and associated orbit. During craniofacial resection the skull base involved with tumor is completely excised.[1-3] The associated orbital involvement would, in most circumstances, be removed as a separate excision. We found that endoscopically resecting the sinonasal component afforded better visualization of the tumor allowing the nonattached tumor to be extensively debulked and the regions of tumor attachment to be accurately identified. This in turn allowed a complete resection of the sinonasal and, if present, the orbital component.

As the experience with anterior skull base tumor resections developed, these techniques could in turn be applied to the resection of malignant tumors involving the skull base and intracranial cavity. Tumors thought to be suitable were tumors with a localized intracranial extension. Because of the infiltrative nature of squamous cell carcinomas these were thought not to be as suitable as adenocarcinoma and esthesioneuroblastoma, which in general have a pushing rather than infiltrative front and are thus more easily addressed

endoscopically. Although the gold standard for resection of these malignancies was a craniofacial resection,[1] there is increasing evidence that for selected patients the wholly endoscopic resection yields comparable results.[2-6] Recently published series have reported similar morbidity and mortality rates and very similar local recurrence rates.[2,3,5,6] In addition, there are significant benefits for the patients undergoing wholly endoscopic resection because uninvolved structures are not removed and this approach avoids skin incisions with improved cosmetic results.[2-6] In addition, those patients who are medically or otherwise unsuitable for a standard craniofacial resection, or who choose not to undergo this procedure, can be offered the endoscopic approach as an alternative. Endoscopic resection of the anterior skull base requires a detailed knowledge of the anatomy of this region.

◆ Anatomy of the Anterior Skull Base

The anterior skull base consists of the orbital plates of the frontal bone with the cribriform plates (part of the ethmoid bone) separating them. These plates attach to the planum sphenoidale (lesser wing of the sphenoid bone) posteriorly (**Fig. 20.1**). The cribriform plate gives rise to the crista galli onto which the falx cerebri attaches anteriorly.

If the anterior skull base is approached endoscopically from front to back the frontal bone (posterior wall of the frontal sinus), foveae ethmoidalis, and intervening cribriform plates can be seen (**Figs. 20.2 and 20.3**). Posteriorly the foveae ethmoidalis and cribriform plates attach to the planum sphenoidale (**Fig. 20.4**). The important vascular structures within the anterior skull base are the anterior and posterior ethmoid arteries. Note how there is a space or cell between the frontal sinus ostium and the anterior ethmoidal artery (**Fig. 20.5**). This is always the case as the artery usually runs in the base of the second lamella which is the upward continuation of the anterior face of the bulla ethmoidalis.

254

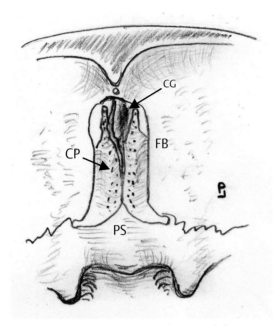

Fig. 20.1 This diagram illustrates the view of the anterior skull base from above (intracranial side). The crista galli (*CG*), cribriform plate (*CP*), orbital plate of the frontal bone (*FB*), and planum sphenoidale (*PS*) of the lesser wing of the sphenoid bone are visible.

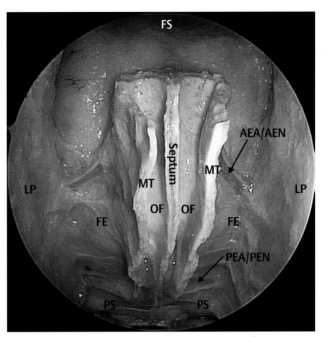

Fig. 20.2 Cadaveric dissection illustrating the anatomy of the anterior skull base following partial resection of both middle turbinates (*MT*) and nasal septum. The communal frontal sinus (*FS*) ostium can be seen anteriorly with both fovea ethmoidalis (*FE*) exposed. The lateral margins are the lamina papyracea (*LP*) and posteriorly the planum sphenoidale (*PS*) can be seen. *OF*, olfactory fossa; *AEA*, anterior ethmoidal artery; *PEA*, posterior ethmoidal artery; *AEN*, anterior ethmoidal nerve; *PEN*, posterior ethmoidal nerve.

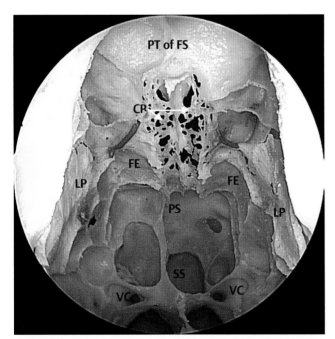

Fig. 20.3 Dry bone specimen following a Draf 3 shows the delicate cribriform plate (*CP*) and fovea ethmoidalis (*FE*). The nasal septum and middle turbinates have been completely resected. The sphenoid sinus (*SS*) can be seen posteriorly with the roof forming the planum sphenoidale (*PS*). The lamina papyracea (*LP*) is still intact. *VC*, vidian canal; *PT of FS*, posterior table of frontal sinus.

Fig. 20.4 Dry bone dissection image taken with a 30-degree endoscope demonstrating the fovea ethmoidalis (*FE*) and cribriform plate (*CP*) junction with the planum sphenoidale (*PS*). This is marked approximately by the posterior ethmoidale artery (*PEA*). *ISS*, intersinus septum of sphenoid sinus; *ON*, optic nerve; *CCA*, anterior genu of the intracavernous carotid artery.

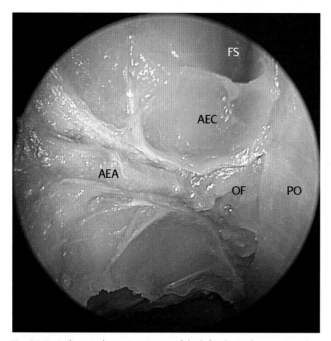

Fig. 20.5 Cadaveric dissection image of the left ethmoid cavity revealing the anterior ethmoidal artery (*AEA*) located one anterior ethmoidal cell (*AEC*) posterior to the frontal sinus (*FS*). *OF*, orbital fat; *PO*, periorbita.

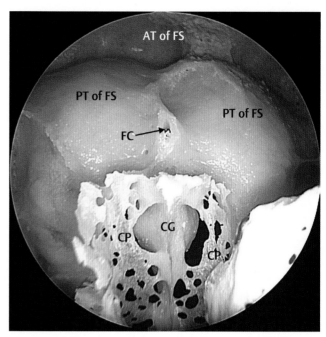

Fig. 20.6 Dry bone specimen following a frontal drillout procedure. This specimen clearly shows the close relationship between the frontal sinuses and the cribriform plate, and hence the advantage of the drillout procedure for anteriorly based lesions. *AT of FS*, anterior table of frontal sinus; *PT of FS*, posterior table of frontal sinus; *FC*, foramen cecum; *CP*, cribriform plate; *CG*, crista galli.

One of the first decisions that need to be made is whether the entire skull base needs to be resected. To determine this, the important landmark is the anterior ethmoidal artery (AEa). If the tumor approaches but does not come further forward than the anterior ethmoidal artery then the posterior skull base can be resected without the need to perform a modified Lothrop or frontal drillout procedure. Once the tumor encroaches past the AEa, a frontal drillout is necessary to be able to achieve the correct angle onto the tumor and be able to delineate the anterior arachnoid/tumor interface. This is necessary so that, once the inside of the tumor has been debulked, the tumor arachnoid plane can be identified and the tumor wall collapsed into the tumor cavity allowing progressive resection of the tumor.

Resection of the skull base is only possible once the entire skull base has been exposed. This requires, as a first step, bilateral sphenoethmoidectomy with exposure of the skull base within the sphenoids, anterior and posterior ethmoids, and visualization of the frontal ostia. If the entire anterior skull base is to be resected the frontal sinuses need to be drilled out with an endoscopic modified Lothrop procedure. The relationship between the cribriform plate and the frontal sinuses is clearly illustrated in this osteology model and illustrates the importance of performing a frontal drillout procedure for more anteriorly based tumors (**Fig. 20.6**). The other important structures that need to be identified are the anterior ethmoidal artery and the posterior ethmoidal artery. Note how the anterior ethmoidal artery has the anterior ethmoidal nerve running adjacent to it and how the lamina papyracea tents into the skull base as the anterior ethmoidal canal is formed (**Figs. 20.5 and 20.7**). This tenting of the lamina papyracea

Fig. 20.7 Cadaveric dissection image demonstrating the left anterior ethmoidal artery (*AEA*) and nerve (*AEN*) running across the skull base toward the middle turbinate (*MT*) attachment. Here it can be seen dividing into several branches including the anterior falcine artery (*AFA*) to supply the falx cerebri. *LP*, lamina papyracea.

Fig. 20.8 Cadaveric dissection image: the skull base has been removed affording a view of the inferior aspect of both anterior cerebral lobes. The olfactory bulbs (*OB*), branches of the anterior cerebral artery (*ACa*), and cut inferior aspect of the falx cerebri (*FC*) can be seen. *FS*, frontal sinus; *AEA*, anterior ethmoidal artery; *LP*, lamina papyracea.

Fig. 20.9 The anterior attachment of the falx cerebri (*FC*) to crista galli (*CG*) is seen. Note the superior sagittal sinus (*SSS*) running in the superior aspect of the falx cerebri within the inferior sagittal sinus (*ISS*) in the lower margin of the falx cerebri. The inferior sagittal sinus becomes the straight sinus (*SS*) after it joins with the great cerebral vein.

is important to understand when exposing and cauterizing the AEa. Our preferred technique is to expose the artery with a diamond burr then to use the suction bipolar to cauterize the artery. However, if the burr is too big or if the exposure is done over the lateral area on the triangular fat invagination, division of the artery with the burr may result in retraction of the artery into the orbit and orbital hematoma formation. This has happened in one case in which an anterior skull base tumor was being removed and required an immediate orbital decompression to relieve the pressure in the eye. The tumor resection continued uneventfully once this had been done. The posterior ethmoidal artery should be addressed in the same manner with exposure with a diamond burr and bipolar cautery. Once this has been done any residual septum is detached from the anterior skull base.

Once the skull base has been dropped down and removed, the anterior cranial fossa can be viewed (**Fig. 20.8**). The two olfactory bulbs and olfactory tracts are seen on the undersurface of the anterior cerebral hemispheres. The major vascular structures are the anterior cerebral arteries and branches from these arteries. The venous drainage of the anterior cranial fossa is via the superior and inferior sagittal sinuses. The superior sagittal sinus runs in the upper border of the falx cerebri whereas the inferior sagittal sinus runs in the lower border of the falx cerebri (**Fig. 20.9**). Large anterior skull base tumors may have large veins draining into the inferior sagittal sinus which if disrupted can bleed significantly.

Vascular Anatomy of the Anterior Cranial Fossa (Video 56)

Tumors that arise in the tuberculum sella region, planum sphenoidale, or posterior olfactory fossa can involve the anterior part of the circle of Willis and anterior cranial fossa vessels as they push posteriorly and superiorly (**Fig. 20.10**). **Figure 20.11** gives an overview of the how the carotids enter the skull base and then form the anterior portion of the circle of Willis and go on to supply the anterior cranial fossa. The most common tumor in this region is the tuberculum sella meningioma but others include craniopharyngiomas and anterior/superior extension of pituitary tumors. When the tumor fills the subchiasmatic cistern, the superior hypophyseal vessels are also at risk and damage to these vessels can lead to ischemic damage of the optic nerves and chiasm with blindness. When the A1–AComm–A2 complex is surrounded by tumor understanding the anatomy of this complex is vital for safe surgery to be performed in this region (**Fig. 20.10**). A detailed description of the anterior cerebral arteries is given in **Fig. 20.12**. A1 (first part of the anterior cerebral artery) is formed when the internal carotid divides into the middle and anterior cerebral arteries. It enters the lamina terminalis cistern and at this point is banded to the lateral aspect of the optic nerves by thick arachnoid bands.[7] The medial lenticulostriate arteries arise from the posterior and superior surface of the first half of A1 and supply the medial septum pellucidum, medial part of the anterior commissure and pallidum, pillars of the fornix, paraolfactory area, anterior limb of the internal capsule, anteroinferior part of the striatum, and anterior hypothalamus. Vessels arising from the second half of A1 are smaller and join the arterial plexus of the optic nerve, chiasm, and optic tract.[7] Once identified the A1 vessel wall can be followed to the anterior communicating artery (AComm) and the recurrent artery of Heubner[8]

Fig. 20.10 **(A,B)** MRI scans show the A1 (*solid white arrow*) leaving the middle cerebral artery juncture toward the AComm (*dashed white arrow*) with the A2s (*black arrow*) progressing superiorly. These vessels are all within the substance of the tumor. The clinical dissection of this tumor is seen in **(C)** and **(D)** with tumor encompassing the perforators (*Perf*) coming off the AComm. Once all tumor had been removed the vascular complex with A1-AComm,-A2 and the important branch of A1, the recurrent artery of Heubner (*RAH*), and the A2 branch, orbitofrontal (*OF*) artery, are clearly visible.

(**Figs. 20.10 and 20.12**). The recurrent artery of Heubner (RAH) is present bilaterally in 85% of patients, unilaterally in 11%, and absent in 4%. It immediately courses posteriorly toward the trunk of A1 before entering the subarachnoid space and penetrating the brain at the junction of the medial and lateral olfactory stria. It is an important vessel to preserve because it supplies the head of the caudate and the anteroinferior internal capsule, anterior hypothalamus, and olfactory region. The other vitally important vessels in this region are the posterior perforating vessels from the AComm. These branches can number from one to six and arise from the superior and posterior surface of AComm and course posteriorly to supply the infundibulum of the pituitary, optic nerve and chiasm, lamina terminalis, anterior perforating substance, corpus callosum, anterior commissure, limbic system, and associated regions of cortex. Deficits associated with injury to these arteries include serious and incapacitating memory deficits, personality changes, and electrolyte imbalances. Occlusion of A1 region can result in paraplegia of the lower extremities with sparing of the upper limbs, incontinence, abulic or motor aphasia, and frontal lobe symptoms.

The A2 (anterior vertebral artery after AComm) has three main branches (**Figs. 20.10 and 20.12**). The RAH originates from the AComm-A2 junction or from the first few millimeters of A2 in 90% of patients (in the other 10% from the upper A1).[7] The other two branches are the orbitofrontal and frontopolar

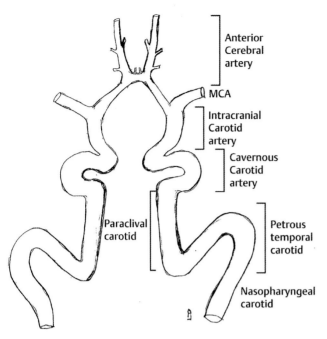

Fig. 20.11 The carotid bends laterally in the nasopharynx before entering the petrous temporal bone. It then swings anteriorly before becoming the paraclival carotid in the floor of the sphenoid and progresses vertically into the cavernous sinus and then enters the anterior cranial fossa giving off the middle cerebral artery (*MCA*) to become the anterior cerebral artery.

branches. The orbitofrontal usually originates from the first 5 mm of A2 at the junction of the lamina terminalis and callosal cisterns and has a downward and forward course crossing the olfactory tract to the gyrus rectus. The frontopolar branch originates after the orbitofrontal branch and travels anteriorly more medially across the subfrontal sulcus.

◆ Surgical Technique (Videos 54 to 56)

The surgical removal of anterior skull base tumors requires a team consisting of an endoscopic sinus surgeon and a neurosurgeon. It is vitally important that both members of this skull base team have endoscopic skills. These are best learnt doing pituitary tumor resections as a team. Here the neurosurgeon learns how to manage the endoscope and how to work from the video monitor in two dimensions rather than with the microscope in three dimensions. The sinus surgeon learns how to manipulate intracranial tumors and surrounding neural and vascular structures. These hours spent on pituitary tumor resection build confidence within the skull base team enabling benign or malignant nasal tumors with intracranial extension to be tackled.

The first steps for access are complete sphenoethmoidectomy with exposure of the entire skull base. If the tumor is relatively posteriorly sited with a relatively small intracranial extension, skull base resection can be performed without a modified Lothrop procedure. In such cases the intracranial extension of tumor must be small and the resection of this extension should be possible without it being necessary to resect across the midline. Surgically, the skull base defect should be clearly delineated and then enlarged to expose uninvolved dura on all sides of the defect. The dura is then excised with a combination of endoscopic skull base scissors* (Medtronic ENT, Jacksonville, FL) or scalpel with a normal margin of dura and the tumor extension and dura delivered into the nose.

However, if a complete resection of the anterior skull base is required then the next step is to perform an endoscopic modified Lothrop procedure allowing the anterior aspect of the skull base to be delineated (**Fig. 20.13**). The nasal septum is separated from the skull base allowing visualization of the entire skull base from the frontal sinuses anteriorly to the anterior face of the pituitary fossa (**Fig. 20.2**). Both laminae

A

B

Fig. 20.12 (**A**) The middle cerebral artery (*MCA*) gives rise to the lateral lenticulostriate arteries (*LLA*) at the bifurcation complex. The medial lenticulostriate arteries (*MLA*) arise from the proximal section of A1. At the juncture of A1-AComm-A2 the recurrent artery of Heubner (*RAH*) is given off. AComm completes the anterior portion of the circle of Willis and has several perforating vessels (*AComm Perf*) that head posteriorly. In the first 5 mm of A2 the orbitofrontal (*OF*) artery is given off with the frontopolar (*FP*) artery staying more medial. (**B**) A clinical picture after removal of a tuberculum sella meningioma with a well-defined display of the anterior cerebral arteries.

Fig. 20.13 Cadaveric dissection demonstrating the completion of a frontal drillout, with a maximized anterior/posterior dimension and complete removal of the intersinus septum. *MT*, middle turbinate; *FS*, frontal sinus.

Fig. 20.14 Cadaveric dissection with osteotomies created using a diamond drill.

papyracea should be on view forming the lateral limits of the resection. Before the skull base can be resected the anterior and posterior ethmoidal arteries need to be identified and ligated or cauterized and divided. The technique of removing lamina papyracea to find the anterior artery as it enters the canal is not preferred as it risks rupture of the artery and with fat prolapse makes identification of the artery very difficult. An easier and safer technique is to run the diamond burr over the region of the anterior ethmoidal artery removing the bone until the artery is exposed in its canal. The bone is removed and the artery identified and exposed. It is then cauterized, and divided. This is done bilaterally before the posterior ethmoidal arteries are also identified using the diamond drill on the skull base. The arteries usually enter the skull base at the junction of the posterior ethmoids and sphenoid and the drill is run over this region of the skull base until the artery is clearly identified, cauterized, and cut on both sides (**Fig. 20.4**).

The next step is to perform an endoscopic modified Lothrop procedure as set out in Chapter 9. A septal perforation (window) is performed and the frontal sinus opened bilaterally and communicated by removal of the intersinus septum (**Fig. 20.13**).

The final preparation step is to disconnect the nasal septum from the skull base. A straight through-cutting Blakesley is used to cut the nasal septum at its insertion on the skull base. This isolates the skull base and allows the osteotomies to be made so that the skull base can be dropped into the nasal cavity (**Fig. 20.14**). A skull base diamond burr 3.2 mm or Stylus high speed 3-mm diamond burr (Medtronic ENT) is used to create the osteotomies along the lines shown in **Fig. 20.7A**. The dura is exposed but can largely be preserved. If necessary a 2- to 3-mm 40-degree forward-biting Kerrison's punch can

also be used to remove any residual bone to maximize the bony osteotomies to improve access for tumors with lateral extension. However, the osteotomies in the planum need to respect the optic nerve canals as their lateral landmarks. Next the dura needs to be incised with a scalpel. The only residual attachment holding the skull base is the attachment of the falx cerebri to the crista galli (**Figs. 20.15 and 20.16**).

Fig. 20.15 Cadaveric dissection demonstrating the skull base scissor cutting the attachment of the falx cerebri (*FC*) to the crista galli.

Fig. 20.16 The skull base is placed under traction and the remaining posterior falx cerebri still holds the skull base. This needs to be cut before the skull base can be dropped into the nose.

Fig. 20.17 The anterior skull base has been removed and both anterior cerebral gyri and olfactory bulbs are visible.

The falx cerebri often has vessels running in it and should be bipolar cauterized before being cut. This is done incrementally with the suction bipolar forceps (Medtronic ENT) before each cut so maximal visualization is maintained during this process. The falx can extend posteriorly for some distance (often more than 1 cm) so care needs to be taken not to damage the vessels lying on each side of the falx. A curved endoscopic skull base scissors* (Medtronic ENT) angled inferiorly is used to cut the falx cerebri and the skull base can then be dropped into the nasal cavity and removed (**Figs. 20.1 and 20.17**).

To perform this maneuver one surgeon puts downward pressure on the mobile skull base, putting any remaining attachments under stretch, thereby allowing the second surgeon to either dissect free or cut any small residual attachments under visualization with magnification. If the posterior osteotomy is not 100% complete, this attachment can be gently fractured through the osteotomy lines but the dura will need to be cut under direct vision. In most cases limited extension of tumor through the skull base will be removed en bloc with the osteotomies placed through normal surrounding bone similar to the technique for a craniofacial resection performed through a craniotomy.[9] Removal of the entire skull base in this fashion exposes the anterior cranial fossa and tumor that remains can now be dissected free. Such a dissection is again very delicate requiring great endoscopic skill from both surgeons. The arachnoid plane needs to be developed and the tumor dissected from the arachnoid. Particularly for meningiomas that extend posteriorly onto the optic chiasm and superiorly and engulf the A1-AComm-A2 complex, dissection of these vessels from the tumor is critical (**Fig. 20.10**). When the A1-A2 complex is engulfed in tumor there are two routes to identifying the vessels and

dissecting them free from the tumor. Once the bulk of the main tumor is removed either with a Cusa Excel Ultrasonic aspirator (Integra Radionics, Burlington, MA) or Sonopet Ultrasonic aspirator (Stryker, Kalamazoo, MI), the arachnoid plane is identified and the tumor wall delivered into the created cavity. This can be done superiorly looking for the frontopolar branch of A2 or for A2 itself or from below delivering the tumor superiorly into the cavity and identifying A1 (**Figs. 20.10 and 20.12**). With either technique once the vessels have been identified, the vessel is dissected free from the surrounding tumor by using a blunt hook (Medtronic endoscopic skull base set) and staying on the vessel wall and gently clearing tumor from the vessel wall. Alternatively, if it is felt that this cannot be safely done either due to the consistency of the tumor, position of the tumor, or endoscopic skill levels of the surgeons, then residual tumor should be left and the vessels not endangered.

Vessels that can be preserved are carefully dissected free from the tumor but vessels supplying the tumor are cauterized with bipolar forceps and divided.

Skull Base Closure (Videos 54 to 56)

If the dura or a large vessel such as the intrasphenoid carotid artery is exposed then coverage of this area is considered important for safe postoperative healing. In most cases this is done with a vascularized pedicled flap or, if this is not available, a free mucosal graft from the nose or fascia lata graft. An exposed carotid artery should not be left unprotected after surgery. All skull base cases have routine preparation of the thigh for the harvesting of fascia lata during the procedure and pituitary tumor cases have either the thigh or

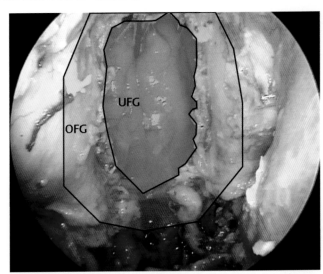

A

B

Fig. 20.18 In dissection (**A**) the fascia lata graft is placed as an underlay (*UFG*) on the inside of the cranial cavity and the edges smoothed out. In dissection (**B**) the second fascia lata graft is placed on the nasal surface of the defect as on overlay graft (*OFG*), again smoothing out the edges to ensure that the graft fits snugly around the entire defect.

abdomen prepared for graft harvesting. In the past when large intra-arachnoid skull base access was needed for tumor resection, the defect was closed in layers utilizing fat then an underlay and overlay fascia lata or the acellular dermal graft AlloDerm (Life Cell, Branchburg, NJ) with a free mucosal graft over the top. In regions where intracranial high flow cerebrospinal fluid (CSF) cisterns have been opened, fat is placed intracranially and used to support the first underlay fascia lata graft or dural substitute graft. The underlay graft needs to extend 5–10 mm past the defect edges circumferentially (**Fig. 20.18**). In the anterior cranial fossa, especially when a Draf 3 procedure had been performed and the defect reaches the posterior wall of the frontal sinus, the underlay graft tends to slip posteriorly and all our leaks have come from the anterior edge of the defect.

We now tend to secure this underlay graft anteriorly by placing two 1-mm holes through the skull base and either passing tails of the graft through these holes and "riveting" the graft or by placing a suture through the underlay graft and passing it through the holes and tying the two sutures together thereby fixing the graft anteriorly (**Fig. 20.19**).[10,11] It is important to ensure that the graft extends beyond the defect edges in all directions. This is best achieved with the malleable skull base probe (Medtronic ENT) as it does not have a ball on the tip and won't drag an adjusted graft back out with it once the graft is properly positioned. It must not have any folds and must be smoothly adherent to the inner surface of the skull base. A thin ring of fat is placed at the defect edges on the underlay graft as a gasket to increase the seal of this layer. In the past a second layer of fascia lata was placed as an overlay on the skull base, again ensuring that there were no folds and that it lay closely approximated to the skull base (**Fig. 20.18**). If a free mucosal graft is available this is placed over the second layer but is not essential. The edges of the overlay graft need to extend beyond the edges of the defect by ~10 mm in all directions and be placed onto bone denuded of mucosa. The edges of the graft are fixed

with oxidized cellulose (Surgicel, Ethicon, Somerville, NJ) and fibrin glue is applied to this layer followed by sheets of Gelfoam (Pharmacia and Upjohn Company, Kalamazoo, MI). The Gelfoam ensures that the nasal pack does not stick to the grafts. The nasal cavity is packed with ribbon gauze soaked in the antiseptic bismuth iodoform paraffin paste (BIPP) or with an inflated intranasal balloon. We do not use the balloon routinely as it is important to do an immediate postoperative CT if the balloon is used to ensure that the reconstruction has not been pushed intracranially by the balloon. This is not necessary with the BIPP pack as it is placed under direct

Fig. 20.19 In this patient two small 1-mm holes (*broken arrow*) have been made through the anterior table anterior to the defect. Tails (*white arrow*) of the underlay fascia lata graft (*FLG*) all pulled through these holes so that the anterior graft is "riveted" into the skull base. This prevents the graft from slipping posteriorly. In our experience this was the most common place for postoperative cerebrospinal fluid leak. *FS*, frontal sinus.

Fig. 20.20 (**A**) The Hadad vascularized septal pedicle flap (*SPF*) is based on the postnasal artery (*PNA*) and encompasses the entire mucosal surface of the septum. In the cadaver dissection (**B**) the postnasal artery (*PNA*) is clearly seen coming through the sphenopalatine foramen. *SO,* sphenoid ostium.

vision and the packing force is at all times is controlled by the surgeon. This technique had a high postoperative CSF leak rate of around 15 to 30%.[10,11]

A recent important innovation by Hadad et al.[12] where the vascularized pedicled septal flap was described has substantially altered the way that intra-arachnoid skull base defects are closed today (**Figs. 20.20 and 20.21**). This flap is based on the branch of the sphenopalatine artery— the postnasal artery (**Fig. 20.22**). This branch leaves the sphenopalatine foramen in its posterior superior aspect and travels along the anterior face of the sphenoid below the natural ostium of the sphenoid before reaching the posterior region of the septum. Here it divides into two main branches which, through the anastomosis with the anterior and posterior ethmoidal artery branches, supply the majority of the septum. The incisions for raising the flap are usually performed after the sinuses have been fully opened and the middle turbinate resected. Be aware that the posterior middle turbinate resection should not compromise the vascular pedicle of the flap. Performing the sinus surgery before raising the flap gives extra space and makes the procedure much simpler. It also allows the second surgeon to put parts of the flap under tension so that using a scissor is easier.

My preference is to use a scalpel blade to make the incision for the flap although others use a Bovey unipolar needle. The superior incision starts at the lower edge of the natural sphenoid ostium and proceeds toward the skull base then coming anteriorly until just behind the mucocutaneous junction. It turns vertically onto the floor of the nose and then proceeds posteriorly to the posterior choana where it is taken along the inferior edge of the choana to the lateral nasal wall (**Fig. 20.21**). A suction Freer is used to raise the flap in the same way that a septoplasty is performed. Where

the incisions have not gone through all the layers the second surgeon places the flap under tension and the primary surgeon uses the skull base scissors to release the flap. In anterior skull base cases the flap is placed in the nasopharynx during the resection. To close the defect either intradural underlay fascia lata graft or a dural substitute such as the collagen matrix Duragen (Integra Life Sciences, Plainsboro, NJ) is used. This underlay graft should extend 5 to 10 mm beyond the bone edges of the defect and, as above, maintain smooth contact with the bony defect edges. The pedicled septal flap needs to be larger than the defect and overlap the mucosa free bony margins of the defect by at least 5 mm. If the septal flap from one side is not large enough, consideration can be given to using the opposite septal flap and resecting the septum. These flaps should then be placed side-by-side with minimal overlap over the bony defect. In some patients this may still not allow complete coverage of the defect and a second layer of fascia lata is then used to create the second layer and may be bolstered by thin strips of fat on joining areas. The flaps are secured with Surgicel and sealed with fibrin glue before being covered with Gelfoam and supported by a BIPP ribbon gauze nasal pack or alternatively an intranasal balloon inflated in the nasal cavity.

One of the morbidities associated with using the pedicled nasal septal flap is the crusting that happens on the donor site of the flap. To overcome this problem we make a U-shaped incision on the opposite septal flap based anteriorly so that the posterior portion of this mucosa can be swung around onto the opposite nostril and used to cover the donor site. This flap is secured with sutures at the beginning of the procedure (**Fig. 20.22**). At times the nose and nasal vestibule can dry out during the procedure making the passage of instruments through this region difficult. To overcome this we place a rectangular piece of silastic over the columella with each

Fig. 20.21 In cadaver dissection (**A**) the inferior incision (*white arrow*) is taken back to the posterior choana. In (**B**) the superior incision (*white arrow*) and donor site (*DS*) of the septum is seen with the rolled

septal pedicled flap (*SPF*) being pushed into the postnasal space. In (**D**) the postnasal artery (*PNA*) is seen entering the elevated septal pedicled flap (*SPF*).

tail going down the nostril and then place a through-and-through suture through the silastic and septum to keep the silastic in place. This helps with the passage of endoscopes and instruments and also protects the rotated and sutured septal flap.

In some patients the tumor involves the septum or in revision patients where the septum has been resected or previously used a septal flap is not available. In these patients the pedicled inferior turbinate flap can be used as an

alternative. It consists of the inferior turbinate and some adjacent floor of nose mucosa pedicled on a branch of the sphenopalatine artery that supplies the inferior turbinate through its posterior attachment. It is raised by performing a vertical incision down the anterior face of the inferior turbinate and then taking this incision onto the lateral nasal wall above the turbinate (the horizontal portion of the uncinate) and running this down the length of the turbinate (**Fig. 20.23**). At the posterior edge this is curved upwards

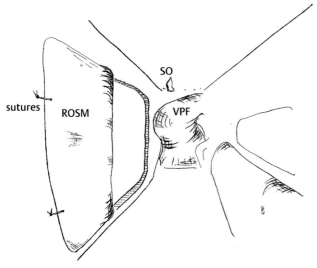

Fig. 20.22 The right-sided opposite septal mucosa (*ROSM*) is rotated from the right onto the left and secured anteriorly with sutures. This covers the donor defect and helps with the postoperative healing. *SO,* sphenoid ostium, *VPF,* vascularized pedicled flap.

toward the sphenopalatine foramen to avoid cutting the artery supplying the flap. The anterior vertical cut is also brought around the anterior end of the turbinate onto the floor of the nose and taken posteriorly and curved up behind the posterior end of the inferior turbinate onto the lateral nasal wall (**Fig. 20.23**). The limitation of this flap is that it, on average, will only cover ~60% of the anterior cranial fossa. However, it will help bring vascularized tissue into

Fig. 20.23 The pedicled inferior turbinate flap is raised by dissecting out the bone of the inferior turbinate and raising adjacent nasal mucosa off the floor of the nose.

the repair area and this with free grafts can be used to successfully close large defects in revision cases.

The anesthetist needs to be aware that, as the patient is recovering from the anesthesia, he or she should be extubated while under relatively deep anesthesia and a laryngeal mask inserted. This allows the patient to be ventilated without the need to use a face mask and also helps to ensure that the patient does not cough or strain during extubation which may precipitate intracranial bleeding and displacement of the reconstruction. The nasal pack is left in place for one week. The patient may be discharged with the pack in place and brought back for pack removal after 1 week.

◆ Case Examples and Surgical Technique

Anterior skull base midline meningiomas are one of the tumors that are suitable for a wholly endoscopic approach. These tumors arise from the dura and bone of the anterior skull base and may present late due to lack of symptoms. Often typical frontal lobe symptoms such as a subtle change in personality or inappropriate uncharacteristic behavior may be the only presenting feature. The intracranial pressure may be raised and the patient may complain of headaches. Meningiomas do have a tendency to recur after removal and recent papers discussing the high recurrence rate of sphenoid wing meningiomas concluded that tumor remnants left in the underlying bone were responsible for the recurrences.[7] The transnasal endoscopic approach overcomes this problem by removal of both the dura and underlying bone from which the tumor has arisen, thereby potentially lessening the possibility of recurrence after surgery.

Example 1 (Video 54)

The first case example is of a young woman who presented with headache. A midline meningioma was diagnosed and initially was monitored with serial MRI scans but the tumor continued to grow (**Fig. 20.24**). She was offered both endoscopic and traditional external approach but chose to have an endoscopic resection.

The surgical plan for this patient was to do a bilateral complete sphenoethmoidectomy with exposure of the frontal ostia. It was not necessary to perform a modified Lothrop procedure as the tumor was located in the posterior region of the anterior skull base. The posterior half of the septum was removed. The next step was to establish the extent of the tumor. With the aid of the computer-aided surgical (CAS) navigation system, the skull base osteotomies were marked out. The osteotomies were performed around the outside of the tumor using diamond burrs and Kerrison punches. A combination of scalpel and endoscopic scissors were used to incise the dura allowing the tumor to drop into the nasal cavity. Arachnoid attachments were carefully dissected free of the tumor and the supplying blood vessels cauterized and divided. The entire tumor and attached dura were removed. The skull base was repaired using the previously described underlay and onlay layers of fascia lata, fibrin glue, and nasal

Fig. 20.24 (**A,B**) Coronal MRI scans in which the meningioma is indicated with a *white arrow*. (**C**) Parasagittal MRI scan in which the roof of the sphenoid is arched upward with the meningioma (*white arrow*) on its roof. (**D**) The meningioma is seen to push between the two cerebral hemispheres in this axial MRI.

pack. This was prior to the development of the pedicled septal flap. The patient was discharged the following day. Postoperative endoscopy shows a well-healed nasal cavity and skull base (**Fig. 20.25**) and follow-up MRI scans over the last 8 years have not shown any recurrence or residual tumor (**Fig. 20.25**).

Example 2

An elderly woman presented with memory loss and headaches. The large anterior cranial fossa meningioma had significant extension intranasally (**Fig. 20.26**). Note the calcification within the tumor and the different consistencies of the tumor in the nose and in the intracranial cavity. Also note that there was substantial brain edema around the intracranial tumor (**Fig. 20.26**).

The surgical approach for this patient was to perform bilateral maxillary antrostomies and complete sphenoethmoidectomies, debulking the tumor during exposure of the sinuses. This debulking should be continued to where the skull base normally would be. An endoscopic modified Lothrop procedure is performed to expose the posterior wall of the frontal sinuses and the bone directly anterior to the tumor edge is removed. The inside of the tumor is carefully debulked, removing most of the inside of the tumor but retaining the outer shell. Once this has been completed, the surgical plane between the tumor and the anterior cerebral lobes are identified and the tumor carefully dissected away from the arachnoid. Neuropatties are placed where this dissection has been performed to maintain this plane and allow adjacent dissection to continue in the same plane. It also protects the underlying brain tissue from inadvertent damage. Any feeding vessels or veins draining from the tumor are cauterized with the suction bipolar forceps* (Medtronic ENT) and divided. In this way the tumor is progressively delivered into the nasal cavity until complete removal is achieved. The cavity is irrigated with warm lactated Ringer's solution and any bleeding vessels cauterized. The skull base is repaired in the manner previously described with two layers of facia lata—the first placed as an underlay and the second as an overlay, followed by fibrin glue, Gelfoam,

Fig. 20.25 (**A**) Endoscopic picture of the region of skull base reconstruction (*black arrow*). Note the two frontal ostia anteriorly (*white arrows*). (**B**) Coronal MRI scan and (**C**) parasagittal MRI in which the region of skull base reconstruction and previous tumor is indicated with a *white arrow*.

and a BIPP ribbon gauze nasal pack. Again this case was done prior to the development of the pedicled septal flap. The pack is removed after 7 days. No lumbar drains are used during the first week but one may be inserted if there is a small leak after the pack has been removed.

Example 3 (Video 55)

The third patient was a middle-aged man who presented with visual symptoms, headaches, and inappropriate euphoria. This midline olfactory groove meningioma was similar to the second case example but significantly larger and there was no nasal or sinus involvement (**Fig. 20.27**).

There are several ways that this meningioma could be tackled. The most common would be the bifrontal and pterional approaches.[13,14] The bifrontal approach gives good access to both sides but results in significant frontal lobe retraction and the important vascular structures are only approached late in the dissection.[13,14] The pterional approach[15,16] is rapid and requires ipsilateral frontal lobe retraction but the opposite frontal lobe does not need retraction and this has an advantage over the bifrontal approach. However, controversy exits as to whether it gives sufficient exposure to the contralateral side in patients with significant bilateral tumor extension.[15,16] In addition it allows access to the skull base vasculature relatively late in the dissection. The attraction of the transnasal approach is that the major arterial supply of the tumor, the anterior and posterior ethmoidal arteries, are ligated before the tumor resection begins. In addition this approach removes the dura and underlying bone of the tumor therefore theoretically lessening the chances of recurrence.[7] A significant advantage of this approach is the complete lack of brain retraction. The downside of the endoscopic approach is the ability of the surgeons to control significant bleeding from the arterial and venous bleeders. It is therefore important to evaluate the arterial blood supply of the tumor preoperatively with an angiogram and assess the arterial supply to the outer surface of the tumor—the so-called "peel" supply. If this is significant then the endoscopic approach may not be suitable. In addition during this procedure any major feeding vessels from the external carotid artery such as the middle meningeal artery can be embolized.

Fig. 20.26 In coronal MRI scans (**A,B**) and parasagittal MRI (**C**) the two consistencies of tumor are visible. The soft tumor is marked with a *solid white arrow* whereas the calcified tumor is marked with a *broken white arrow*. In coronal CT scan (**D**) the calcified part of the tumor is clearly seen (*white broken arrow*). (**A,B**) Brain edema is indicated with a *solid black arrow*. The other important feature seen in (**C**) is the close approximation of the tumor to the posterior wall of the frontal sinus (*broken black arrow*). This means that the anterior osteotomy should be through the posterior wall of the frontal sinus.

Image guidance is essential for a patient such as this as it allows the tumor to be "seen" through the skull base so that the anterior osteotomy can be placed through bone directly adjacent to the tumor. Correct placement of the osteotomies allows the surgeon to identify the surgical plane between the outer surface of the tumor and normal brain tissue. This helps both with the removal of the core of the tumor while preserving the outer layer as well as when this outer layer is dissected from the arachnoid and brain. The standard preparation for resection of this tumor is bilateral maxillary antrostomies, complete sphenoethmoidectomies, and the endoscopic modified Lothrop procedure on the frontal sinuses. Once this is complete the anterior and posterior ethmoidal arteries are identified or cauterized and divided. The posterior osteotomies are performed with the diamond burr and the lateral osteotomies in the fovea ethmoidalis with either a diamond burr or Kerrison punch. The skull base is dropped into the nasal cavity after the fibrous attachment between the crista galli and falx is

cut. It can then be removed from the nose and the base of the tumor exposed. In a tumor such as this, it is crucial that the tumor should be for the most part removed from the inside out thereby allowing the tumor to be collapsed inward on itself. If the tumor is soft this can be done with the skull base suction dissection instruments* (Medtronic ENT) or with the 2.7-mm microdebrider blade.

Great care must be taken when using the microdebrider blade with the intracranial cavity as it can be very aggressive when removing soft tissue. The suction should be placed on a suction regulator to minimize the amount of tissue sucked into the cutting region. In addition, the oscillating speed of the blade should be below 1000 rpm and the entire extent of the blade should be visible during use. The blade is generally used facing superiorly so that the endoscope is looking at the opening when in use and the blade can be stopped if too much tissue is sucked into the opening or the tumor that is being resected is thought to contain a vessel. The second technique for removing the core of

Fig. 20.27 MRI scans (**A**, coronal; **B**, parasagittal; **C**, axial) in which the tumor is indicated with a *white arrow*. (**B**) Note how the tumor closely approximates the posterior wall of the frontal sinus.

the tumor involves using the blades of the suction bipolar forceps to grasp the fibrous threads within the tumor and, while gentle traction is placed on these, the bipolar is activated further, shrinking the tumor and causing the tumor to collapse inward.

Finally, new ultrasonic aspirators now have endonasal attachments (Cavitron ultrasonic aspirator [CUSA; Radionics, Burlington, MA] and Sonopet [Stryker, Kalamazoo, MI]) which allow the inside of the tumor to be removed. This can be useful especially when there is bone inside the tumor as may be found in meningiomas.

Once it is felt that only a relatively thin shell of tumor remains, the surgical plane between the arachnoid and the brain is established and developed. A combination of malleable probes, suction Freer elevator, and neuropatties are used to mobilize the tumor from the brain. Vessels that are seen are mobilized and preserved or cauterized with the bipolar forceps before being divided. In this patient the surgery went relatively uneventfully until a relatively large vein draining the tumor into in the inferior sagittal sinus was avulsed from the sinus. Ligar clips controlled the bleeding from the sinus

and the remaining surgery was uneventful. This would not have been possible without two surgeons working simultaneously in the intracranial cavity. Skull base reconstruction was performed with an underlay and onlay fascia lata graft, fibrin glue, Gelfoam, and a BIPP nasal pack. Again this case was done prior to the development of the vascularized pedicled septal flap. The pack was removed after 1 week. Postoperative MRI shows complete removal of the tumor (**Fig. 20.28**).

◆ Conclusion

Endoscopic transnasal intracranial surgery is a new and exciting development in sinus surgery. However, this surgery requires a high level of training and skill from both the sinus surgeon and the neurosurgeon. To perform such surgeries, sinus surgeons and neurosurgeons need to form a skull base team. Such a team should develop their endoscopic skills by

Fig. 20.28 Postoperative MRI scans (**A**, coronal; **B**, parasagittal; **C**, axial) in which the region where the tumor was resected is indicated with a *white arrow* and the reconstructed skull base with a *black arrow*.

doing numerous endoscopic pituitary tumor dissections. As the level of expertise develops the team can tackle smaller selected intracranial tumors. Case selection and preparation are vitally important to the success of the surgery and the team should always be mindful that surgery with the highest likelihood of success and least morbidity should be chosen. One of the most important aspects of this surgery is the two-surgeon approach. Having two surgeons operating at the same time has huge advantages for both the ability of the surgeons to remove the tumor by placing traction on it and for the management of complications especially if significant hemorrhage occurs. The exact role of endoscopic cranial base resection in the management of malignancies is still not clear but it is likely that endoscopic techniques will increasingly play a role in the management of these patients. Finally, there is no substitute for a sound knowledge of anatomy and this chapter (and book) focuses on presenting the surgical anatomy in detail. This should be augmented with multiple cadaver dissections until the surgeon has extensive and detailed knowledge of the anatomy in this region.

References

1. Howard DJ, Lund VJ, Wei WI. Craniofacial resection for tumors of the nasal cavity and paranasal sinuses: a 25-year experience. Head Neck 2006;28(10):867–873
2. Batra PS, Citardi MJ, Worley S, Lee J, Lanza DC. Resection of anterior skull base tumors: comparison of combined traditional and endoscopic techniques. Am J Rhinol 2005;19(5):521–528
3. Castelnuovo PG, Belli E, Bignami M, Battaglia P, Sberze F, Tomei G. Endoscopic nasal and anterior craniotomy resection for malignant nasoethmoid tumors involving the anterior skull base. Skull Base 2006;16(1):15–18
4. Leong JL, Citardi MJ, Batra PS. Reconstruction of skull base defects after minimally invasive endoscopic resection of anterior skull base neoplasms. Am J Rhinol 2006;20(5):476–482
5. Buchmann L, Larsen C, Pollack A, Tawfik O, Sykes K, Hoover LA. Endoscopic techniques in resection of anterior skull base/paranasal sinus malignancies. Laryngoscope 2006;116(10):1749–1754
6. Snyderman CH, Kassam AB. Endoscopic techniques for pathology of the anterior cranial fossa and ventral skull base. J Am Coll Surg 2006;202(3):563
7. Hernesniemi J, Dashti R, Lehecka M, et al. Microsurgical management of anterior communicating artery aneurysms. Surg Neurol 2007;70:8–29
8. Uzün I, Gürdal E, Cakmak YO, Ozdogmus O, Cavdar S. A reminder of the anatomy of the recurrent artery of heubner. Cen Eur Neurosurg 2009;70(1):36–38

9. Pieper DR, Al-Mefty O, Hanada Y, Buechner D. Hyperostosis associated with meningioma of the cranial base: secondary changes or tumor invasion. Neurosurgery 1999;44(4):742–746, discussion 746–747

10. Zanation A, Thorp B, Parmar P, Harvey R. Reconstructive options for endoscopic skull base surgery. Otolaryngol Clin N Am 2011;44(5):1201–1222

11. Jardeleza C, Seiberling K, Floreani S, Wormald PJ. Surgical outcomes of endoscopic management of adenocarcinoma of the sinonasal cavity. Rhinology 2009;47(4):354–361

12. Hadad G, Bassagasteguy L, Carrau RL, et al. A novel reconstructive technique after endoscopic expanded endonasal approaches: vascular pedicle nasoseptal flap. Laryngoscope 2006;116(10):1882–1886

13. Hentschel SJ, DeMonte F. Olfactory groove meningiomas. Neurosurg Focus 2003;14(6):e4

14. Spektor S, Valarezo J, Fliss DM, et al. Olfactory groove meningiomas from neurosurgical and ear, nose, and throat perspectives: approaches, techniques, and outcomes. Neurosurgery 2005; **57**(4, Suppl)268–280, discussion 268–280

15. Turazzi S, Cristofori L, Gambin R, Bricolo A. The pterional approach for the microsurgical removal of olfactory groove meningiomas. Neurosurgery 1999;45(4):821–825, discussion 825–826

16. Babu R, Barton A, Kasoff SS. Resection of olfactory groove meningiomas: technical note revisited. Surg Neurol 1995;44(6):567–572

21 Endoscopic Surgery of the Craniocervical Junction

Surgery on the craniocervical junction (CCJ) is complex due to its location behind the nasopharynx and difficult to access through traditional techniques. The traditional approach has been the transoral approach.[1] This involves placing retractors in the mouth, opening the jaw, and retracting the tongue. Additionally the soft palate is split and portions of the hard palate are resected, depending on the access required. The disadvantages of this approach are the need for a pre- and postoperative tracheostomy to secure the airway, contamination of the surgical field with oral bacteria, the potential postoperative dysfunction of the soft palate in swallowing and phonation, and the need to feed the patient through a nasogastric tube postoperatively.[2]

The endoscopic approach avoids these problems as the surgery site is out of the swallowing mechanism, swelling is usually limited and does not threaten the airway, and oral bacteria are avoided.[3]

◆ Pathology

There are several pathologies that can be addressed with this approach.

Rheumatoid Arthritis

The most common condition affecting the CCJ is the development of a rheumatoid pannus in patients with rheumatoid arthritis. The inflammatory process in the rheumatoid pannus causes ligament laxity, bone erosion, and then, because the odontoid peg is no longer supported, it migrates into the brainstem causing compression by either direct pressure or by cervical subluxation.

Congenital Disorders

There are several congenital odontoid malformations, basilar invagination syndromes, and anomalies of the skull base that may affect the CCJ. Basilar invagination occurs when the tip of the odontoid moves more than 4.5 mm above a line drawn from the back of the hard palate to the base of the occiput (McGregor's line).[2]

Chordoma

Chordomas arise in the bone of the clivus and upper cervical spine from notochord remnants and are the most common tumor of the mobile spine.[2] These tumors rarely metastasize but are locally aggressive with bone destruction and neurologic involvement. Complete resection with postoperative proton beam irradiation provides the best long-term survival.

Nasopharyngeal Carcinoma

These patients are treated initially with radiotherapy and usually respond well to this treatment. However, there are a small group of patients that fail multiple courses of radiotherapy and may need salvage surgery if the tumor involves this region. In addition, multiple courses of radiotherapy may result in radio-osteonecrosis of this region, which in turn may require surgical debridement.

◆ Anatomy

The CCJ consists of the region of the upper spine (C1 and 2) and the skull base (occiput) that articulates with C1. C1 (atlas) does not have a vertebral body or spinous process which in turn allows significant movement between the atlas and the skull base. This movement accounts for over half of the head's axial rotation.[4] The atlas has two thick lateral masses which articulate with the occipital condyles. The odontoid peg is positioned where the vertebral body of the atlas would normally be and fixed to the clivus by the apical and alar ligaments.

Fig. 21.1 Cadaveric dissection following the removal of the mucosa and pharyngobasilar fascia. The middle third of the clivus has been removed to reveal the pons. The longus capitis (*LC*) muscles insert broadly onto the floor of the sphenoid sinus (removed in this specimen). The pharyngeal raphe (*PR*) can be seen attaching to the pharyngeal tubercle (*PT*) of the occipital bone. *ET*, eustachian tube; *BA*, basilar artery; *PCA*, paraclival artery.

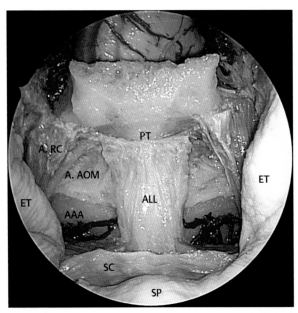

Fig. 21.2 Cadaveric dissection following the removal of the longus capitis muscles. This step reveals the anterior longitudinal ligaments (*ALL*), the anterior atlantooccipital membrane (*A. AOM*), and the anterior rectus capitis muscle (*A. RC*). Note how the superior constrictor (*SC*) muscle finishes at the level of the soft palate (*SP*). *AAA*, anterior arch of the atlas; *ET*, eustachian tube; *PT*, pharyngeal tubercle.

As most surgery in this region involves exposure and resection of the odontoid, the ligamentous attachments and layers of the CCJ are important to understand. When this region is approached anteriorly the first layer encountered is the nasopharyngeal mucosa followed by the pharyngobasilar fascia,

the longus capitis, and, more inferiorly, the longus coli muscles, atlanto-occipital membrane, anterior longitudinal ligament, atlanto-occipital ligaments, arch of the atlas, and odontoid peg (**Figs. 21.1**, **21.2**, **21.3**, and **21.4**). The peg is supported by the apical and alar ligaments which form a secure attachment

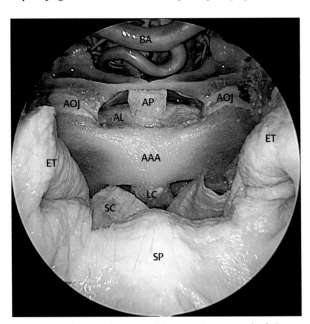

Fig. 21.3 Cadaveric dissection following the removal of the anterior atlantooccipital membrane, anterior longitudinal ligament, the longus capitis muscles, and the anterior rectus capitis muscles. This reveals the joint capsule of the atlantooccipital joint (*AOJ*). This joint capsule has been removed to reveal the joint surfaces. The superior constrictor (*SC*) has been split to show the insertion of the longus coli muscle (*LC*). The apical ligaments (*AP*) and alar ligaments (*AL*) can be seen clearly. *SP*, soft palate; *ET*, eustachian tube; *AAA*, anterior arch of the atlas; *BA*, basilar artery.

Fig. 21.4 Cadaveric dissection following the removal of the apical and alar ligaments, and the odontoid process has been drilled away (*OP*). This reveals the strong and thick transverse portion of the cruciform ligament (*CL*). Behind this is located the tectorial membrane (*TM*). *ET*, eustachian tube; *SP*, soft palate; *HC*, hypoglossal canal; *VA*, vertebral artery; *BA*, basilar artery.

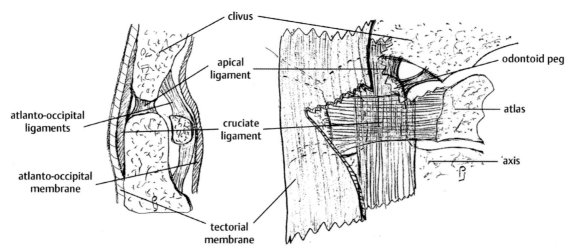

Fig. 21.5 An illustration of the CCJ in the sagittal plane (*left*) and viewed from posterior with the tectorial membrane and cruciate ligaments partly cut away to reveal the underlying structures.

to the occipital bone/clivus (**Fig. 21.5**). Posterior to the odontoid, the cruciate ligaments (vertical and horizontal elements) provide strong support for the odontoid and prevent posterior displacement (**Fig. 21.6**). The cruciate ligaments are commonly affected by the rheumatoid pannus and weakened by the associated inflammation. Behind the cruciate ligaments is the tectorial membrane (**Fig. 21.5**). In **Fig. 21.5** the anatomy is viewed from posterior with the tectorial membrane partially cut away to give a view of the cruciate ligaments. The superior aspect of the cruciate ligament is cut away to give a view of the apical and alar ligaments of the odontoid peg (dens).

A parasagittal view is also provided demonstrating the layers from anterior to posterior in this complex area.

As the intracranial cavity is approached the lower region of the brainstem and lower cranial nerves are exposed. The medullary pyramids face the clivus with the hypoglossal nerve arising from the upper medulla. This series of rootlets then converge on the hypoglossal canal which lies above the occipital condyles (**Figs. 21.6** and **21.7**). The accessory nerve has a cranial component whose rootlets hitch onto the vagus (**Fig. 21.6**). Its spinal portion arises from a series of rootlets from the lower medulla and upper spinal cord and

Fig. 21.6 Cadaveric dissection with image taken just above the skeletonized hypoglossal canal (*HC*) at the cerebellopontine angle. The anterior inferior cerebellar artery (*AICA*) can be seen intimately associated with the vestibulocochlear nerve (*CN VIII*), facial nerve (*CN VII*), and the nervus intermedius (*NI*). The posterior inferior cerebellar artery (*PICA*) can be seen running between the vagus (*CN X*) and spinal and cranial portions of the accessory nerves (*CN XI – S, CN XI – C*).

Fig. 21.7 Cadaveric dissection image showing the hypoglossal nerve exiting the hypoglossal foramen with its corresponding vein that communicates the internal jugular vein with the basilar plexus. *HC*, hypoglossal canal; *CN XII*, hypoglossal nerve and rootlets; *FM*, foramen magnum; *VA*, vertebral artery; *PICA*, posterior inferior cerebellar artery; *BA*, basilar artery; *CN X*, vagus nerve.

Fig. 21.8 Cadaveric dissection following removal of the tectorial membrane and the odontoid process. The anterior arch of the atlas has been drilled away centrally to reveal the upper cervical spinal cord behind. C1 and C2 spinal nerves can be seen clearly. *AAA*, anterior arch of atlas; *VA*, vertebral artery; *BA*, basilar artery.

then is the only cranial nerve to pass through the foramen magnum. The vertebral arteries pass lateral to the lateral masses in the axis and enter the upper cervical region and then pass behind the occipital condyles to join anterior to the medulla to form the basilar artery (**Figs. 21.8** and **21.9**).

Fig. 21.9 Cadaveric dissection image shows the close-up view of the upper cervical spinal cord. The image clearly shows the C1 and C2 nerve rootlets, the dentate ligaments (*DL*), and the vertebral artery (*VA*) as it enters the foramen magnum. *ASA*, anterior spinal artery.

The vertebrobasilar junction is usually at the pontomedullary junction (**Fig. 21.8**). The main branch of the vertebral artery is the posterior inferior cerebellar artery (PICA; **Fig. 21.6**).

◆ Preoperative Preparation

Preoperatively patients have both a computed tomography (CT) scan and a magnetic resonance imaging (MRI) scan with contrast. This allows the soft tissue, bony landmarks, and vasculature to be accurately identified. The CT and MRI are merged on the image guidance machine (**Fig. 21.10**) and the toggle is used to move on a single image between bone windows and soft tissue windows. The contrast MRI also allows accurate identification of the vasculature so surgical approaches can be planned with minimum risk to the vasculature. The extent of resection of the anterior arch of the atlas and odontoid is decided on the scans and plans are made as to whether fixing of the CCJ is needed and if this is better done preoperatively or postoperatively. The thigh is prepared for harvesting of fat and fascia in case this may be needed in the reconstruction of the surgically created defect.

◆ Endoscopic Surgical Approach to the Odontoid Peg

The first step is to decide to what extent resection of the clivus is needed. In patients with a chordoma extending down into the atlas, it may be necessary to resect the clivus from the floor of the pituitary fossa down to the base of the arch of the atlas (**Fig. 21.8**). If the pathology is an invagination of the odontoid, opening of the sphenoid may not be required and the resection can be limited to the nasopharynx. To maximize the access the inferior turbinates are lateralized or resected. To improve the postoperative healing a pedicled septal flap is elevated and placed in an opened maxillary sinus to move it out of the operative field. A posterior septectomy is performed and the mucosa from the opposite posterior septal region is folded anteriorly to cover the donation site of the pedicled septal flap and secured anteriorly with sutures.

Image guidance is used to map out the cervical carotid arteries to ensure that they are not in the surgical field. In addition the clivus, anterior arch of the atlas, and body of the axis are identified. The arch of the atlas is at the most caudal region that can be reached through the transnasal approach. If it is necessary to increase the caudal exposure the posterior superior edge of the hard palate can be drilled away but care should be taken to preserve the oral mucosa under the hard palate. The next step is to remove the mucosa and longus capitis muscles over these structures as far lateral as the Eustachian tubes (as this is usually medial to the carotids) until the atlantooccipital membrane is identified. No attempt is made to raise a flap as doing this is difficult and

Fig. 21.10 This merged CT/MRI shows the tumor (*red dot*) at the base of the clivus and abutting the atlas and odontoid peg in the region of the CCJ in coronal, sagittal, and axial planes. Note the contrast in the vessels allowing clear identification of the major vessels.

the raised flap compromises the access. Instead the Coblator (ArthroCare, Sunnyvale, CA) or unipolar diathermy is used to remove these structures down to and including the atlanto-occipital membrane. The bone of the anterior arch of the atlas and the odontoid is exposed. A high-speed drill is used to remove the bone of the anterior arch up to the lateral masses. This increases the exposure of the odontoid peg (dens).

To begin the odontoid resection, the superior aspect of the dens is exposed by cutting the apical ligament. Care should be taken not to open the dura. This allows the dens to be removed from top down by using a high-speed drill to gently remove the center of the dens leaving a posterior egg shell behind. This egg-shelled bone is then carefully dissected free of the alar ligaments and cruciate ligament. Traction is placed on the bony fragments to lessen the intradural compression during dissection. The bony fragments and

any associated rheumatoid pannus is dissected free of the tectorial membrane. In some patients the pannus may contribute to the compression so this should be removed until underlying pulsatile dura is seen ensuring a complete decompression. The defect is covered with the pedicled septal flap with the edges of the flap covered with a layer of Surgicel (Ethicon, Somerville, NJ) and fibrin glue. No other packing is placed.

Other pathologies can also be addressed in this area. In some patients clival chordomas may localized to the CCJ and the surgical access is similar to what has been described previously (**Fig. 21.10**). In this patient the chordoma is at the lower end of the clivus and involves the arch of the atlas and extends laterally to the occipital condyles. In **Fig. 21.11** a much larger chordoma extends from the base of the pituitary all the way to the atlas and involves the atlas and upper

Fig. 21.11 A large clival chordoma with involvement of the entire clivus and extending inferiorly into the CCJ, abutting the atlas and odontoid peg (*white arrow*).

aspect of the odontoid peg. This patient would require a full clival exposure and a CCJ exposure to ensure complete resection of the tumor.

◆ **Key Points**

- Multiple different pathologies occur in the region of the CCJ
- Imaging with both CT and MRI is important for assessment of the pathology, vasculature, and for planning of the surgical approach
- A decision needs to be made before surgery as to the need of cervical fixation either pre- or postsurgery
- A pedicled septal flap is raised before a posterior septectomy is done
- All soft tissues and ligaments anterior to the peg and arch of the atlas are removed

- The peg and anterior arch of the atlas are removed with a high-speed drill with the posterior wall egg-shelled before being dissected free.

References

1. Hadley MN, Spetzler RF, Sonntag VK. The transoral approach to the superior cervical spine. A review of 53 cases of extradural cervicomedullary compression. J Neurosurg 1989;71(1):16–23

2. Wu JC, Mummaneni PV, El-Sayed IH. Diseases of the odontoid and craniovertebral junction with management by endoscopic approaches. Otolaryngol Clin North Am 2011;44(5):1029–1042

3. Kassam AB, Snyderman C, Gardner P, Carrau R, Spiro R. The expanded endonasal approach: a fully endoscopic transnasal approach and resection of the odontoid process: technical case report. Neurosurgery 2005;57(1, Suppl):E213, discussion E213

4. Cardosa ACC, Brock R, Martins C, de Alancastro LP, Rhoton AL. Microendoscopic anatomy of the craniocervical junction. In: Aldo C. Transnasal Endoscopic Skull Base and Brain Surgery. New York: Thieme; 2011

22 Carotid Artery and Major Vascular Injury during Endoscopic Sinus Surgery

The incidence of injury to the internal carotid artery (ICA) during endoscopic sinus surgery (ESS) is very low, with only 29 cases been described in the literature.[1] Injury during endoscopic skull base surgery, however, is more common with an incidence during pituitary surgery of around 5% and higher in parasellar and post fossa surgery.[1] One of the limitations of endoscopic skull base surgery for tumors involving the carotids has been the ability of the surgeon to be able to endoscopically control and repair major vascular hemorrhage. Major vascular injury has a significant and probably underestimated mortality of 15% and permanent morbidity of 26%.[1] Significant tumor involvement of the major vasculature has in the past been considered a relative contraindication to the endoscopic approach. However, with training courses on animals duplicating the conditions of vascular rupture during surgery,[2] skills have been developed that allow skull base teams to now tackle such cases.

◆ High Risk Patients

Patients at high risk are those with previous radiotherapy, hormone-secreting pituitary tumors (particularly prolactinomas), and growth hormone–secreting tumors. Acromegalic patients will at times have ectatic carotids often with the tumor in contact or surrounding the carotid.[3] Any tumor including meningiomas, clival chordomas, and craniopharyngiomas that contact or envelop the carotids places the patient at higher risk during dissection of the tumor.[1]

◆ Management

Surgical Field

A major vascular injury creates the most challenging surgical field possible in endoscopic surgery. The high-volume and high-pressure blood flow quickly contaminates the end of the endoscope leaving the surgeon without a view.[4] No safe maneuvers can be performed if the surgeon cannot see. It is usually not possible for the surgeon to both obtain a surgical view and perform an effective maneuver if he/she is alone. The two-surgeon approach allows one surgeon to control the bloodstream and direct it away from the endoscope and this allows the second surgeon to obtain sufficient view to perform the maneuvers necessary for achieving hemostasis.[4] There are several principles for surgical field control. First two large bore (10 French) suctions are needed and, if available, the endoscope should have a lens cleaning system that enables the end of the endoscope to be washed immediately it is contaminated. This means that the endoscope does not be need to be removed to clear the view. The first step is to decide in which nostril to place the endoscope. Usually the bloodstream is directed predominantly into one side of the nose (**Fig. 22.1**).[4]

This should be assessed and the endoscope should be placed down the opposite nostril. The second surgeon should place the suction down the side of major flow while the primary surgeon places the endoscope and second suction down the opposite nostril. The primary surgeon should push the pedicled septal flap out of the way and clear the nostril of blood ahead of the endoscope. We have found that in these situations the flap floats and if only one suction is used, it quickly becomes blocked as the flap is sucked into the end of the suction and the surgical field is lost. Once the flap is pushed into the nasopharynx the second surgeon can place their large bore suction directly over the bleeding vessels and guide the bloodstream into their suction thereby providing the primary surgeon with the visualization necessary to perform the surgical maneuver for hemostasis (**Fig. 22.2**). If the endoscope and the suction are placed down the same nostril when this guiding of the bloodstream is attempted, the bloodstream will often track alongside of the suction with immediate soiling of the endoscope and loss of the surgical field (**Fig. 22.3**).

Fig. 22.1 **(A)** The vascular stream can be seen coming predominantly out of the right nostril and, when the endoscope is placed into the nose **(B)**, the stream (*white arrow*) can be seen going into the right nasal cavity and the endoscope is protected from the stream by the back of the septum.

Hemostasis

Muscle Patch

In the past the first response of surgeons in this very challenging situation was to attempt to pack the bleeding vessel to achieve hemostasis. Raymond et al.[5] reviewed 12 cases in which a carotid injury had occurred. In 8 of the 12 the nasal packing resulted in complete occlusion of the internal carotid artery (ICA), 4 had stenosis of the ICA, and 1 patient

partial occlusion of the middle cerebral artery as well as the ICA. The authors concluded that overpacking contributed to both the morbidity and mortality of the patients.[5]

In skull base surgery there is often wide exposure of the surgical field with a large amount of brain and associated critical vessels, such as the basilar and brainstem perforators from the circle of Willis, exposed. Packing in this situation can contribute significantly to the morbidity and even mortality of the patient and should only be done on the bleeding vessel alone rather than on the surgical area being operated

Fig. 22.2 **(A)** The suction is down the left nostril (*S*) and hovering over the vascular injury and guiding the stream up the suction while the endoscope and vascular clamp are placed down the right nostril. **(B)** The suction (*S*) continues to draw the stream of blood away from

the endoscope allowing the vascular clamp to be placed. The technique of placing the open clamp on either side of the suction and pushing the suction of the lesion is preferred.

Fig. 22.3 (**A**) The suction and endoscope are placed in the same nostril attracting the vascular stream to the suction. (**B**) The vascular stream tracks up the suction and will soil the endoscope with loss of vision.

upon. In our department we have developed an animal model of carotid artery injury and assessed the various materials commonly available for management of a significant vascular injury. These included oxidized cellulose, thrombin-gelatin matrix, and crushed muscle patch. Valentine et al.[2] showed the only effective agent was crushed muscle, which succeeded in achieving hemostasis in all cases. The other materials did not achieve hemostasis with resultant exsanguination of the animal model. The techniques of using the muscle patch repair is for the muscle to be harvested from either the thigh (usually preprepared in skull base cases for taking of a fascia lata graft) or from the sternomastoid muscle in the neck. A $2 \times 1.5 \times 1$ cm piece of muscle is harvested and then crushed between two metal kidney dishes. The primary surgeon uses a Blakesley forceps to guide the muscle patch toward the bleeding vessel. The second surgeon keeps the surgical field clear by continually guiding the bloodstream up a large bore suction. The suction is hovered just above the site of injury. If the suction gets too close it will suck onto the wall of the vessel and result in loss of the surgical field. These techniques are now taught in our workshops. The sheep animal model of carotid injury is used[6] with the nasal model to re-create the exact clinical situation with the very challenging surgical field and teach how to maintain the surgical field and be able to place the muscle patch and achieve hemostasis. Such courses are recommended as the skills attained in this way will more effectively allow surgeons faced with this very difficult situation to achieve better outcomes for their patients.

Direct Vascular Repair

In the situation where there has been considerable dissection of the vasculature and the vascular lesion is not enclosed by bone or in a difficult to access location, direct repair of the injury is possible. We have developed in conjunction with Medtronic

ENT (Jacksonville, FL) a series of endoscopic vascular clamps that can be endoscopically placed (**Fig. 22.4**). These clamps have been designed to side clamp the vessel lesion while still allowing patency of the vessel during suturing of the lesion (**Fig. 22.5**). The sutures used have been the Medtronic U-clips which have a nitinol self-knotting end which does away with the need to tie the sutures (**Fig. 22.5**). This is a technically

Fig. 22.4 The series of endovascular clamps, clip appliers, and suturing forceps* developed in conjunction with Medtronic ENT to manage vascular injuries during endoscopic skull base surgery.

Fig. 22.5 (**A**) The carotid artery is side-clamped with blood still passing behind the clamp. (**B**) The self-knotting suture is passed through the lesion and the suture released. (**C**) The U-clip self-knotting sutures have successfully closed the carotid lesion and the vessel remains patent.

demanding technique that should be practiced on the animal model courses before being attempted on patients. Laws et al.[7] have also described direct repair of a vascular lesion but again it is stressed that to do this requires considerable technical skill, the correct equipment, experience, and training.

Intravascular Techniques

In some patients it may not be possible to achieve hemostasis and the patient should be immediately transferred to the endovascular suite for either stenting, balloon occlusion, or coiling. Stenting is the preferred technique but can be very difficult in the siphon of the cavernous carotid. Distal migration may also occlude the ophthalmic artery with subsequent blindness. A balloon occlusion should ideally be done with an awake patient to test to see if there is sufficient collateral circulation to allow perfusion of that side of the brain

without neurologic deficit. The balloon occlusion test (BOT) is usually performed for 30 minutes and if there are no neurologic sequelae the vessel is occluded. This is not possible in the emergency situation where vascular control has not been achieved and occlusion techniques may be the only way that the patient's life can be saved. In addition there is 4% risk of a stroke in the 30 days after stent placement.[8] Antiplatelet therapy may be needed for up to 3 months after placement.[9]

◆ Postoperative Complications

Once hemostasis has been achieved and the surgery completed, the patient should be transferred directly to the endovascular suite for an angiogram. The repair is assessed and if necessary further endovascular intervention can be performed. The most common postoperative complication is the formation of a pseudoaneurysm and this occurs in up 60% of patients.[1] A pseudoaneurysm is a defect through all layers of the vessel wall with flow of blood into a contained space outside the walls of the vessel. The aneurysm commonly forms in the first 6 weeks postsurgery but can form even years later. If the immediate postoperative angiogram is normal the patient is monitored in intensive care until the packing is removed and a further angiogram is performed, usually a week later. If this is normal the angiogram is repeated again at 6 weeks, 3 months, and 1 year. If a pseudoaneurysm is detected it is treated by either stent graft placement or if this is not possible by coiling the aneurysm opening or occluding the vessel either with coiling or balloons. Coiling the aneurysm opening has a higher complication rate as the pseudoaneurysm does not have a wall against which the coil can sit and rupture may still occur.[10] Coiling the aneurysm opening is reserved for patients who fail the balloon occlusion test as extracranial/intracranial carotid artery bypass surgery has a high complication rate and is the only alternative. The other major complication is a carotid-cavernous sinus fistula (CCF) which occurs between the carotid defect and cavernous sinus. The endovascular treatment is the same as for a pseudoaneurysm. However, in this situation, detachable balloons may be used to occlude the fistula while maintaining parent vessel patency.

◆ **Major Vessel Injury Management Training**

As major vessel injury is the next major frontier for endoscopic surgeons, the availability of realistic animal model training in the management of this significant complication is a major advance. Adelaide now runs these courses twice a year and encourages skull base teams (ENT and neurosurgeons) to attend and learn the techniques of surgical field management, muscle patch, and direct vessel suturing (www.adelaidesinussurgery.com).

References

1. Valentine R, Wormald PJ. Carotid artery injury after endonasal surgery. Otolaryngol Clin North Am 2011;44(5):1059–1079
2. Valentine R, Boase S, Jervis-Bardy J, Dones Cabral JD, Robinson S, Wormald PJ. The efficacy of hemostatic techniques in the sheep model of carotid artery injury. Int Forum Allergy Rhinol 2011;1(2):118–122
3. Hatam A, Greitz T. Ectasia of cerebral arteries in acromegaly. Acta Radiol Diagn (Stockh) 1972;12(4):410–418
4. Valentine R, Wormald PJ. Controlling the surgical field during a large endoscopic vascular injury. Laryngoscope 2011;121(3):562–566
5. Raymond J, Hardy J, Czepko R, Roy D. Arterial injuries in transsphenoidal surgery for pituitary adenoma; the role of angiography and endovascular treatment. AJNR Am J Neuroradiol 1997;18(4):655–665
6. Valentine R, Wormald PJ. Controlling the surgical field during a large endoscopic vascular injury. Laryngoscope 2011;121(3):562–566
7. Laws ER Jr. Vascular complications of transsphenoidal surgery. Pituitary 1999;2(2):163–170
8. Wholey MH, Wholey MH, Jarmolowski CR, Eles G, Levy D, Buecthel J. Endovascular stents for carotid artery occlusive disease. J Endovasc Surg 1997;4(4):326–338
9. Leung GK, Auyeung KM, Lui WM, Fan YW. Emergency placement of a self-expandable covered stent for carotid artery injury during transsphenoidal surgery. Br J Neurosurg 2006;20(1):55–57
10. Higashida RT, Halbach VV, Dowd CF, Barnwell SL, Hieshima GB. Intracranial aneurysms: interventional neurovascular treatment with detachable balloons—results in 215 cases. Radiology 1991;178(3):663–670

Index

Note: Page numbers followed by *f* and *t* indicate material in figures and tables, respectively.